MATHEMATICS RESEARCH DEVELOPMENTS

FOCUS ON SYSTEMS THEORY RESEARCH

MATHEMATICS RESEARCH DEVELOPMENTS

Additional books and e-books in this series can be found on Nova's website
under the Series tab.

MATHEMATICS RESEARCH DEVELOPMENTS

FOCUS ON SYSTEMS THEORY RESEARCH

MANUEL F. CASANOVA
AND
IOAN OPRIS
EDITORS

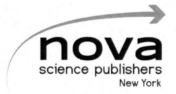

Copyright © 2019 by Nova Science Publishers, Inc.

All rights reserved. No part of this book may be reproduced, stored in a retrieval system or transmitted in any form or by any means: electronic, electrostatic, magnetic, tape, mechanical photocopying, recording or otherwise without the written permission of the Publisher.

We have partnered with Copyright Clearance Center to make it easy for you to obtain permissions to reuse content from this publication. Simply navigate to this publication's page on Nova's website and locate the "Get Permission" button below the title description. This button is linked directly to the title's permission page on copyright.com. Alternatively, you can visit copyright.com and search by title, ISBN, or ISSN.

For further questions about using the service on copyright.com, please contact:
Copyright Clearance Center
Phone: +1-(978) 750-8400   Fax: +1-(978) 750-4470   E-mail: info@copyright.com.

NOTICE TO THE READER

The Publisher has taken reasonable care in the preparation of this book, but makes no expressed or implied warranty of any kind and assumes no responsibility for any errors or omissions. No liability is assumed for incidental or consequential damages in connection with or arising out of information contained in this book. The Publisher shall not be liable for any special, consequential, or exemplary damages resulting, in whole or in part, from the readers' use of, or reliance upon, this material. Any parts of this book based on government reports are so indicated and copyright is claimed for those parts to the extent applicable to compilations of such works.

Independent verification should be sought for any data, advice or recommendations contained in this book. In addition, no responsibility is assumed by the publisher for any injury and/or damage to persons or property arising from any methods, products, instructions, ideas or otherwise contained in this publication.

This publication is designed to provide accurate and authoritative information with regard to the subject matter covered herein. It is sold with the clear understanding that the Publisher is not engaged in rendering legal or any other professional services. If legal or any other expert assistance is required, the services of a competent person should be sought. FROM A DECLARATION OF PARTICIPANTS JOINTLY ADOPTED BY A COMMITTEE OF THE AMERICAN BAR ASSOCIATION AND A COMMITTEE OF PUBLISHERS.

Additional color graphics may be available in the e-book version of this book.

Library of Congress Cataloging-in-Publication Data

Names: Casanova, Manuel F., editor. | Opris, Ioan (Medical research personnel), editor.
Title: Focus on systems theory research / editors, Manuel F. Casanova and
    Ioan Opris (University of South Carolina School of Medicine Greenville,
    Greenville, SC, US, and others).
Description: Hauppauge, New York: Nova Science Publishers, Inc., 2018. |
    Series: Mathematics research developments | Includes bibliographical references and index.
Identifiers: LCCN 2018047552 (print) | LCCN 2018049902 (ebook) | ISBN
    9781536145625 () | ISBN 9781536145618 (hardcover)
Subjects: LCSH: System theory. | Medical care--Quality control.
Classification: LCC Q295 (ebook) | LCC Q295 .F6285 2018 (print) | DDC 362.101/1--dc23
LC record available at https://lccn.loc.gov/2018047552

Published by Nova Science Publishers, Inc. † New York

CONTENTS

Preface		**vii**
Chapter 1	Biases in the Process of Designing a System *Helmut Nechansky*	**1**
Chapter 2	Mathematical Theory of Reliability and Biological Robustness: Reliable Systems from Unreliable Elements *Vitaly K. Koltover*	**49**
Chapter 3	Quantum Models of Complex Systems *Miroslav Svítek*	**81**
Chapter 4	Model-Order Reduction with H_2/H_∞ Performance *Salim Ibrir*	**101**
Chapter 5	Systems Thinking in Health Care: From Theory to Implementation *Sheuwen Chuang and Peter P. Howley*	**115**
Chapter 6	Applications of Genome-Scale Metabolic Models and Data Integration in Systems Medicine *Ali Salehzadeh-Yazdi, Markus Wolfien and Olaf Wolkenhauer*	**131**
Chapter 7	Reality is Hierarchically Organized: The Recursive Foundations of Living Systems and Beyond *Patrick Connolly*	**151**
Chapter 8	New Directions in Occupational Roadway Safety Grounded in Complex Systems Theory and Simulation Modeling *Michael Kenneth Lemke and Yorghos Apostolopoulos*	**171**

vi   *Contents*

Chapter 9   The Part-Systems Continuum in Medicine   **191**
                   Patrick Finzer

Chapter 10   Systems Theory and the Cerebral Cortex   **205**
                   Manuel F. Casanova, Ioan Opris, Estate M. Sokhadze
                   and Emily L. Casanova

Chapter 11   From Quorum Sensing to Dynome through Mitochondria   **221**
                   Jean Ciurea and Tatiana Ciurea

Chapter 12   The Nutrition System and the Brain   **259**
                   Cosmin Sonea and Ioan Opris

Chapter 13   A Modular Approach to the Organization of Brain Functions **287**
                   Ioan Opris, Estate M. Sokhadze, Emily L. Casanova,
                   Cosmin Sonea and Manuel F. Casanova

About the Editors   **315**

Index   **317**

PREFACE

This book is divided into two sections: one dealing with the theoretical background and another with the practical applications of systems theory. Developments along both of these pathways have transpired, for the most part, independent of each other with few attempts at integrating them. We have been fortunate to have had the contributions of leading experts in their fields who have delved into those critical aspects faced by practitioners. The ultimate aim of the book is to provide a set of tools allowing for better understanding of natural organizations as they exist in equilibrium with their environment. These systems live in dynamic interactions with other systems on which they may depend in order to continue functioning. In this manner, we may examine conceptual or actual, living or non-living, natural or man-made, organizations from the standpoint of living organisms. This perspective accrues regardless of whether we are focusing our attention on wide-ranging problems such as traffic (vehicular) congestion on highways or debating the philosophy of consciousness. Curiously, the comprehensive nature of subjects covered in this book warmly reminds us how all of the contributors themselves were part of a system; wherein they acted as modules that taken together may ultimately give rise to unpredictable new ideas from our readership.

A basic understanding of systems theory often helps simplify messy problems. It allows us to anticipate potential complications and think away from limiting organizational conceptual frameworks. In essence, systems theory is a way of looking at the big picture and, with a new gained understanding, optimize the chance for long-term success. It is hoped that this new understanding will guide us to create and manage systems that will surpass capabilities presently observed in the living world. This optimistic outlook is reflected in the multidisciplinary nature of this book. Indeed, system theory was born from the ideas of von Bertalanffy who in the 1930's introduced the concept as a way of accommodating the interrelationships of disparate fields of study. This was a conceptual approach at creating a Common Law that would apply similarly to the natural, social, and formal sciences. It may thus be possible that in a future edition of this book we could expand our perspectives by including contrasting points of view like biochemistry or physical chemistry and see how we could apply those to analyze a variety of natural situations.

The editors (MFC and IO) are grateful to NOVA Science Publishers as they were the ones that initiated the idea of writing this book. Their vision formalized our goal-seeking behavior while their suggestions provided our initial input. NOVA allowed us to take ownership of our work and to fulfill our vision. We appreciate the fact that they were not micromanagers and trusted the opinions of the editors and contributors as professionals. Hopefully the book, in its present format, serves as the appropriate "output" whose quality will be evaluated by "feedback" from the readers. It may be posited that the book itself enjoyed a measure of "self-organization" as its resultant order was born out of an initially disordered system. We just hope that, in editing this book, we have not reached a regulated state or equilibrium as we believe that there is much more to learn and hope that we may push our boundaries a lot further in the immediate future. Finally, we are extremely grateful to all of the contributors, some of whom complied with stringent deadlines while battling through sickness. The book, in this regard, was borne out of the interdependence of all contributors whose efforts and ideas have affected each of us in a positive manner.

In: Focus on Systems Theory Research
Editors: Manuel F. Casanova and Ioan Opris
ISBN: 978-1-53614-561-8
© 2019 Nova Science Publishers, Inc.

Chapter 1

BIASES IN THE PROCESS OF DESIGNING A SYSTEM

Helmut Nechansky[*]
Nechansky - Engineering Efficiency, Vienna, Austria

ABSTRACT

System design is mostly considered as a rational process running from a set goal to a final design. Yet this paper analysis system design in a wider context and identifies 7 biases which influence it: (1) The educational/environmental/cultural base of the goal-setter and the system designer; (2) material constraints; (3) the explicit goal-setting for the design, coming with implicit material, ethical, moral and political valuations; (4) the specific knowledge, creativity and intuition of the system designer and (5) actual decisions based on that, determining investigated solutions; (6) the acceptance criteria, determining when a design is 'good enough'; (7) the dominating educational/environmental/cultural context-specific paradigms, which determine how a design is received in a larger context. So the paper concludes that systems design is not purely rational and value-free, as mostly assumed. Instead, it is a highly biased process depending primarily on a material base, related interests, and power in the relevant context.

Keywords: system design, system design methodologies, system context, context dependence, bias, truth

---

[*] Corresponding Author Email: hn@nechansky.co.at.

1. INTRODUCTION

"One option is to maintain the spirit of the classical laboratory by collecting just those data that appear relevant and can be obtained objectively [...]. The other option, the harder one, is to recognize that the unpredictable human is an essential aspect, and to begin to invent a methodology in which human bias is a central aspect. Will this methodology be 'scientific'? No, if we doggedly stick to the assumption that the classical laboratory is the basis of science. Yes, if 'science' means the creation of relevant knowledge about the human condition." C. West Churchman (1979, 62)

System design is mostly considered as a purely rational process running from a set goal to a final design.

Yet in this chapter, our objective is to follow Churchman's consideration quoted above and to investigate system design in a larger context than usual. We will analyze how this context influences the design process and particularly how biases resulting from individual actors, societal settings and stakeholder interests shape its outcome.

Before, we start reviewing a few selected approaches to system design. This selection is far from complete, and cannot do justice to the many thinkers in the field. But we think it provides a sufficient overview on the field by presenting widely complementary views.

In the following summaries we will primarily focus on the highly original core contributions of the various authors. But secondarily we will discuss important aspects, which are not clarified in these selected approaches. This is an unjust procedure, because it tends to neglect what is clarified. But we think that is necessary to develop the starting point for our investigation below. There we will try to integrate important aspects of the presented approaches, as well as to address some important aspects of system design, which were often left out so far.

1.1. Mesarovic and Takahara's General Systems Theory

We start the discussion of approaches to systems design with the work of Mesarovic and Takahara (1975, 4), a classical text on mathematical systems science. According to these authors, just four steps are necessary to design a system:

1. A verbal description;
2. A block diagram;
3. A set theoretical "general systems model";
4. Preferably a detailed mathematical model consisting of (differential) equations, or otherwise a computer simulation.

Mesarovic und Takahara (1975) consider the verbal description and the block diagram as imprecise preliminary steps, and consider even their own set theoretical "general systems model" as mathematically trivial, while they see only a mathematical model as an "exact" method.

We think this approach reflects widespread current thinking in science. Here the whole process seems quite simple, short and straightforward. What is sought is a fast track to mathematical formulae. Once these are formulated, then "exact" science must have occurred. What seemingly does not occur on this route are any epistemological questions, e.g., how a certain design is influenced by the goals pursued, or by decisions to include or exclude variables, etc.

1.2. Systems Engineering

Systems engineering uses much more detailed schemes for system design (see, e.g., Patzak, 1982, Winzer, 2013). Here the main steps are:

1. A prime step of goal-setting specifies what should be achieved.
2. Then follow some steps of sketching and then increasingly detailing the system design. After each step, some tests are carried out to evaluate, if the current detailing of the design might be appropriate to realize the goals.

   Should some of these tests fail, then the design is reworked and changed, till one is found that passes the tests.
3. Finally, if a sufficiently detailed design passed all theoretical tests, the system is realized.
4. Then all parts of the design are realized, and are again tested and evaluated.
5. When all the parts passed the tests, the whole structural design is realized, and a planned start up procedure is carried out to test the function of the whole system; if all tests are passed the system is released to normal use.
6. Finally the planners evaluate the whole design process and consider 'lessons learnt', i.e., which of the recent experiences can be generalized and can contribute to the design process, so that it will be improved, if a comparable systems has to be designed again in the future.

Here we find a much more detailed and considerate view of the very system design process, than in Mesarovic and Takahara (1975).

We find the prime act of goal-setting, a step-by-step detailing of the design, the evaluation of each step, and a variety of conceptual tools, which need not be mathematical formulae, but my be technical drawings, flow-sheets, organograms, etc.;

4   *Helmut Nechansky*

and, finally, we find a rail to generalize any insights, which might be useful for future projects.

We do not find here any considerations of the goal-setting process itself and of the evaluative steps; nor do any persons, like clients, system designers, or users play an explicit role.

1.3. Klir's Architecture of Systems Problem Solving

A different and quite complex general approach was elaborated by Klir (1985; for a useful short summary see Flood, 1989). He developed a multi-level bottom-up approach to system design, and he even found a place for the role of the investigator or investigating team in the design process.

Let us try to briefly summarize Klir's scheme:

Klir starts with the "formulation of a source system". Here an investigator or an investigating team observe an "object" within the "environment" of the investigator(s). Their consideration of the object is guided by the "purpose" and by "constraints" of the investigation. From these considerations the investigator(s) derive(s) a "hierarchy of epistemological types of systems", which consists of at least five basic levels, but may have more, when complex issues are investigated. The five basic levels are:

Level 1: The lowest level is the "source system". It consists of a set of the variables, which are considered, a set of ranges of validity of these variables, and operations to characterize these variables when observing their occurrence in reality.

Level 2: Then follows the "data system"; it provides the actually observed data for the variables defined a level 1.

Level 3: This is the "generative system" containing the models, which are applied to generate the data of level 2.

Level 4: This is the "structure system" defining the relations between the models of level 3.

Level 5: This is the "metasystem" describing the relations between the relations on level 4.

There may be more levels starting with a "meta-metasystem", and so on, to characterize more levels of relations between complex systems.

So, Klir (1985) addresses the role of the system designer(s) and the goal-setting in the design process, and acknowledges that constraints may decisively limit it.

Klir reflects the important fact that any integration of two (or more) elements or subsystems into a larger system always requires a higher meta-level containing meta -

decision rules how to combine them. And Klir's system designers create, fill and modify these epistemological levels moving up and down within their system design.

What remains open in Klir's bottom-up approach is how the system designers can create any additional level of their design, without having already an even higher level how to combine the elements making up the additional level.

1.4. Van Gigch's Metamodeling

Van Gigch (1993) developed a more-level approach, too, less detailed than Klir's (1985) approach, but with some resemblances and additions.

Let us briefly describe van Gigch's levels bottom up:

Level 1: This is the "lower level" of "practice", where "evidence" of "organizational problems" forms the input. To these problems "scientific theories and models" are applied, which lead to planned actions. These actions lead finally to the output of "solutions" to the problems.

Level 2: This is the higher "object level" of "science", where "evidence" of "scientific problems" is the input. To these problems "paradigms" are applied, and theoretical considerations and research activities are derived from them. These lead to the output of "scientific theories and models", which are applied later on level 1 to solve practical problems.

Level 3: This is the "meta level" of "epistemology", where "evidence" of "epistemological questions" forms the input. To these questions some "philosophy of science" is applied and thought processes are derived from it. These, in turn, lead to the output of epistemological and scientific "paradigms", which are applied on level 2 to resolve scientific problems.

What van Gigch (1993) emphasized more clearly than Klir (1985) is that there are continuous cyclic processes; these consist, first, of normative top-down processes, followed later by corrective and innovative bottom-up processes:

System designers implicitly apply paradigms (van Gigch's level 3) which determine scientific theories (level 2), which they use to solve practical problems (level 1). Whenever that does not work and there remain unsolved practical problems (level 1), they move to a higher level, trying to develop new scientific theories (level 2), while applying given paradigms (level 3). Then they move down again, and test the new scientific theories (level 2) applying them again to practical problems (level 1). Whenever that does not work (level 1), too, and there remain unsolved scientific problems (level 2), they move to an even higher level, trying to develop new paradigms (level 3), while applying a "philosophy of science" (an even higher level not numbered by von Gigch). Then they move again down one level and apply these new paradigms (level 3) to develop new scientific theories (level 2), which are tested again on the lower level when applied to practical problems (level 1).

According to van Gigch (1993) the "metalevel" of "paradigms" (his level 3) is decisive for system design, because it contains the "design foundations of modeling", which "consist of reasoning processes, guarantees of truth, proofs, axioms of validity, or any other logic which underlies a methodology."

So, we find in van Gigch what we missed in Klir's bottom-up approach (1985), namely that the design process starts top-down by applying some given (levels of) theories (like "paradigms" and a "philosophy of science") to problem solving.

Yet surprisingly van Gigch fails to explain why his unnumbered highest level, the "philosophy of science", which directly or indirectly *determines* the content of *all* his lower levels including his "metalevel", is not the most important one. And he does not explain, too, where this determining "philosophy of science" might come from and how it is formulated.

1.5. Churchman's Design of Inquiring Systems

Churchman (1971; for a very good summary see Linden et al., 2007) started with the interesting observation that system design always has to begin with limited, *preliminary knowledge*, for it is exactly this limitation that makes the investigative process necessary (p. 4).

Then he continues with a preliminary description of the design process (without ever giving a final one) suggesting that it has at least five characteristics (Churchman, 1971, 5 - 8):

1. The design process has to distinguish between different possible behaviors (distinguishing *what* can be done).
2. The design process has to try to evaluate which behavior will best serve previously defined goals (answering *when* something should be done).
3. The aim of the process is to provide a design in a form that can be communicated to others, so that these can realize it, and actually serve the previously defined goals (telling *how* something should be done).
4. Furthermore, the design process aims at generality, too, to provide guidelines for other system designers facing similar problems (answering *why* something should be done).
5. The system designer defines the elements considered in the design process and the interrelations between them; and with that he or she determines the limits of the design, too.

Now this design process can be applied to design five types of "inquiring systems", which start from different presuppositions, and are designed to serve different notions of "truth" (van Gigch, 1988). We follow here widely the crisp summary of Linden et al. (2007):

- Leibnizian inquiring systems:

  Here "Knowledge of *a priori* law predominates knowledge of *a posteriori* fact";

  And "Knowledge of *a posteriori* fact does not predominate knowledge of *a priori* law" (Linden et al., 2007, 839).

  Leibnizian or "rationalist" inquiring systems "begin with some given propositions, postulates, or axioms and use deductive logic to drive the process. Empirical facts are meaningful only in so far as they fit into or inform the logical scheme" (Linden et al., 2007, 839).

  Here "Truth is analytical, that is, the truth content of a system is associated entirely with its formal content"; and: "Systems can be represented by formal models whose validation rests with their ability to offer theoretical explanations of a wide scope of phenomena" (Churchman, 1971, 9).

- Lockean inquiring systems:

  Here "Knowledge of *a priori* law does not predominate knowledge of *a posteriori* fact";

  And "Knowledge of *a posteriori* fact predominates knowledge of *a priori* law" (Linden et al., 2007, 839).

  Lockean inquiring systems or "empiricism" "begin with elementary observations or facts which drive the process by becoming the raw material input for inductive generalizations. Laws are meaningful only in so far as they help explain the data" (Linden et al., 2007, 839).

  Here 'truth' is only obtained from observations, facts and data.

- Kantian inquiring systems:

  Here "Knowledge of *a priori* law predominates knowledge of *a posteriori* fact";

  And "Knowledge of *a posteriori* fact predominates knowledge of *a priori* law" (Linden et al., 2007, 839).

  Kantian inquiring systems place "laws and facts on equal footing" and seek "to find the best model to fit the data often moving back and forth until an adequate synthesis is found" (Linden et al., 2007, 839).

  Here 'truth' is approached in an approximating process where *a priori* knowledge is applied to make empirical investigations, which in turn are applied to improve the previous knowledge, and so on, to achieve an increasing fit between the two. So, Kantian inquiry systems combine aspects of Liebnizian and Lockean ones.

- Hegelian inquiring systems:

    Here "Knowledge of *a priori* law does not predominate knowledge of *a posteriori* fact";

    And "Knowledge of *a posteriori* fact does not predominate knowledge of *a priori* law" (Linden et al., 2007, 839).

    Hegelian or "dialectic" inquiring systems relegate "both laws and facts to a secondary role" and stress "the dialectical arguments that drive the process toward a synthesis" (Linden et al., 2007, 839).

    Here 'truth' is sought by confronting opposing views, a thesis and an antithesis, attempting to find a more encompassing synthesis; this may get confronted again with an antithesis to drive the process further on towards an all-encompassing *Weltanschauung*.

- Singerian inquiring systems (named after the American philosopher E. A. Singer):

    Churchman finally developed a fifth type of Singerian inquiry systems trying to unite the advantages of the other four, while overcoming their weaknesses, particularly when dealing with complex systems.

    Here again "Knowledge of *a priori* law does not predominate knowledge of *a posteriori* fact";

    And "Knowledge of *a posteriori* fact does not predominate knowledge of *a priori* law" (Linden et al., 2007, 839); so, in a way Singerian inquiry systems are Hegelian.

    But Singerian or "pragmatic" (Linden et al., 2007, 840) inquiry systems do not consider observations as unequivocal facts (like $X = P$), but as attributions (like $X \rightarrow P \pm p$), because P always depends on measurement (Churchman, 1971, 202); and it may depend on the context of a changing larger system. Furthermore Singerian inquiry systems start to question any laws and any given knowledge, whenever correspondence between laws or knowledge and observations is observed too often. Therefore, they ask when it is time to refine knowledge and/or even to reconsider previous goals for system design, to get to an ever more differentiated picture of the world and to be able to serve ever more individual interests of different "users".

    So, whenever the other inquiry system approaches might have led closer towards a final 'truth', Singerian inquiry systems move in the opposite direction, start to question their knowledge and to differentiate it, developing ever more measurement-, context-, goal- and user-specific system designs.

Churchman (1971) is not very specific on the process of designing a system, but he adds the decisive insight, that designs may strive towards different notions of 'truth', which may be sought in the following alternative options:

- Leibnizian 'truth': The correspondence with a given body of thought;
- Lockean 'truth': The correspondence with observed facts;
- Kantian 'truth': The approximative development of an increasing correspondence of a continuously improved body of thought with increasing numbers of observed facts;
- Hegelian 'truth': The integration of opposing views into an encompassing agreement;
- Singerian 'truth': The development of ever more problem- and user-specific solutions.

So, put very shortly and in more profane language, we can say that Churchman (1971) addresses the important question: When is a system design 'good'?

Only when we agree that a system design is 'good', we know we are on the right track, and can proceed on the chosen way. Churchman tells us that a system design might be 'good', when it fits a holy text or scientific paradigm, or fits some facts, or fits facts better than a previous system design, or enables agreement, or enables individual solutions.

1.6. Jackson's Systems Paradigms

Jackson (2003) reviews approaches to system design for management applications and orders these approaches in a "system of systems methodologies".

From Jackson's numerous insights we take here only the point that system design can happen in different contexts, where parties can pursue different systems of goal-values, and therefore can get in different relations with which each other:

(1) Parties can pursue diverging goal-values. In such contexts we usually find some powerful and coercive actors, which can establish hierarchical relations and can enforce the realization of their goals, against the interests of others.
(2) In these contexts, where parties pursue diverging goal-values, we find, accordingly, victims of coercion, too, which are subordinated to coercive actors, who ignore or suppress their interests.

(3) Parties can pursue pluralistic goal-values, i.e., they have different, but somehow compatible views. This allows peaceful coexistence, and searching for possible mutual endeavors, which can be realized with means all parties can agree on.

(4) Parties can pursue unitary goal-values, i.e., they widely agree on what they want to achieve. This is the base for cooperative relations and mutual optimization of outcomes.

So, Jackson (2003) shows that system design can happen in different contexts coming with different relations, or we would say different modes of coexistence (Nechansky, 2016a, 2016b, 2017), between the parties concerned. And Jackson's analysis adds to the system design literature that the context can decisively influence the design process, and particularly the goal-setting process. Additionally he suggests that the system design process should be modified in accordance with the context to enable the involvement of many and ideally all parties concerned; if that does not prove possible, system design will only lead to the satisfaction of few.

1.7. Summary of the Selected Approaches to System Design

After this review of some selected approaches to system design let us try to bring order into the variety we found. We start trying to show some *common* elements:

- Mostly there is agreement that the whole process of system designs starts with setting goal-values, describing what should be achieved.
- Then there is wide agreement that system design proceeds in steps:
  – Here first parts of the system are conceptualized.
  – Then the parts are evaluated.
    When the parts passed the evaluation the design process can proceed: First to the next parts, then to the integration of the parts into subsystems, the evaluation of the subsystems, and so on, till finally the whole system is conceptualized and evaluated.
- There may be alternative solutions for the design of the whole system, which may be evaluated to finally choose the best system design.
- There may be a realization phase of the system (if the system is not a purely conceptual one), using similar steps of making and testing parts, putting these together, testing, etc.

Let us remark at that point, that even if most approaches acknowledge the necessity of goal-setting and evaluative processes, surprisingly little is said about how these processes actually work.

Then there are some aspects of the design process, which seem to apply generally, but are highlighted only in *some* approaches:

- Usually there are material constraints limiting system designs (Klir, 1985).
- Some preliminary (Churchman, 1971) or higher level knowledge (van Gigch, 1993, Klir, 1985) is needed, which determines the decisions, which parts and subsystems should enter into and make up the final system design.
- Different notions of 'truth' (Churchman, 1971) can be applied, each giving a system design process a different direction, to satisfy different criteria evaluating when a design might be considered as 'good'.

Finally there may be different contexts in which system design can take place:

- Jackson (2003) points out that system design can take place in contexts with different modes of coexistence (Nechansky, 2007, 2016), with coercive, suppressed, indifferent, or agreeing parties, showing different degrees of correspondence about the goal-values, which should be pursued.
- Churchman (1971) implicitly adds that parties might not only differ in their views about goal-values, but additionally in their notions of 'truth', too, i.e., how to evaluate if a goal or system design is 'good'.

So, from the approaches we reviewed here, we get a quite unclear and complex picture of the many aspects of system design. As far as we know, it was never tried to unite all these aspects to develop a unified theory. In the following we will investigate the interrelations between these aspects, to move towards such a unified description of system design.

Before we start with that investigation, we have to clarify some notions.

2. SOME BASIC NOTIONS AND SOME IMMEDIATE CONSEQUENCES

2.1. Definition of Core Notions

We will use the following notions in our analysis of system design:

- We take our notion of a system from Klir's (1991) simple and pragmatic definition:

A system is defined by a set of elements and relations between these elements.

We will try to remain as general as possible, so we will not give any more detailed description of either elements or relations, leaving open if they are just abstract concepts, or certain physical or social entities. We will occasionally give examples to illustrate our general considerations.

- We understands *states* as patterns or sequences of patterns, which an individual can observe in the external world around him or her, or which may be the result of thought processes modifying previous observed patterns or sequences of patterns.
- We name a *goal-value* (or sometimes shortly a goal) a certain state which should be achieved with a system design.

  That means the goal-value describes these pattern or sequences of patterns, which should be observable once the system is finished. So, a goal-value may describe a scientific conceptual understanding of a chain of causes and effects, or a technical function fulfilled, or a social interaction enabled, etc.
- We understand as *knowledge* any representation of states available to a human individual, i.e., patterns and/or sequences, which have been either observed, or created in thought processes.

  Particularly we distinguish between the following:
  - o *Passive knowledge* consists only of observed or created patterns and sequences.
  - o *Active knowledge* contains decision rules, which combine patterns or sequences with particular actions effecting and changing these patterns or sequences.
- We understand as *system designer* the human individual carrying out the design process, i.e., the person in charge of the decisions, which states should become elements and relations making up the system.

  (That means we rule out here some automatized system design with computers; we consider this as a second rated problem, because any computer was initially programmed by a system designer according to our definition.)

  We will consider only single system designers, leaving out any conflicts or coordination problems, which might occur when more are involved.
- We understand as the *design process* that sequence of activities of the system designer, which leads from a given state towards the state described by the goal-value.
- Finally we understand as *bias* any decision criteria of persons concerned with the design process, which are applied during the design process and give a systems design a more personal form rather than a universal character.

Such decision criteria may result, e.g., from personal views, personal interests, group interests, or group- or culture-specific accepted models of thought, etc.

2.2. Some Consequences Derived from the Definition of Core Notions

Already from that very general definition of a system taken from Klir (1991) we can derive some basic aspects of the process of system design:

1. If the selection of the elements and relations, which shall make up a system, is not an arbitrary choice from the sets of all possible elements and relations, then a system has to be the result of a *goal-orientated* design process. Here the goal-value delivers the criterion to investigate, understand, model and/or realize some states.

2. The goal-value serves primarily as the criterion to select appropriate elements (while leaving out others), which are the smallest units of investigation and are characterized by having certain properties.

   These elements are not further analyzed within a certain systems approach. The properties, which they are supposed to have, are not explained within that systems approach. But these properties have to explain at least the kind of relations, which can be established between the elements.

3. A system has certain *limits*, constituted by the fact that only selected elements belong to it. With these limits comes the definition of an *environment* or *context*, containing everything not considered as part of the system.

4. The goal-value serves secondarily as the criterion to select certain relations (while leaving others out), which connect the elements of the system. Relations can be any kind of connections, static or dynamic, uni- or bidirectional, able to transport matter, energy and/or data, etc.

   Inputs are ingoing relations leading from the environment to elements of the system.

   Outputs are outgoing relations leading from elements of the system into the environment.

5. The sum of all elements and the considered relations, inputs and outputs constitute the *structure* of the system. It determines the actual complexity of the system.

After these definitions of key terms, we can now turn to our analysis of system design.

3. OUTLINE OF THE DEVELOPED APPROACH
TO SYSTEM DESIGN

Above we reviewed various approaches to system design and the different aspects, which they highlight. Now, let us outline what we take from these approaches, what we add to them and how we additionally investigate interrelations between all aspects considered. We will proceed as follows:

- System design happens in a *context*. We take that view from Jackson, but differentiate it:

  We start with the investigation of the core actor(s): There is at least one system designer; but additionally there may be a client, ordering a design, and an employer employing a system designer.

- System design has a necessary *material base*. Surprisingly this is only mentioned by Klir.

  System design requires material resources, at least to support one system designer and to document the final design. But, of course, requirements can be enormous. Anyway, the available resources always limit what can be done.

- A *process of goal-setting* initiates a system design. Practically all approaches agree on that.

  But usually goal-setting is simply taken for granted as starting point, but never investigated. Yet we think it is decisive to understand where goal-values actually can come from, how they are related to actors, are restricted by the material base, and determine the whole design process.

- Goal-setting is necessary, but not sufficient to evaluate the design process. We need additionally *goal-orientated evaluation criteria*, to decide, first, if the design process is '*good*' and leads towards the goal (this was the focus of Churchman, 1971), and, secondarily, to decide when it is '*good enough*', to know when the mission is accomplished; this latter point is practically never considered.

- Once the previous points are clear, at least one system designer can carry out the core design process.

  Most approaches focus on the *steps* of this process (and particularly systems engineering). But we will emphasize the related activities and particularly the *decisions* of the system designer(s), and how his or her knowledge and assumptions, as well as the goal-setting process influence the design process.

- Finally we will consider the *wider context* of the system design.

  Here we investigate how the design of the core actors may be received in a wider context, where various parties may be concerned, which may be coercive, suppressed, indifferent or cooperative, according to Jackson's (2003) approach (discussed in section 1.6.).

So, we will take a wider look on the process of system design: We will ask where goals may come from, and how they determine the whole design process; we will consider the influence of the designer and of a wider context. And particularly we will investigate how these factors can amount to *biases*, which can crucially determine the final design and can make it something quite different than the result of purely rational process to optimally realize a certain goal. So, let us analyze these factors in turn.

4. THE CORE CONTEXT FOR SYSTEM DESIGN

Following Jackson (2003), we have to consider the context of system design. However, we will differentiate and supplement his approach:

We will focus here on a *core context*, where core actors a directly involved in a design process. We will consider only later a *wider context* (see section 9), where more parties with different power may be concerned, which may be coercive, suppressed, indifferent or united (Jackson, 2003).

In the core context *core actors* have to accept clear goal-values so that a design process can start:

1. In the simplest case, there is just a single actor, a *system designer* making a system for himself or herself.
2. More often, we will find additionally a second core actor, namely at least one *client* ordering a system designer to make a design.
3. Additionally we find often that a client addresses an *employer*, who employs the system designer.

So there may be one or up to three different types of core actors.

How these core actors can work and realize their system design in the *core context* depends on their positions according to Jackson the *wider context*. If they are part of coercive parties, they will have a more easy play. But if they belong to suppressed ones, they will have to consider the coercive parties throughout the process, from goal-setting, via the design process to some final realization. Furthermore, the whole process can be complicated, if the parties forming the context apply different criteria for 'truth' according to Churchman. We will consider the effects of such settings in section 9 below.

5. The Material Base for System Design

Next we have to consider the material base for the system design. Surprisingly only Klir (1985) acknowledges that this may be a major constraint.

5.1. The Material Needs for System Design

There are two material demands for designing a system:

The first concerns the material needs of the system designer. Obviously, like every human, the system designer needs an income securing at least his or her existential needs (i.e., at least food, shelter and health care). Here the available material means determine the amount of time and effort the designer can spend on the project.

The second material needs concern the design process itself. Here the available material means determine the support that can be offered to the designer (like technical equipment, information, personal services, etc.).

The overall availability of material means for both, designer and design process, limit the scope and the sophistication of any design. This *material constraint* is one *bias* limiting the system design.

5.2. The Sources of the Material Base for the System Design

Now there are different possibilities to provide for the material need of design and designer, which depend on the core context (as discussed in section 4 above):

- The system designer may cover all material needs from personal wealth;
- The system designer may get a personal income and a budget for the design process directly from some client, who entrusts him or her with the systems development.
- The system designer may get a personal income from an employer, who gets a budget for the designer and the design process from some client.

Again, the activities of the core actors as well as their use of their means, may be influenced by the larger context, e.g., if they have to act against coercive parties, or may work freely (see section 9).

Let us consider next how the source of the material base that can influence goal-setting and can introduce further biases in the design process.

6. THE GOAL-SETTING PROCESS

So far, we have clarified possible core contexts for system design. And we have addressed material needs, which may be served by different sources, which can vary again with the core context. These are major determinants, which influence the decisive goal-setting process specifying what a system design should be all about. We turn now to this process.

We start considering the options for goal-setting, i.e., which of the core actors may actually set the goals, and which interests come with that. Next, we highlight the interrelations between goal-setting, interests and material constrains, before we turn to the goal-setting process itself.

6.1. The Options for Goal-Setting

In our scheme with three possible core actors, which may be involved in the system design, there are only two sources where goal-values may come from:

- First, the system designer can set the goal-values, if, and only if, he or she has a secure material base (ideally from own personal wealth, or from some guaranteed personal income) to provide for himself or herself as well as for the design process.

  Only in that case there are no external goal-conflicts or conflicts of interest during the design process.

  Here remains just the question, if the system designer is driven by impersonal professional interests (like scientific rigor) or by prevailing personal interests (like fame).
- Secondly, a client can set the goal-values for the system and provides the material resources for the design process.
  - Here the client may enter in a direct relation with the system designer.

    Then we have an implicit conflict of interests between client and designer.
  - Or, the client enters in a relation with an employer, who cares for the design process and provides for the system designer.

    Here we have an implicit conflict of interests between client, employer and designer.

These are the basic settings for system design. And here we have to emphasize one decisive point, which most approaches to system design, which neither consider the material base nor where goals may come from, do not even touch:

The right of goal-setting for a system design is mostly linked to the ability to provide the necessary material resources.

The ideal case seems to be the first case, the single, wealthy researcher driven by impersonal professional interests and pursuing own goal-values. Yet with scientific, technical and organizational systems getting ever more complex, the reach of a single individual seems too limited to achieve very much alone. So other settings become increasingly important, particularly the third one, which may include many system designers working under one head. Yet with these settings come conflicts of interests, at which we have a closer look next.

Anyway, to think that system design may be just a linear, rational, value free process leading from a goal-value to an optimal solution, without any intervening diverging interests, is at best possible for the single wealthy system designer. Yet much of the literature on system design leaves out the context of goal-setting, the source of the material base, as well we the resulting interrelations of interests and the related biases creeping in.

6.2. Contexts of Goal-Setting and Resulting Biases Influencing the Design Process

Depending on the number of core actors, as well as on the source of the material base and of the goal-values for the design project, we get ever more complex interrelations of different interests playing into a design process.

When we consider the core actors alone, without considering a wider context yet (to which we turn in section 9 below), we find the following constellations for system design:

- There are always the interests of the system designer.

    These consist of continuously securing an income (at least for existential needs like food, shelter and health), and maybe a prevailing impersonal professional interest in the quality of the system design, or maybe prevailing personal interests in fame, quick income, etc.

    Additionally there are probably long-term interests in stable social relationships with a community (probably including family and friends), i.e., a wider context (see section 9).

- There may be additionally interests of a client.

    Of course, the interests of the client have to include, too, continuously securing an own income (at least for existential needs like food, shelter and health).

The client's goal-values for the system design may directly serve his or her material interests (maintaining or increasing income); or, provided these are served, the client may want to pursue any other personal goals. Anyway, independent of the content of the selected goals, he or she will probably demand a material optimality, i.e., he or she will wish to get a maximum of value with minimal effort.

The interests of the client will probably include, too, long-term interests in stable social relationships with a community (probably including family and friends), i.e., a wider context (see section 9), and/or eventually with the system designer.

And here, when working for a client, the system designer's interests may include the wish to provide a system design that is a good compromise between value for the client and value for him- or herself. This may include the trial to use or to fit in available information, know-how from previous approaches, or to reuse other designs for the design for the actual client, etc. Additionally the system designer's own professional and personal interests, as well as his or her social interests may be moderated by long-term interests in stable social relationships with the client, to secure long-term income.

- And there may be additionally interests of the employer of the system designer.

Of course, the interests of the employer have to include, too, continuously securing an own income (at least for existential needs like food, shelter and health).

Additionally the interests of the employer may include the wish for a system design that is a good compromise between value for the client and value for the employer. This may include the trial to use or to fit in available information, know-how from previous approaches, or to reuse other designs for the design for the actual client, etc.

The interests of the employer will probably include long-term interests in stable social relationships with a community (probably including family and friends), i.e., a wider context (see section 9), too, and/or eventually with the client to secure long-term income and/or additionally the system designer to secure long-term services to clients.

And here the client's interests may be moderated by long-term interests in stable social relationships with the employer.

And here the system designer's interests may be moderated by long-term interests in stable social relationships with the employer.

We think it is important to make explicit all these possible and likely interests that may be involved in the core design process alone. And we think it is particularly important, to emphasize the obvious, i.e., that humans continuously have material existential needs. Only if they have an income to serve these needs, then they can engage in anything else. So system design either directly aims at securing someone's income; or otherwise we will find behind it a solution securing the income of the core actors, that allows them to pursue the design. Ignoring these existential dependencies means turning away from the divergent material interests, which may influence or even shape a system design process.

In sum these interests of the core actors can amount to the following *goal-setter biases*:

There are always *explicit objectives for the design* (a necessary bias), usually determined by the provider of the material base for the systems design. The pursuance of these objectives may be influenced by the *interests of a system designer* (a first occasional bias) and additionally by the *interests of an employer* (a second occasional bias).

So, considering system design as a rational, scientific, value-free process may apply at best to the single and wealthy researcher, but seems to be fairy tale in the most usual settings today.

6.3. Goal-Setting

So, there may be two sources for setting the goal-values what to achieve with the system design: The system designer, or a client.

And there may be three different contexts for the system design: With a system designer alone, or one hired by a client, or one hired by an employer working for a client.

Most approaches to system design do not even distinguish these different settings. They just agree that the whole process starts with some goal-values, and simply take them for granted, without asking where they might come from. And they only ask how to realize the set goals.

We consider that as a technically valid move, if one just wants to get an overview on the steps of the design process. But that means leaving out the decisive questions of systems design, which are:

- What is a goal-value at all?
- What is a goal-value for?
- And how does a goal-value come about?

We suggest the following answers to these questions:

- A goal-value is a *description of some future states*, which currently do not occur, or at least do not always occur (i.e., it is "teleological" as Churchman, 1971, has put it.)
- A goal-value includes the assumption that *the described states are 'better' for somebody in some way* than the currently given states.

  We strongly suggest that we can widely ignore cases where something should not be 'better'; we will shortly come back to that below.

  Now, from our analysis of the role of the core actors above we can say that the crucial guiding assumptions *'better for whom'* and *'better in which way'* depend on the person setting the goal-values; and that is normally, too, the person providing the material resources, i.e., paying for the system design.

  That means that system design usually aims at something, which is 'better' either for the wealthy system designer, or for the wealthy client.
- Finally, as an assumption of some future 'better' states, a goal-value is itself sort of a system design:

  But such a goal-value is only *an intuitive and vague system concept*, a quick and brief sketch, delivering a simple outline of some 'better' goal-states, which seem possible and feasible.

So, we suggest that actually an *intuitive* system concept delivering goal-values precedes the systematic, rational and technical system design process trying to realize these goal-values. This intuitive concept includes the assumption that something might be better for somebody, usually the system designer or the client. And the role of system design is to investigate and, if possible, to validate, if the intuitive assumptions of possibility, feasibility and betterment actually do hold.

We cannot overemphasize that point:

There are no problems in the world per se, *there are only problems because of goal-values, i.e., because of intuitive, imaginative concepts and assumptions that something might be 'better'.*

If you are always satisfied with the world as you find it, there are no problems. You might happily walk to the next spring to drink water, pluck fruits wherever you find them, and sleep under trees. Perhaps you traveled that way sometime, when you were young, or still occasionally do it when you take holidays. You might even experience a welcome relaxation in such times. Why that: Because problems occur only if you start to imagine that something could be any different, e.g., that water should be available out of a pipe near you, fruits should be delivered on order via mobile phone, sleep should be protected by an air-conditioned house, etc., etc. Whenever you select such an imagination and try to realize it, you have set a goal-value, you have declared some current state as unsatisfactory and you have *created* a problem. And only after that you can enter the realm of system design as it is understood by most thinkers - as starting once a goal is *set*.

But actually, once the goal is set the decisive decisions determining the whole design process have already been made.

So, we strongly suggest that setting goal-values for system design unites two features, which are usually not associated with systematic developments and even less with science:

- *Setting goal-values is an intuitive act.* (And actually it is only the first important place of intuition in system design; we will identify a second one in section 8.1.1. below).

  We follow here Bergson (1912, 89), whose work dealing with intuition was acclaimed in philosophy, but was never closely observed in science:

  "But the simple act, which started the analysis, and which conceals itself behind the analysis proceeds from a faculty quite different from the analytical. This is by its very definition intuition."

  In the goal-setting act *one somehow promising option* is selected from available knowledge. If this option actually will be promising is an open question, but that is evaluated as worth investigating.

  So the goal-setting act, consisting of the selection of one option as well as the evaluation of the worth to investigate it, is not and cannot be 'rational' in the sense, that it could be explained completely with available clear and unequivocal arguments. Since it is not known that the option will really turn out promising, there cannot be such arguments; so both, the selection and the evaluation derive from intuition.

  And the lack of unequivocal arguments for the goal-values is exactly what makes the investigative system design process necessary.

- And setting goal-values comes with a notion of 'better'.
  Again we can follow Bergson (1912, 41):

  "We do not aim generally at knowledge for the sake of knowledge, but in order to take sides, to draw profit – in short to satisfy an interest."

  There seems to be no reason, why the states described in the goal-value should have been selected, if not because they are promising, i.e., 'better' in some regard, than the given states. (Even masochists, sadists and suicide bombers, which tend to select states, which most people consider as objectively 'bad', do that because they consider them as subjectively 'better' in some, fortunately, only unusual and personal way.)

But where does this notion of being 'better' come from:

First, it is the privilege of the person setting the goal-value, i.e., the system designer or the client, not only to determine what shall be tried to achieve, but additionally, *implicitly, but inseparable included*, to decide what is considered as 'better' in some way, for somebody, what is worth trying, worth working for, important to realize.

Second, let us emphasize that this notion of 'better' can have only one ultimate source:

Any *ongoing* activities of humans (leaving aside activities like personal sacrifice, suicide, suicide bombing, etc.) require that persons continuously secure their existential needs. (These include primarily existential goal-values, like physiological necessities of maintaining a certain body temperature and levels of nutrients; humans can survive deviations from these existential goal-values only for short periods of time. So they need secondarily the material supply of air, water and food to maintain that; and tertiary usually an monetary income is needed to provide for that. And they can decide just once to ignore that, as in an act of personal sacrifice or in a suicide.)

So any notion of 'better' usually will at least *include* the provision not to endanger the existential goal-values of the person defining it. Only if that is secured, then 'better' may concern anyone or anything else.

So, the act of goal-setting relevant for system design is ultimately derived from the existential interests of the goal-setter, who has an intuitive, sketchy idea of something 'better'. Or put the other way round: 'Better' is something normally only then, when it does not endanger existential material requirements of the goal-setter.

That means that the act of goal-setting does not provide just a technical, rational and unbiased answer to the question of what shall be done. The act of goal-setting allows the person, which has the privilege and the discretion to carry it out, to implicitly make the following decisions going beyond the mere content of the goal:

- Goal-setting comes with an implicit *material* decision for something, which at least does not endanger (if not improve) the existential conditions the decider (but may have other, positive or negative, effects on the material conditions of others).
- Goal-setting comes with an implicit *ethical* decision, what the decider considers as 'better' than the status quo, as worth spending his or her material resources for, and as worth investigating.
- Goal-setting comes with an implicit *moral* decision that pursuing a selected goal-value can be justified in relation to others (which might have other views of what

might be 'better', or other material interests), which do not profit or even might suffer from the 'better' states aimed at.

- Goal-setting comes with an implicit *political* decision, that there are no more important goal-values within a community, than the particular goal-values selected for a certain system design.

The relation between goal-values and ethics was already observed by Aristotle (1984) at the very beginning of the Nicomachean Ethics, where he writes that goals always point towards some "good", behind which we finally find some "ultimate good". Churchman stated practically the same the other way round, when he claimed that ethics is "the theory of the appropriate goals of a system" (Churchman, 1979, 21).

Yet surprisingly this knowledge of the interrelation of goal-setting and ethics never really became a main concern in the consideration of system design:

The process of system design, understood solely as a process running from a set goal to the desired end product, may seem to be a widely straightforward, rational, un-biased, value-free process. (We will look more closely at this process shortly.) But the goal-setting, from which it all started, is definitely neither un-biased nor value-free, and with that the very end product, the realization of the goal-value towards which that whole process runs, is, of course, neither un-biased nor value-free, too. So, focusing narrowly on the process in between leaves out the decisive biases and values, which drive the whole development.

The value judgment that goes parallel with goal-setting comes implicitly with the exclusion of other projects. Deciding for certain goal-values is a material decision excluding to fund other projects, is an ethical decision personally excluding alternative activities, is a moral decision to confront others with certain developments and results, and a political decision to withhold alternative ends from a larger community.

A simple example may illustrate the point:

The steps of system design may be quite similar, if a system designer gets the order to make a tank or an ambulance car. But the questions of ethics, morals and politics are concentrated in the act of goal-setting, in ordering the one or the other. The system designer with the order to construct a tank may have some freedom to apply own biases and to make it a more defensive, and less threatening and deadly weapon. But he or she has not the freedom to leave out any means for killing and even less to turn out an ambulance car. So, can we say that the process leading from the goal-setting to make a tank to the final weapon would be 'value-free' anyway?

Western philosophy and science seemingly ever lived happily with a focus on the 'value-free' and 'rational' process between goal-setting and goal-realization, neglecting that neither the first nor the second are.

Let us mention here in passing that Graham (1989) sees a main difference between Western and Chinese philosophy in their different focus on goal-realization versus on goal-setting:

> "[…] and the crucial question for all of them [the Chinese philosophers] is not the Western philosopher's 'What is the truth' but 'Where is the way?', the way to order the state and conduct personal life." (Graham, 1989, 3)
>
> "We might sum up the Chinese attitude to reason in these terms: reason is for questions of means, for your ends in life listen to aphorism, example, parable and poetry." (Graham, 1989, 7)

So, in Chinese philosophy, there is a focus on the prime question of how to determine "ends", i.e., on setting goal-values, and how to justify them in relation to a larger whole, i.e., in relation to the material, ethical, moral and political questions, which implicitly come with goal-setting. Therefor the core of Chinese philosophy is not, cannot and does not want to be 'rational' in the Western sense (see Ames and Hall, 1987, 1995, 1998), because it tries to stimulate the *intuition*, which we identified above as a part of goal-setting; and this can be achieved, e.g., by listening to "aphorism, example, parable and poetry". With that comes a vague, but wide-ranging knowledge what really might be worth to be done, worth to serve whom in particular, and, with that, worth to be considered as really 'better' within a larger whole.

Bergson (1912, 92) tried to approach this question of the vague knowledge of a larger whole, which he called the "integral experience", which "has nothing in common with a generalization of facts". We think that nicely and shortly grasps the core issue. What science transmits is the "generalization of facts". Yet what cannot be transmitted completely from individual to individual is the "integral experience", which contains those particulars, which may decisively deviate from the generalizations in certain contexts. Individual intuition can consider such particulars and in that way may be superior to scientific prognoses.

Only more recently Western systems theory turned to this vague knowledge, addressing questions of holism, and trying to overcome the increasing separation of the ever more specialized fields of science. But perhaps its most important insight is to make aware that an all-encompassing holism cannot be achieved, because, due to the limited capacities of humans, we have always to work with restricted models trying to somehow represent the whole. Ulrich (1994, 35) summarized that crisply:

> "The implication of the systems idea is not that we must understand the whole system but rather that we need to deal critically with the fact that we never do."

So, questions of holism, of the vague knowledge of a larger whole, have at least arrived in Western thought, too. But the relation between the currently available vague knowledge (i.e., Bergson's "integral experience") and goal-setting was, to the best of our knowledge, never systematically addressed.

And while the relation between goal-setting and ethics was early acknowledged in Western thought, it is still hardly considered. Instead it concentrates on "means" (as Graham put it, see above), on the alleged 'value-free' process of a science, of system design, which excluded the consideration of goal-values from its agenda, and with that their personal and material sources, and their implicit ethical, moral and political justifications. Western science and following it, Western technology, simply accept goal-values and their definitions of something 'better', and focus on a 'rational' way running towards them, whoever may have formulated them, to whatever end they may lead and whomever they may finally serve.

So, we have to conclude here, that the goal-setting process not only sets an explicit objective (the bias discussed in section 6.2. above), but with that provides an implicit notion that this objective is 'better' in some way than other options, and therefor comes with an *implicit bias containing material, ethical, moral and political valuations*.

6.4. Summary: The Goal-Setting Process

In consideration of the described philosophical and scientific background our previous analysis tried to shed more light on the relation between knowledge, goal-setting, ethics, morals, politics - and the material requirements to pursue a system design project.

We suggest that the setting of far-reaching goal-values (i.e., which go beyond immediate existential needs) depends on:

- A person in control of secured material means to pursue such a far-reaching endeavor (which may be the system designer, but is mostly a client).
- The entire knowledge that is currently available to that person, which constitutes the current state of 'holism' (i.e., Bergson's, 1912, "integral experience"), from which goal-values can be derived.
- An act of intuition, in which that persons singles out a subset of states contained within this personal knowledge; these states are assumed to be 'better' in some way than some currently given states, in a way that is important to that person.
- An evaluation by that person, that these singled out states are worth to be pursued as the goal-values for a system design project.

     With that evaluation implicitly material, ethic, moral and political decisions are made, too. These implicit decisions come about by excluding to fund other projects, excluding alternative personal activities, and excluding alternative results for concerned others and alternative priorities for a larger community.

We want to emphasize explicitly that we link at that point material personal well-being with what can become a goal-value for system design. So, we suggest a relation how economic facts determine what can become scientific, conceptual, technical and social facts.

In sum all the discussed interests can amount to the following *biases related to goal-setting*:

There is always *a first goal-setter bias in the form of explicit goal-values*; with that comes *a second goal-setter bias in the form of an underlying implicit value system, containing material, ethical, moral and political valuation*, which justifies the explicit goal-values. The pursuance of these explicit goal-values may be moderated if a system designer and an employer are involved; that can introduce a *bias of designer interests* and a *bias of employer interests*.

As practical implications of this section we suggest that considering a system design should always start with the following questions:

- What exactly is the goal-value, at which the system design aims?
- For whom should that be 'better', and in which way?
- And: Who paid for it?

7. THE PREREQUISITES OF SYSTEM DESIGN

So far we addressed the context, the material base and the goal-setting for system design. But before we can proceed to the very design process we have to clarify a problem, which we introduced when we discussed goal-setting.

Above we said that goal-setting is a form of system design, even if only an intuitive, sketchy and conceptual one. Now we cannot investigate the process of system design and say it starts with some process of system design, without clarifying where that beginning comes from.

Therefore we will suggest in the following the way of the development of knowledge, from *a priori* given human abilities towards that preliminary knowledge that enables intuitive goal-setting and which is the base of system design, too.

7.1. *A Priori* Knowledge

We suggest that humans are born with quite a lot of '*a priori*' knowledge. This is based on internal controller structures, which provide knowledge in the form of decision-rules to control the fulfilling of existential needs; and it is based on externally orientated controller structures, which provide knowledge in the form of basic decision-rules how to interact with the environment.

The internal controller structures provide the following main functions:

- They provide the highest existential goal-values of the individuals (concerning basically body temperature, and necessary level of air, water and food supply).
- They provide sensors to measure the current internal states in relation to these existential goal-values.
- They provide a basic inbuilt notion of what is 'better' for the individual, and that is basically anything that is closer to the goal-value for temperature, and above the necessary level of air, water and food supply.
- They start externally orientated controller structures for protection and for search mechanisms, whenever the individual tends to leave one or the other range of what is defined as 'better', in the way stated in the previous point.

Now these externally orientated controller structures consist of the following main elements (for the basic principles of the processes involved here see the ongoing series of Nechansky, 2012a, 2012b, 2013a, 2013b):

- They provide sensors (eyes, ears, sensors for touch, smell, taste) directed towards the environment.
- They provide structures, which enable a constant spatial and temporal mapping and storing of sensor data (in terms of left - right, up - down, and before - after).
- They provide effectors to act on the environment (hands and arms, feet and legs, and a mouth).
- They enable pattern and sequence recognition in observed data.
- They enable the formation of decision-rules, how to combine sensor data, patterns and/or sequences to steer particular actions of the effectors.
- They enable immense abilities to deal with stored sensor data, patterns and sequences to recombine them, to derive generalizations and particularizations from them, to find similarities in them, etc., to arrive at conceptions of sensor data, patterns and sequences, which have never been observed in the environment.

The last three points are usually summarized under the heading of 'learning', consisting of (1) observing and storing of patterns and sequences, as well as of (2) combining these with actions to form decision-rules how to change observed patterns and sequences and (3) reusing and recombining patterns, sequences and decision-rules for future applications.

This is a very short sketch, how the '*a priori*' knowledge coming with the inborn human controller structures enables the acquisition of that preliminary knowledge, which is needed for both, goal-setting and system design.

7.2. From *A Priori* Knowledge to Preliminary Knowledge

Now humans apply the '*a priori*' knowledge, as sketched above, to their environment, primarily to find out what serves their existential needs (i.e., what keeps them warm, what they can drink and eat). But the better these interests are served, the more individuals are free to learn anything else by observing, playing with and acting on anything that may come to their attention.

From observing the basic objects of their experience (like stones, sticks, flow of waters, and plants, animals, and other humans) they will store patterns and sequences. Then they will try to interact with some of them. And they will evaluate, if the results of these interactions are 'better' for them, primarily in relation to their existential goal-values, and secondarily in relation to any other personal interests. And so they will develop decision-rules combining observed patterns, tried actions, and achieved results, i.e., the resulting changed patterns; and they will remember that for future application, particularly if the achieved results are 'better' in some existential or other way.

All that leads primarily to a passive knowledge of observed patterns and sequences, and secondarily to an active knowledge containing decision rules, how particular observed patterns or sequences can be changed with particular actions.

And finally, the third ability of learning, which we identified above, is applied to all that. Generalizations, particularizations, and similarities are derived from observations, using the processes of induction, deduction and abduction. From known decision-rules possible future decision rules are conceptualized.

So, from the observation of and the interaction with basic objects, individuals can derive assumptions about what can be done with somehow similar objects (e.g., from stones, sticks, flows of water to other solid elements, connections, flows of other media). And they will notice that other objects, which seem quite similar on the surface (e.g., plants, animals and other humans) do not allow the same degree of coherence and consistence, when making assumptions and conceptions about seemingly similar ones.

So humans can develop an increasing body of preliminary knowledge consisting of observations, of decision rules and of derived likely assumptions and conceptions about two different kinds of objects, which we can classify as follows:

- A first body of knowledge deals with material, strictly *law-bound systems*.

  This consists of quite precise observations and decision-rules, which allow a high degree of predictability when dealing with comparable patterns (like stones, sticks, flow of waters, etc.) in comparable contexts.

  This knowledge is additive: New experiences add to the existing knowledge.

- A second body of knowledge concerns living, only *constraint-bound systems*.

  This consists of vague observations and decision-rules, which allow only an occasional and approximate predictability when dealing with seemingly comparable patterns (like plants, animals and other humans) in seemingly comparable contexts.

  This knowledge is cumulative, but not additive: New experiences enter into a collection of case-specific knowledge, with imprecise differentiation and overlap.

These bodies of knowledge contain the base on which any system design has to be built.

And combining any element of these bodies of knowledge with some notion of something 'better' is all we need for the intuitive and sketchy process of goal-setting:

We can start with one pattern or sequence that occurred in one context. Then we may apply a thought process of induction, deduction or abduction. Based on that, we may conclude that a somehow similar pattern or sequence may work in another context to make something 'better'. Then we have created a possible goal-value. And when we decide to pursue such a goal, decide to strive for that idea of 'better', then we enter into the core process of system design. Then we have to apply again such preliminary knowledge - either our own or that of a hired system designer - to systematically approach that goal.

Now, even if all this knowledge is difficult to describe in general terms and we had to remain vague here, we think we provided a valid outline of the way leading from inborn human '*a priori*' knowledge to that 'preliminary' knowledge, which is the base for the intuitive goal-setting for a system design (as discussed in section 6.3. above).

Since this 'preliminary' knowledge is the product of all the previous experiences of the goal-setter, it reflects the education, the environment and the cultural setting, which he or she got to know. Therefor we call it the *educational/environmental/cultural bias* influencing the system design.

7.3. The Preliminary Knowledge of the System Designer and Its Necessary Scope

So, we have clarified above the way leading to the kind of intuitive knowledge needed for goal-setting.

Now we suggest that the system designer, of course, starts with some preliminary knowledge, too, reflecting his or her educational/environmental/cultural background. We call it 'preliminary knowledge', because it is not sure at the outset of system design, that this knowledge will be sufficient to realize a set goal-value; in many cases it turns out to be not sufficient.

And even if we cannot say at the outset if that preliminary knowledge will be sufficient, we can specify, what minimum knowledge a system designer does need, in case he or she is hired by a client who set the goal-values. Or, put the other way round, we can specify, what kind of minimal knowledge a client must demand, when selecting a system designer. We suggest the system designer has to have the knowledge to understand at least the following:

- The system designer has to understand the goal-values, i.e., the states described by it.
- The system designer has to understand the problem that is constituted by setting the goal-value, i.e., the difference between the goal-states and some given states, and why these problem-states are considered as 'worse' than the 'better' states named with the goal-value.

  This includes the knowledge of an evaluation process, which includes at least a step function (or, better, a continuous function), which can characterize the difference between the given 'worse' problem-states and the 'better' goal-states, and any states in between.

  Notice that as this point the system designer must be able to apply an evaluation function, which is *goal-specific*, because it distinguishes and judges *all* possible states considered during the design process *in relation to the set goal-value*. Here our entire material, ethic, moral and political considerations come in, as discussed in section 6.3. above, and that *permanently during the whole design process*.

  So the system designer must be ready to continuously subordinate his or her activities to such an evaluation function which is derived from the set goal-values. He or she must be ready to act neither unbiased nor value-free, but always focused on the goal-values and the criteria, which determine what the goal-setter considers as 'better'.

- The system designer has to have some understanding of the context of the problem.

  The context concerns all those states with currently or during a realization of a system design might play a role, which might hinder or endanger the realization of a goal-value. This necessary understanding of the context is the most difficult to define.

So the preliminary knowledge of the system designer, acquired within his or her educational, environmental and cultural setting, has to include the goal-states, the derived problem states and a measure for the difference between them, as well as relevant states separating the two.

The degree, how far the preliminary knowledge of the system designer covers that, forms his or her *educational/environmental/cultural bias*.

8. THE CORE PROCESS OF DESIGNING A SYSTEM: FROM THE PREREQUISITES AND GOAL-VALUES VIA PRELIMINARY KNOWLEDGE TO THE FINAL DESIGN

Now we have addressed all the preparatory issues that play a role and have a determining influence already before the very core process of system design can start: The context, the material sources, the goal-setting process with its implicit material, ethical, moral and political assumptions, and the sufficient preliminary knowledge of the system designer.

All these issues are widely neglected in most of the literature on system design., e.g., Mesarovic und Takahara (1975) seem to think that all of them play *no* role on their way to their "general systems model" (as discussed in section 1.1.).

Anyway, assuming that all these issues are sufficiently provided for in some way, we can move now to the core process of system design in the more narrow sense, in which it is usually understood. So, we come now to the construction of a system consisting of certain elements and relations (according to the definition we derived from Klir, 1991, in section 2.1. above).

We suggest that this core design process is usually carried out in some steps, many of which may be repeated. These steps lead from selecting elements and relations, to combining them to parts and subsystems, etc., testing and evaluating all these intermediate components till a final design is available; this has again to be tested, and eventually modified, till it can be accepted.

We look now closer on these steps, without going into too much detail. We think the technical aspects of this core design process are completely covered in systems engineering (see, e.g., Patzak, 1982, Winzer, 2013).

8.1. The Core Process of System Design: From Elements and Relations via Subsystems to a Complete System Design

Faced with the task to find a way from a given problem-state to the wanted goal-state the system designer has to make decisions what might be relevant and what not. We suggest that these decisions usually amount to a process carried out in steps of increasing detailing, with each step consisting of the following parts:

1. The system designer derives assumptions from his or her preliminary knowledge, about what might be relevant.
2. Based on these assumptions he or she selects particular elements and relations to make up parts or subsystems of the system.
3. Then he or she applies some test and evaluates the result, to decide if the elements, relations, parts and/or subsystems seem sufficient for reaching the goal.

These steps are repeated until a complete system design is finished.

Whenever the test (point 3) is not passed, other elements and/or relations will be selected (moving up to point 2), whenever that does not work either, other assumptions have to be made (moving up to point 1).

We find here principally the leveled process described by van Gigch (1993, see section 1.4. above) or in a more detailed way by Klir (1985; see section 1.3.). Yet we suggest the highest level of this order is not a "Philosophy of Science", as van Gigch (1993) assumes. We strongly suggest:

At the top of this order stands the preliminary knowledge of the system designer.

This preliminary knowledge will *probably contain* a "Philosophy of Science", understood as knowledge that is derived from the context in which the system designer learned, and that is shared with others in that context. Yet we cannot say for sure that it is only or just primarily such knowledge that will be applied in a certain design process. Quantum leaps in human development often occurred exactly when such shared knowledge of a certain "Philosophy of Science" was *not* applied.

What we can say is that if this preliminary knowledge is not sufficient to drive the whole process, then the system designer is not fit for this system design. Then he or she has to move to a playful and experimental way of developing improved preliminary knowledge (as discussed in section 7.2. above) to become able to enter into a straightforward design process later on.

Let us discuss in the following what has to happen generally in each step of the design process, without considering if we discuss a selection of elements, relations, parts or subsystems.

8.1.1. Assumptions

Since system design is a process searching for a way from a given problem state to a goal-state, it has always to start from preliminary knowledge. For if we had complete knowledge, we would not need any investigative design process, but could go immediately to the realization of the goal. This is an important point, mostly overlooked, mentioned only by Churchman (1971, 4). But Churchman did not elaborate his observation. It means that we have to make assumptions when we go into the design process.

And when making such assumptions the personality of the system designer is in three ways crucial for the whole process:

- First, his or her *preliminary knowledge* sets the frame and the limit from which solutions can be derived. (This is the "integral experience" of the systems designer, in the sense of Bergson, 1912, which we mentioned in section 6.3. above).
- And, second, his or her *creativity* to relate parts of the preliminary knowledge to the goal-value determines the number of possible solutions, which the system designer can consider.
- And, third, his or her *intuition* leads to assumptions, which of these possible solutions might work best and should be primarily tried, detailed and tested.

It is important to notice here that a system designer with a lot of preliminary knowledge need be one with much creativity, nor with much intuition, and *vice versa*.

Anyway, we find here intuition for a second time. All we said about intuition in relation to goal-setting applies here, too. When making assumptions about details of the system design, then again *one somehow promising option* is selected from the available ones. If this option actually will be promising is an open question; but that is intuitively evaluated as worth investigating.

So, intuition not only determines the goal-setting process. It determines making assumptions when detailing the system, too, when selecting possible solutions, which have to be elaborated and tested; so it decisively determines the effort, which has to be put into the project, and how fast and accurate it can proceed, as well as its chances for success.

Based on his or her preliminary knowledge, creativity and intuition the system designer has to make *assumptions* concerning at least the following issues:

- Which states within the context do exactly make up the 'problem'?
- Which details might be important to exactly characterize the goal-states, which might not be provided by the sketchy and intuitive formulation of the prime system concept?

- Which elements, relations, parts and/or subsystems might be important to get to a system that can realize the goal-values?

The results of these assumptions determine what will be elaborated, tested and evaluated in the next steps.

Ashby (1970, 178) nicely summarized this problem of approaching a goal by making assumptions derived from preliminary and incomplete knowledge:

> "The fundamental principle of decision on a finite quantity of information may be expressed thus: Use all that you know to shrink the range of possibilities to their minimum; after that, do as you please."

Hylton (2007, 84) formulated the same problem in more positive words:

> "Creating good hypotheses is an imaginative art, not a science. It is the art of the science."

That said we have to emphasize again, that the searching of the preliminary knowledge to derive assumptions is a goal-orientated process, solely driven by goal-values, which have been set before for the system design.

So, based on our previous analysis, we have to emphasize the following:

The art of science, of making assumptions for hypothesis, follows and is dependent on the art of goal-setting, which in turn depends on the art of providing the material base to pursue all that.

Finally, we want to suggest at that point, that we think it would be important to always make explicit the core determinants of system design: And these are the goal-values, towards which the whole process should run, and the assumptions made and the options considered to realize them. All that is seldom made explicit. But it would be an act of intellectual honesty to let others explicitly and completely know these determinants, to explain and justify the own approach and to open its base for critical and scientific questioning.

Anyway, these implicit assumptions, which determine the next step, the selection of elements and relations, form a *decision bias* of the system designer.

8.1.2. Selecting Elements and Relations

Now, based on his or her intuitive assumptions the system designer has to decide what to include in the system and what to leave out.

These decisions determine directly which elements and relations should make up the system. At the same time they determine the internal structure of the system, and its limits.

In the simplest case these decisions make up a linear process leading directly to a layout, or it might be a parallel process leading to parts and/or subsystems, which are put together later on (as was investigated by Klir, 1985). This adds to the complexity of the sequence, but does add not any new aspects; it is always a repetition of the goal-orientated decision process. Therefore, for our purposes we need not consider these more complex processes.

8.1.3. Intermediate Evaluation

Once certain elements and relations have been selected, sooner or later an evaluation process has to be carried out. Here the question has to be clarified, if the system designer is on the right track, i.e., if his or her design fulfills the specifically demanded criteria of 'better', which come with setting the goal-value (as discussed in section 6.3.).

Now, to determine if any current development of the system design fulfills this criterion of being 'better', the current state of the design can be compared either to the problem state, or to the goal-value.

It is at that point that the system designer needs the evaluative function we talked about in section 7.3., which has to be at least a step function to evaluate, if different intermediate designs actually move away from the problem state and towards the goal-state. Here that solution will be accepted, which comes in 'best' in this evaluation, i.e., leads farthest away from the problem state, or closest to the goal-state.

This evaluation is a widely objective and rational process, particularly if measurements based on empirical data or at least empirical observations can be applied, i.e., if we can use the criteria for 'truth' of Leibnitzian or Kantian inquiry systems according to Churchman (1971); for other inquiry systems that evaluation remains vague.

But, we have to emphasize again, even than the objectivity and rationality of these measurements depends on the acceptance of the goal-value for the whole design, as something that is better (as discussed in section 6 above). This applies, of course, too, to the decisive evaluation process, when a final decision is made, if an element, a relation, a part, or subsystem can sufficiently serve that goal and should enter into the design or not.

If these tests fail, we have to move up again (as indicated in the introduction to section 8.1. above), and have to search for other elements and relations (as discussed in 8.1.2.), or, if this repeatedly fails, too, we have to make different assumptions (as discussed in 8.1.1.). If all that repeatedly fails, we have to question the preliminary knowledge of the system designer, and make him or her research for further preliminary knowledge. Or we might fire him or her and engage another one. An interesting and open question is here, how much failures have to occur so that we speak of 'repeated' failure. Material constraints may play a role in determining that.

Anyway, to whatever level we have to move up at that point, we have to move down to testing any new trials again.

Let us emphasize that this evaluation of elements, relations, parts or subsystems, or even complete system designs does not define the end of the design project. We address that next.

8.2. From a Complete Design to the Final Design or When Is a System Design 'Good Enough'?

During the evaluation processes applied to the selected elements, relations, parts, and subsystem, we continuously ask, if they promise a system that is 'better' than the problem state. So we get finally to the point when we have a first complete system design fulfilling that criterion.

Now we have to make a *different evaluation*, not only asking if it is really 'better' than the problem state, but if it is *'good enough'*. Here the first question delivers just the information that the system design is on the right track. But the second question, which is less clear but more important, has to deliver the information, if the system design was successful and can be accepted, or if the work must be continued till delivering something really 'good enough'.

And the first question can probably be objectively answered by anyone with sufficient preliminary knowledge. Yet the second question can only be answered by that person, which had set the goal-values for the system design, i.e., in our approach either the system designer, if acting alone, or the client. Only that person can decide, if his or her expectations are fulfilled or not.

Now the decision, if the system design is 'good enough' may be restricted by material constraints, e.g., if further improvement simply cannot be paid; then the person setting the goal-values would have to accept whatever he or she got (we are not interested here in processes like suing to get the material input back).

Otherwise the decision on the acceptance of a system design is the expression of the *satisfaction* of the person setting the goal-values with what has been achieved. This is a freely and individually determinable decision criterion.

Let us explicitly point out that we discuss her two different criteria, and that that even applies to empirical scientific work. Let us detail that:

The criterion to evaluate a scientific theory is the correspondence of theoretically predicted data and empirical data. To determine the correspondence we use statistical methods, mostly regression analysis and calculation of a regression coefficient (which may lie between 0 and 1); here one theory (a form of system design) delivering a higher regression coefficient (closer to 1), means that it is 'better', than another theory delivering a lower value. But this does not touch the question, if we consider any of these theories as 'good enough'. For that we have to deliberately choose a *'level of significance'*, which says, which kind of correspondence we want to achieve. In the natural sciences most often a 'level of significance' of 0.95 is demanded, while anything below 0.9 is usually seen as no correspondence. In social sciences even a 'level of significance' of 0.6 may be seen as a good result. Anyway, the point is that, *if a scientific theory is considered as 'good enough' depends on the previous decision for a goal-value for a 'level of significance'*. Let us emphasize that in this context 'good enough' is equal to the notion 'true'. So if we demand a higher 'level of significance' we may have to reject some theory and may get a *different* 'scientific truth'.

So, while the decision what is 'better' is rational in regard to the goal-value for the system design, the decision of what is 'good enough' results from the individual view of the person setting the goals. In terms of Churchman's inquiry systems the question what is 'better' is mostly part of a Lockean or Kantian system, dealing with facts, while the second one, what is 'good enough' is part of a Leibnizian system: here a necessary, but arbitrarily determined, *a priori* set individual demand determines what will be accepted.

We cannot overemphasize that point:

1. First a widely *objective* criterion is determined, how far a system design is 'better' than a problem state, i.e., in which properties it is closer to the goal-state; this is objectively 'rational' in relation to the goal-values set for the whole design.
2. And then a purely *subjective* decision criterion is applied, reflecting if that system design can be considered as 'good enough', i.e., if its properties are that close to the goal-state that it is acceptable for the person setting the goal-value. This second criterion depends only on the individual desires and preferences of the goal-setter; it is only subjectively justifiable in relation to these individual desires and preferences.

Based on that, we want to express again our doubts, that *any* system design could be considered as value-free. We found that already goal-setting is an individual and value-loaded process; now we find that ending and accepting a design is an even more individual evaluation act. This is another goal-setter bias: the *acceptance criteria*.

8.3. A Byproduct: An Increase in the Preliminary Knowledge of the System Designer

No matter, how good the result was, which was achieved with a first complete system design, one thing already increased: And that is the preliminary knowledge of the system designer, with which he or she can start the next time.

Now, at least, he or she does know, what does not work. Given that, he or she has a more accurate base for his or her intuition enabling to make better assumptions next time. The amount of this increase depends on the issue of the project, and if it is in the realm of additive or cumulative knowledge (as distinguished in section 7.2.).

8.4. Redesigning a System

Finally, let us briefly address the case that the system design was not 'good enough'.

Then, given a sufficient material base to proceed, of course, a redesign has to start. Then the system designer has to move up again, on the scale discussed in sections 8.1. and 8.1.3. So, he or she has to reconsider selected elements, relations, parts and/or subsystems. Here using a design with parts or subsystems can strongly ease a redesign, if changing and improving of one can be done without having to change any other. If that does not work, again, assumptions and eventually the sufficiency of the preliminary knowledge have to be questioned.

Anyway, after moving up, the whole steps discussed in sections 8.1. and 8.2. have to be carried out top - down again.

8.5. Summary of the Core Design Process

In sum the core of system design is an approximating process leading from assumptions towards a final system design. This process is guided by permanent reference to the goal-values for the design. Here the following aspects are particularly important:

- The preliminary knowledge, creativity and intuition of the system designer determine the scope, number and selection of assumptions, which guide the design process.
- These assumptions determine what exactly is considered as the problem and as the characteristics of the goal-state;
- And these assumptions lead to the selection of elements and relations, parts, etc., which are included in the design and elaborated.
- These elements and relations, parts, etc., have to be tested and evaluated, if they contribute to a design that is 'better' than the problem state; if not they have to be reworked or exchanged.

- Once a complete system design is available, it has to be tested, if it is 'good enough', i.e., if it meets the individual criteria of the person setting the goal-values, and therefore can be accepted.
- During the whole process, the system designer subordinates all activities to the question, if they might lead towards the goal, or not. So the presumed 'rationality' of this process depends completely on the acceptance of the goal and the implicitly included ethical, moral and political valuations (see section 6.3. above).

As practical implications of this section we suggest that the first questions when considering a core system design process should always be:

- What assumptions have been made and what options have been considered?
- What were the criteria to consider the system design as 'good enough'?

9. PUTTING A SYSTEM DESIGN IN A WIDER CONTEXT

In section 8 we discussed the core process of system design, running from a given goal-value to a final design considered as 'good enough'. There we focused on the work of a system designer, working either for him- or herself, or for a client, or eventually for an employer. So, till now we focused on activities of the core actors, as defined in section 3.

Now we assume that we got a system design that is considered as 'good enough' by these core actors. And we ask, what may happen, if these core actors have to introduce their design into a larger context. This may mean to publish a theoretical concept, to realize a technical system, or to intervene in an organization, etc. Anyway, here the system design enters in one of the contexts, which we identified in section 1.6., following Jackson (2003).

So, we have to consider now what can happen, if the system design has to face a public, while being forwarded from one of the different possible positions, and what that means for the chances to be still considered as 'good enough'. Additionally we will consider Churchman's (1971) different criteria for 'truth' (see section 1.5.), where appropriate:

(1) The core actors may belong to the coercive parties (following Jackson, 2003; see section 1.6.).

Then they dominate other parities in the context and will have an easy play to forward their design, whatever its content.

In case there is disagreement between the coercive parties point (3) below does apply.

(2) The core actors may belong to the suppressed parties and are victims of coercion (following Jackson, 2003, section 1.6. above).

Here their chances to forward their design will depend on which of Churchman's criteria for 'truth' the design does fulfill:

- If it fits in the dominant ideology or paradigmatic position of the coercive parties and meets their criteria (i.e., fits the Lockean criteria of what the suppressors consider as 'truth'), there is a change that they may go ahead with their design.

- If it forwards evidence that might challenge the dominant ideology or paradigmatic position or derived criteria of the coercive parties (i.e., does not fit their Leibnitzian criteria of 'truth'), their chances are usually slim.

This is sort of a Bayesian aspect of system designs coming to the public: Anything coming up in opposition to dominant views is not only surprising, but must contain some remarkable aspect of (Leibnitzian) 'truth', i.e., point to facts that must be difficult to deny.

(3) The core actors and other parties may have different, but somehow compatible goal-values (following Jackson, 2003, section 1.6. above).

Here again Churchman's criteria may play a role:

- There is a good chance that an approximation and some compromise are possible.

  Then the parties arrive at a mutual definition of a Hegelian criterion of 'truth' and the result is probably a modified system design that acknowledges and takes care of the different interests.

- But it may turn out, too, that the differences cannot be overcome.

  This can be the case, e.g., if some (maybe coercive) parties see a challenge to their dominant ideology or paradigmatic position, while others see non; or, e.g., if a scientific community, united by an approximate overall consensus, faces a new theory challenging an established theory or paradigmatic position. Then a conflict may arise, if the new system design can be accepted or not. And at that point no agreed on, mutual decision criteria are available to settle the conflict. This is the case in times of "paradigm changes", as Kuhn (1970) called that.

  In Churchman's (1971) scheme this is a Kantian problem, where the question arises if new facts or previous assumptions should be the standard to evaluate future work. Unless the parties do not reach a new agreement (finding to a Hegelian definition of a new mutual 'truth') this question cannot be solved. Or, as Kuhn (1970, 94) put it:

> "As in political revolutions, so in paradigm choice - there is no higher standard than the assent of the relevant community."

(4) The core actors and all concerned parties may share mutual goal-values. Then, finally, a system design will be easily accepted.

These considerations are particularly important for the following reasons:

- There is an interrelation between the context and the kind of system designs, which can come to the surface in a society and can be realized.
  Correspondence to the prevailing views, interests, and ideological and paradigmatic positions within a society (i.e., to the Lockean criteria of what is generally accepted as 'truth') will ease the acceptance of a system design.
- The previous point together with the fact that system design can only be carried by those who can afford it (see section 5), suggests that system designs, which are easily accepted within a society, will probably show a correspondence with the interests of the wealthy, as well as with the prevailing views, ideological and paradigmatic positions within the society.
- Realized or published system designs, which were accepted at one point in time, form the pool of exemplary, easily available and accessible solutions in a certain context. These solutions will be used in education and in the development of the preliminary knowledge of future goal-setters and system designers.
- So there may be a reinforcing effect, since the previous acceptance of system designs influences what kind of preliminary knowledge a system designer will develop in that context. And this in turn influences what forms of system designs become possible in future.
- So, the carrying out of system designs mainly depends (1) on a goal-setter providing material wealth, and (2) on the preliminary knowledge of system designers; then (3) the reception and acceptance of system designs depends widely on the correspondence with prevailing interests, views, and ideological and paradigmatic positions; and (4) future knowledge of systems designers depends partly on such accepted system designs.

Together these points mean:

We should rather expect a reinforcement of the correspondence of interests of wealthy persons, existing knowledge, and dominating interest and prevailing views in the society than a questioning of them all.

In sum, in the context, where a system design is applied, the core actors will face parties with own views, interests, and ideological positions. These will introduce another bias, i.e., the *bias of context-specific prevailing paradigms*. If the core actors face suppressors that will take a particularly severe form, namely *bias of the paradigms of the suppressors*. Anyway, the intentions pursued with the system design may be in accordance or in opposition to these biases; and that will influence the chances of acceptance.

As practical implications of this section we suggest to ask the following prime questions, when considering the reception and the evaluation of a system design in a certain context:

- What is the position of the core actors in relation to other parties in the context of the system design (coercive, suppressed, indifferent, or united)?
- What are the prevailing interests, views, and ideological and paradigmatic positions, which are relevant to evaluate a system design?
- Is the system design in accordance with or deviating from prevailing views, interests, and ideological and paradigmatic positions in the context or society?

SUMMARY AND CONCLUSION

In this chapter we suggested to take a wider look at system design than usual. We did not just consider the core process running from a set goal to a final design.

Instead, we looked at a wider context including core actors, which set the goal-values for a system design, provide the material means and carry it out. And particularly we asked which influence these core actors can have on the design process, and at which point their influence and their decisions become decisive for the final design. Furthermore, we asked which role other parties, which may be concerned about the results, might play in the acceptance or rejection of a design.

From this analysis, we suggest that system design is the result of the interplay of the following factors. And, returning to our quotation of Churchman (1979) at the beginning of this paper, we suggest that these factors introduce different biases influencing system design:

- A given context influences what can easily become the preliminary knowledge of goal-setters (*Bias 1: Educational/environmental/cultural standards of the goal-setter*; see section 7.2.).
- An available material base limits which goal-values for system design can be pursued (*Bias 2: Material constraints*; section 5.1.).

- Usually the provider of the material base has the right to set the goal-values for system design (*Bias 3a: Goal-setter bias I - explicit objectives*; section 6.2.).

  The goal-values for a certain system design come with implicitly contained material, ethical, moral and political valuations (*Bias 3b: Goal-setter bias II - implicit value system*; section 6.3.), which come from the fact that pursuing one goal excludes alternative design projects.

  Only if the system designer can provide the material base, then goal-setting and design process are in the same hands.

  Otherwise a client, providing the material base and setting the goal-values, has to engage a system designer (*Occasional bias 3c: Designer interests*; section 6.2.). Here an employer (*Occasional bias 3d: Employer interests*; section 6.2.) of a system designer may play an intermediate role.

- When goal-values are explicitly accepted, the core design process can start:

  Then the actual preliminary knowledge, the creativity and the intuition of the system designer (*Bias 4: Educational/environmental/cultural knowledge of the designer*; section 7.3.) determine what can be achieved in the design process. Together they lead to assumptions (*Bias 5: Designer decisions*; section 8.1.1.), which possible designs might work best and should be elaborated and tested.

- Tests determine first, if possible designs actually are 'better' than the problem states and lead towards the goal-values. These evaluations use rather objective criteria.

- Final tests of a complete design determine, if it is 'good enough' to meet the goals, and if the core design process can be finished. These decisions use subjective criteria determined by the person setting the goal-values (*Bias 6: Goal-setter bias III - acceptance criteria*; section 8.2.).

- So, the whole core design process is subordinated to the goal-values and the acceptance criteria of the person setting the goal-values.

  It is 'rational' only in relation to the achievement of these goal-values; it does not ask, if it is 'rational' to pursue these goals at all, seen from any other point of view.

  And the design process is not value-free because it accepts the implicit material, ethical, moral and political valuations coming with the goal-value, and because the final acceptance criteria, when the design is considered 'good enough', are purely subjective.

- The larger context determines how a system design is received.

  Here it is decisive, if the system design is in accordance with prevailing interests, views, and ideological and paradigmatic positions (*Bias 7a: Context-specific prevailing paradigms*; section 9), or is deviating from, or even in opposition to these views.

In this larger context the position of the core actors (system designer, client and/or employer) has a modifying effect: If they are coercive parties they will meet little resistance; if they belong to suppressed parties and forward opposing views they will face more difficulties (*Occasional bias 7b: Paradigms of suppressors*; section 9); if there are diverging, but somehow compatible views of concerned parties the result is open; and only if there are uniform views there will be no difficulties.

These factors and the related biases 1 to 7 are always at work: Bias 3a (goal-setting for the system) is the most obvious, while the others go widely unnoticed. Only when bias 7b eventually shows (paradigms of suppressors), it is often criticized from persons outside a society holding a different ideological position. Yet these factors and biases seem to influence strongly, which system designs can surface within a society, i.e., will be pursued, elaborated and accepted:

- Prevailing interests, views, and ideological and paradigmatic positions (bias 7a/7b) will not only strongly influence what system designs can be realized in a society, and so can become a model solution available to future systems designers; they determine, too, what is generally taught in education, too (bias 1). So, the final point of the list above leads us back to the first one.
- Furthermore system designs that are in opposition to the interests of wealthy persons as well as to dominating interests and prevailing paradigms seem less likely to emerge, because they lack an educational base (bias 1), will get less material support (bias 2) and will meet more resistance (bias 7a/7b).
- And, turning the previous point upside down seems to suggest the fast track to a 'career': Alignment to educational standards (bias 1), to the interests of the wealthy (bias 2), and to dominating interest and prevailing paradigms (bias 7a/7b) will open material sources and reduce resistance.

In sum, we should rather expect a reinforcement of the correspondence of interests of wealthy persons, existing knowledge, and dominating interests and prevailing views in the society, than a questioning of them all.

We suggested a number of practical questions, which might be useful to get quickly to these core aspects of system design and the related biases. Ideally we should demand that answers should be published with any systems design, clarifying at least the most important questions (The goal-values of the system; For whom and why should that be 'better'; Who paid for it; What are core assumptions, and what alternative options have been considered/rejected; What were the acceptance criteria for 'good enough'). But, anyway, applying these questions personally and trying to get the answers to them may help to get an impression of the biases at work in any system design.

So, in our analysis we tried to consider system design in a very general way and in a wider context than usual, to show factors and biases which strongly influence it, even if they do not directly show in the core design process. Proceeding that way we left out many details, which were a concern of those authors, whose approaches we surveyed in the introduction. Yet we strongly suggest that the biases coming with the larger context we analyzed here may have a greater influence on system design, than many of these details.

REFERENCES

Ashby, W. Ross (1970), Chance favors the mind prepared, in Conant, R. (Ed.), *Mechanisms of intelligence - W. Ross Ashby's Writings on Cybernetics*, pp. 177 - 179, Intersystems Publications, Seaside (published in 1981).

Aristotle (1984), "Nicomachean Ethics", trans. Ross, W.D., revised by J.O. Urmson, in *The Complete Works of Aristotle, The Revised Oxford Translation, vol. 2*, Jonathan Barnes, ed., Princeton University Press, Princeton.

Bergson, Henri (1912), *An Introduction to Metaphysics*, trans. Hulme, T. E., Putnam, New York.

Churchman, C. West (1971), *The Design of Inquiring Systems*, Basic Books, New York.

Churchman, C. West (1979), *The Systems Approach and Its Enemies*, Basic Books, New York.

Flood, R. L. (1989), Six Scenarios for the Future of Systems "Problem Solving", *Systems Practice*, 2 (1): 75 – 99.

Graham, Angus C. (1989), *Disputers of Tao*, Open Court, Chicago.

Hall, David L. and Ames, Roger T. (1987), *Thinking through Confucius*, State University of New York Press, Albany.

Hall, David L. and Ames, Roger T. (1995), *Anticipating China*, State University of New York Press, Albany.

Hall, David L. and Ames, Roger T. (1998), *Thinking from the Han*, State University of New York Press, Albany.

Hylton, Peter (2007), *Quine*, Routledge, London.

Jackson, Michael C. (2003), *Systems Thinking - Creative Holism for Managers*, Wiley, Chichester.

Klir, George J. (1985), *Architecture of Systems Problem Solving*, Plenum Press, New York.

Klir, George J. (1991), *Facets of Systems Science*, Plenum Press, New York.

Kuhn, Thomas S. (1970), *The Structure of Scientific Revolutions*, The University of Chicago Press, Chicago.

Linden, Lars P., Kuhn, John R., Parrish, James L., Richardson, Sandra M., Adams, Lascelles A., Elgarah, Wafa, and Courtney, James F. (2007), Churchman's Inquiring Systems: Kernel Theories for Knowledge Management, *Communications of the Association for Information Systems*, 20, pp 836 - 871, http://aisel.aisnet.org/cais/vol20/iss1/52 (retrieved 13.05.2015).

Mesarovic, M. D. und Takahara, Y. (1975), *General Systems Theory: Mathematical Foundations*, Academic Press, New York.

Nechansky, H. (2012a), Elements of a Cybernetic Epistemology: Sequence Learning Systems, *Kybernetes*, 41 (1/2): 157 - 176, DOI:10.1108/03684921211213007.

Nechansky, Helmut (2012b), Elements of a Cybernetic Epistemology: Pattern Recognition, Learning and the Base of Individual Psychology, *Kybernetes*, 41 (3/4): 444 - 464, DOI:10.1108/03684921211229514.

Nechansky, Helmut (2013a), Elements of a Cybernetic Epistemology: Elementary Anticipatory Systems, *Kybernetes*, 42 (2): 185 - 206, DOI: 10.1108/03684921311310567.

Nechansky, Helmut (2013b), Elements of a Cybernetic Epistemology: Complex Anticipatory Systems, *Kybernetes*, 42 (2): 207 - 225, DOI:10.1108/03684921311310576.

Nechansky, Helmut (2016a), The Interaction Matrix: From Individual Goal-Setting to the Four Modes of Coexistence, *Kybernetes*, 45 (1): 87-106, DOI: 10.1108/K-09-2014-0192.

Nechansky, Helmut (2016b), The Four Modes of Coexistence in Psychology and Group Dynamics, *Kybernetes*, 45 (3): 371 - 392, DOI: 10.1108/K-09-2014-0193.

Nechansky, Helmut (2017), The Four Modes of Coexistence in Social Systems, *Kybernetes*, 46 (3): 433 - 449, DOI: 10.1108/K-10-2015-0268.

Patzak, G. (1982), *Systemtechnik - Planung komplexer innovativer Systeme* [*Systems engineering - Planning of Complex Innovative Systems*], Springer, Berlin.

Winzer, Petra (2013), *Generic Systems Engineering*, Springer, Berlin.

Ulrich, Werner (1994), Can we secure future-responsive management through systems thinking and design? *Interfaces*, 24 (4): 26 – 37.

van Gigch, John P. (1988), Design of the modern, *Systems Research*, 5: 267 – 269.

van Gigch, John P. (1993), Metamodeling: The Epistemology of System Science, *Systems Practice*, 6 (3): 251 – 258.

In: Focus on Systems Theory Research
Editors: Manuel F. Casanova and Ioan Opris

ISBN: 978-1-53614-561-8
© 2019 Nova Science Publishers, Inc.

Chapter 2

MATHEMATICAL THEORY OF RELIABILITY AND BIOLOGICAL ROBUSTNESS: RELIABLE SYSTEMS FROM UNRELIABLE ELEMENTS

Vitaly K. Koltover, PhD[*]

Institute of Problems of Chemical Physics,
Russian Academy of Sciences, Chernogolovka,
Moscow Region, Russia

ABSTRACT

In engineering, reliability is defined as ability of a device to perform its function for a given time under given specific conditions. The foundations of the mathematical theory of reliability were laid in the 1950s due to the needs of aeronautic machinery, electronics and problems of communication and management. Biological systems perform their functions in presence of a great number of random factors which disturb all functional strata, starting from the molecular level of organization ("nanobioconstructs") to ecosystems. Therefore, similarly to technical devices, biological constructs are not perfectly reliable in operation, namely, normal operation acts alternate with random malfunctions or failures. The field of systems biology, in dealing with the problem of reliability, incorporates investigations of: systematization and classification of failures in biological systems of different levels of complexity; quantitative characteristics of failures; mechanisms of failures; possible ways to evaluate molecular failures in functional breaks; mechanisms of renewal processes; and an elaboration of methods for testing reliability and predicting failures in biological systems. The regular conferences on reliability of biological systems, starting from the first one in 1975, Kiev, Ukraine

---

[*] Email: koltover@icp.ac.ru.

(former USSR), have given the strong impetus to research in this direction. A quarter of a century after, it has spurred similar biological studies under the style of "robustness." In this review, in order to illustrate the ideas of the reliability trend, I present several examples of analysis of reliability of biological systems at different functional levels, starting from the level of biomolecular nanoreactors. The main line of assuring the high systems reliability is the preventive maintenance, i.e., unreliable elements should be timely replaced for novel ones ahead the phase of their wear-out begins. This prophylaxis of failures proceeds under control of functional elements of the highest level of hierarchy, designated as supervisors or longevity-assurance structures. The problem of reliability of biological systems has direct bond to the problem of aging. The systems reliability approach, which was developed in our papers, is based on several general postulates. First, all biological constructs are designed in keeping with the genetic programs in order to perform the preset functions. Second, we believe that all constructs operate with the limited reliability, namely, for each and every biological device normal operation acts alternate with accidental malfunctions (recurrent failures). Third, the preventive maintenance, i.e., the timely replacement or prophylaxis of unreliable functional elements through the metabolic turnover that follows the pattern preset in the genome, is the main line of assuring the high systems reliability. Forth, there are a finite number of critical elements of the highest hierarchic level which perform the supervisory functions over the preventive maintenance ("the power structure"). And, five, the supervisors also operate with the limited, genetically preset, reliability. On the systems reliability basis, the universal features of aging of living organisms, such as the exponential growth of mortality rates with time and the correlation of the longevity with the species-specific resting metabolism, are naturally explained. From the reliability point of view, aging occurs as the inevitable consequence of the genetically preset deficiency in reliability of biomolecular constructs while the free-radical redox-timer, located in specialized neurons of the central nervous system, serves as the effective stochastic mechanism of realization of the aging program. Furthermore, the systems reliability approach serves as the heuristic methodology for preventive medicine including the antioxidant therapy.

Keywords: systems biology, reliability, robustness, bioreliability, failures, prophylaxis, preventive maintenance, bioconstructs, aging, longevity, life testing, program, determinism, genetics, stochastic, oxygen, free radicals, antioxidants

INTRODUCTION: HISTORICAL SYNOPSIS

The foundations of mathematical theory of reliability were laid in the 1950s due to the needs of aeronautic machinery, electronics, and problems of communication and management [1-4]. The problem of reliability of biological systems was first put forward by D. Grodzinsky and his collaborators [5, 6]. The regular conferences [7-9], which were initiated by Ukrainian Academy of Sciences, in cooperation with the special commission on reliability of biological systems at the scientific council on biological physics of USSR Academy of Sciences, D. M. Grodzinsky as the chairman of the commission, V. K. Koltover and Y. A. Kutlakhmedov as the vice-chairmen of the commission), to deal with the problem of reliability of biological systems, have given a strong impetus to research in this direction [10-34].

Not long ago, a new wave of the analogous research has been spurred under the style of "biological robustness" (see Refs. in [35-40]). This term, "robustness," is now often used in biological articles and databases instead of the term "reliability." Meanwhile, the term "reliability," but not «robustness», has been universally accepted in the scientific literature on engineering, communication, management and so on [1-4]. The term "reliability," not «robustness», has been used in the pioneering works on biological reliability [5-18]. In engineering, reliability is recognized and defined as a probability to work without failures during the given period of time. As a matter of fact, it is the probability to work robustly, i.e., without failures. It might be said that the reliability is the robustness exerted in course of the work. Yet, "robustness," as the term, is slang, smacked of the terms like "serviceability" or "Robusta coffee." There is the mathematical theory of reliability, and mathematicians consider this theory as the part of the probability theory. Hence, there is no need to contrive "biological robustness" or any other quasi-novel approaches to the problem of reliability of biological systems. As said by Immanuel Kant, "in any partial doctrine of nature, one can find as much genuine science as there is mathematics in this doctrine and no more."

In this mini-review, in order to illustrate the basic ideas of the reliability trend, I present several examples of analysis of reliability of biological systems at different functional levels, starting from the level of biomolecular nanoreactors. Besides, the results of application of ideas and methods of the mathematical theory of reliability to the problem of aging of living systems are presented. The reliability-theory approach clearly demonstrates that aging is a stochastic consequence of the limited reliability of biomolecular constructs, the reliability of which is predetermined by the genetic program. In addition, it is demonstrated that the systems reliability approach serves the heuristic methodology for development of biomedicine, including the antioxidant therapy.

BASIC TERMS AND IDEAS

Similarly to technical devices, biological objects are constructs, i.e., all of them are designed accordingly to special genetic programs with the aim to perform predetermined functions. Besides, they all, starting from the molecular level of organization and to ecosystems inclusive, perform their functions in the presence of a great number of random factors which disturb all functional strata. Therefore, biological constructs are not perfectly reliable in operation: for each and every device normal operation acts alternate with random stochastic malfunctions or failures. The field of systems biology, in dealing with the problem of reliability, incorporates investigations of: systematization and classification of failures in biological systems of different levels of complexity; quantitative characteristics of failures; mechanisms of failures; possible ways to evaluate molecular failures in functional breaks; mechanisms of renewal processes; and an elaboration of methods for testing reliability and predicting failures in biological systems.

To study reliability of a device, it is necessary first of all to specify a function of the device, i.e., we need to know what this device has been designed for. However, in many instances, a biological object performs not a single function but several functions and, moreover, some of the functions may be mutually exclusive. For example, in any population, an individual should perform two functions: he should survive in the given conditions and he should afford an advantage to the survivorship of his population or even the species as the whole. Thus, even this very first step of the bioreliability analysis can meet difficulties. Nevertheless, one of the operation functions of the object may be allocated to a first approximation as the main, or "quasi-main," function.

The next thing to be done is to define what a normal operation of the biological device under study is and what its failure is. The simplest way of the definition is to introduce a time-dependent random vector $Y(t)$, each k-element of which ($k = 1, 2, ..., m$) corresponds to the relevant functional parameter of the device, and to introduce the relevant m-dimensional admissible limits of the functional parameters. If values of the functional parameters (Y_k) are in the limits, then the state of the device is defined as the normal operation. If any of the functional parameters occurs beyond the limits, then we say that the device is in the state of the failure. Inasmuch as the object performs its functions in the presence of random factors, all Y_k are random functions of time. Moreover, the admissible limits of the functional parameters may also be time-dependent and stochastic.

Accordingly, the quantitative characteristic of reliability is the probability, R, of the non-failure operation in the given interval of time $(0, t)$:

$$R(t) = P(\tau > t),$$

where τ is a random value of the failure-free operation time [1-4, 6, 31]. In reliability tests, this probability is experimentally estimated as the ratio $n(t)/n_0$, where $n(t)$ is a number of the objects which are alive (normally operate) in the moment t, and n_0 is the initial size of the sample. The graph of the function R with time is named the reliability function. The probability of a failure in the same time-interval is correspondingly defined as the probability of the opposite event, $G(t) = P(\tau \leq t) = 1 - R(t)$, with the probability density function $g = dG/dt$.

Another important characteristic of reliability is the so-called hazard or failure-rate function:

$$h(t) = -R'/R = -d(\ln R)/dt$$

This parameter has the meaning of the conditional probability of failure per unit time provided the object operated failure-free up to the given moment. The sequence of the random moments of time in which the failures take place is named a flux of failures. Of special importance in the theory of reliability are the so-called elementary or Poisson fluxes of failures. In the case of a Poisson-type flux, the probability of the failure-free operation during the given time t follows an exponential distribution with the time-independent parameter $\lambda > 0$:

$$R(t) = P(\tau > t) = \exp(-\lambda t)$$

In this case, the failure rate h is constant (λ) and reliability of the device does not depend on the operation time. Hence, a device, the reliability of which is described by the exponential distribution, does not age. Moreover, if there are a great number of fluxes of random events, each being of low intensity and mutually independent, then the sum of them asymptotically converges on a Poisson flux (so-called Khinchin-Palm's in-limit theorem) [3]. It works for complex systems with a large number of component elements none of which contributes very heavily to the total failure probability, even if the distributions for the individual components are not exponential. Among other processes, it applies to the distribution of the time between failures for a complex system when the failed element is replaced immediately by another element of the same type. Therefore, the exponential distribution plays a central role in engineering and in biology too.

Figure 1 shows a graph of a hazard function for a typical technical device. Inasmuch as some functional elements of the device can be defective, the failure rate in the first period of life can be rather high. It is the time of the so-called initial failures ("breaking-in period"). As for the "breaking-in" of biological systems, it has obviously accomplished at the earliest evolution phase or even before the beginning of evolution. At least it should be true for the simplest biological constructs like enzymes, ribosomes, and mitochondria of cells. For modern technical devices such as large-scale integrated circuits, the initial failure rates are negligible as well. As the defective elements are replaced with the good ones, the failure rate goes down and stabilizes at a rather low constant level. It is a period of normal operation when rare failures come unexpectedly, for example, due to the accidental overloading. It is, correspondingly, a Poisson flux of failures with the constant failure-rate parameter. With time, when wear-out of functional elements comes into play, the failure rate of the device begins to grow up. It is a period of the wear-out failures.

An analogy between failures of technical devices and deaths of living systems is appealing. The reliability function $R(t)$ for the probability of the failure-free operation during the given time is quite analogous to the survival function, i.e., the probability of being alive at a moment t, while the probability density function $g(t)$ is analogous to the so-called death-rate function and the failure-rate function $h(t)$ is analogous to the mortality rate function. Therefore, the same mathematical theory of reliability is essentially applicable to the mathematics of mortality [6, 12, 17].

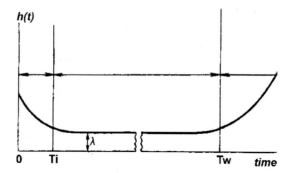

Figure 1. A graph of the failure-rate function $h(t)$ versus time for a typical technical device. The intervals $(t < T_i)$, (T_i, T_w), and $(t > T_w)$ correspond to the phases of initial failures ("breaking-in period"), normal operation and wear-out, respectively (compiled from [31]).

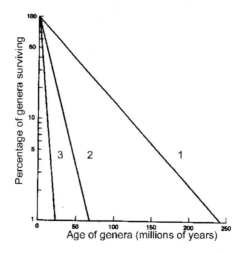

Figure 2. Survival functions for extinct genera of the clams (1), Mesozoic rudists (2), and mammals (3) plotted using a logarithmic ordinate (compiled from [41]).

The breaking-in period for technical devices is formally similar to the period of the infant mortality for people, marked by the high mortality rates. There is also a formal analogy between chance failures of technical devices during normal operation period and deaths of wild animals. Namely, for technical devices the exponential distributions of failures take place with the constant failure-rate parameters. In the similar manner, survival curves of wild animals fall exponentially with the constant mortality-rate parameters. It means that the wild animals die mostly not because of senescence but owing to random accidents. Moreover, the mortality of people killed in accidents also follows the exponential distribution with the time-independent constant λ that reflects random environmental influences on the mortality. Furthermore, the failure rates of technical devices begin to grow up with time when the wear-out of functional elements comes into play. Similarly, aging of people and animals results in growth of the mortality rate.

Here, it is pertinent to call attention to the survival functions of genera of the extinct animals from the paper of Van Valen [41]. Figure 2 shows these curves for three groups of the specialized Mesozoic animals. It is quite clear that the logarithm of the percentage of surviving for all three genera linearly falls with time. Hence, it appears that the kinetics of the survivorship follows the exponential distribution. From the reliability-theory point of view it means that the species have succumbed due to "chance failures." This finding corresponds to the well-known idea of A. Weissmann, who stated in 1882 that the germ cells of species can be considered as potentially immortal compared to an aging soma (a review of Weismann's ideas can be found in [42]).

In biology, as well as in engineering, there are several lines of creating reliable devices from unreliable functional elements. One of them is redundancy, when the elements of the same type are introduced in the system to fulfill one and the same function. In engineering, there are different kinds of redundancy, among them – the structural redundancy (insertion of superfluous amount of functional elements), the functional redundancy (exploitation of elements capable to carry out additional functions besides their basic ones), the informational redundancy (surplus information supplement), and the temporal redundancy (superfluous time of functioning) [1-4]. The same kinds of redundancy take place in biology. All essential biomolecular constructs are present in cells in superfluous amounts. The redundant amounts of enzymes, mitochondria and other organelles represent the examples of the structural reservation. The elimination of hydrogen peroxide (H_2O_2) and organic peroxides from cells by two different enzyme systems, catalase and glutathione peroxidase, is the example of the functional reservation. The nucleotide sequences of DNA coding certain histones are repeated in tallies of ten per genome in some animal cells, up to the hundred times in the Sea hedgehog's genome. This is the example of the information type of reservation in biology. There are many other examples of redundancy in biological systems (see Refs. in [5, 31, 39, 43]).

Another line of enhancement of reliability is to supply the repair and the replacement of functional elements. The repair and renewal processes proceed in all complex biological systems starting from the cell level. The template principle of organization of living systems implies that the information DNA structures are of the first operation importance in the cell hierarchy. Hence, of importance is the special enzyme system of reparation of DNA from damages induced by ionizing radiation and other deleterious environmental factors. The special antioxidant enzymes, the function of which is to catch the active forms of oxygen in aerobic cells, should be mentioned as another important case of the repair system.

The template synthesis provides cells with the novel molecular constructs in place of ones which have been damaged. In engineering, however, the failure rate of the system may become intolerably high if functional elements are replaced only as they have been damaged or wearied-out. In order to provide the level of failures as low as possible, functional elements are to be replaced for novel ones ahead the phase of their wear-out begins. In engineering, the preventive maintenance replacement, i.e., a schedule of the planned maintenance actions to guarantee the prophylaxis of the wear-out failures, may increase the reliability as great as 100-fold [1]. It is naturally to assume that the well-known turnover of cell components enables the similar preventive maintenance. Moreover, the quantities of proteins, lipids and other biomolecules in cells are too large to discriminate the damaged molecules from undamaged ones promptly. Hence, the preventive replacement of functional elements which follow the pattern preset in the cell genome seems to be the main line of providing the high reliability of biological systems.

RELIABILITY OF ENZYMES

The function of an enzyme, as a molecular machine, consists in catalyzing a specific biochemical reaction. From the point of view of the reliability theory, an enzyme is actually a "robot" specialized in accelerated assembly and disassembly of specific molecules. By way of derivation, it is interesting to note that this common word, "robot," was originally proposed by Czech writer Isaac Azimov. It comes from the Slavonic word for "work" ("*rabota*" in Russian), which is further derived from the Slavonic word for "slave" ("*rab*" in Russian). Any enzyme catalysis is performed as a process of step-by-step electron-conformation interactions which are induced by attachment of a substrate molecule to the enzyme molecule. Regarding the membrane electron-transfer enzymes, this approach was supposedly formulated first in [44]. The electron-conformation interactions represent the sequences of displacements and reorientations in enormous quantities of atomic groups. One can suggest that temperature fluctuations and fluctuations of other "environmental parameters" bring about the possibility of random accidents in the sequences of electron-conformation interactions, in other words, the possibility of conformational changes in incorrect directions. Such accidents may develop in one or another functional violation of the enzyme (inactivation, violation of selectivity, etc.), i.e., – the failures. Thus, the conformational fluctuations may set a limit to the enzyme reliability.

The analogy between the inactivation of enzymes and failures of technical devices is self-obvious. Yet, the thermal inactivation of enzymes does not directly concern the problem of reliability of living systems. A hen obviously lays her eggs not for the later use them in an omelet. Of more importance seems to be another kind of the enzyme failures, namely – the violation of selectivity when an enzyme catalyzes a reaction with an analogue of the enzyme substrate instead of the reaction with the "substrate-in-law" [15, 17].

From the general principles of the theory of reliability, one can expect that the definite conformation and the optimal conformation lability must correspond to the given conditions of the enzyme functioning in cells and tissues, so that to provide not only the high efficiency but also the high reliability of the enzyme. Conversely, any environmental factors, capable of tuning the enzyme conformation away from its physiological optimum, should increase the probability of malfunctions thereby decreasing the reliability of the enzyme. This "theorem" may serve as a guide-line for designing special experiments on the problems of bioreliability [17, 31]. In this respect, it would be of interest to study malfunctions of the enzymes which are known that play the key roles in controlling the long-term stability of cells, such as the enzymes of the translation apparatus. For example, a malfunction in selectivity of aminoacyl-tRNA synthase may produce errors in translation of the genetic information from DNA into the proteins. It is worth remembering also numerous potentialities regarding the temperature "tuning" of enzymes which may be used for the adaptation of bacteria, plants and poikilotherms to temperature conditions of the environment. Such effects of "tuning" may be observable in the presence of other variable factors such as pH, concentrations of salts, etc. These questions have not been explored to date.

Energetic demands of every operations in living systems are met by the molecules of adenosine triphosphate (ATP), most of which are synthesized during the oxidative metabolism in cellular mitochondria. The normal functioning of electron-transport chains (ETC) of mitochondria lies in the transport of electrons from the oxidation substrates to cytochrome oxidase and then to oxygen with the reduction of oxygen molecules to water and synthesis of ATP [45]. The mitochondrial nanoreactors have very ancient evolutionary origin and, hence, seem to be ones of the most reliable molecular machines. But, after all, their reliability characteristics are not perfect. Namely, normal elementary acts of the electron transfers alternate with the accidental malfunctions which result in the formation of the so-called superoxide radicals ($O_2^{\bullet-}$). Next, hydrogen peroxide (H_2O_2) is formed as the product of the reaction of dismutation of the $O_2^{\bullet-}$ radicals and, then, $O_2^{\bullet-}$ reacts with H_2O_2 with the formation of $OH^{\bullet}$ radical, the so-called reaction of Haber-Weiss:

$$O_2^{\bullet-} + O_2^{\bullet-} + 2H^+ \Rightarrow H_2O_2 + O_2 \, .$$

$$O_2^{\bullet-} + H_2O_2 \Rightarrow OH + OH^{\bullet} + O_2 \, .$$

From chemistry, it is known that $OH^{\bullet}$ radical is the strong oxidant which initiates the free-radical reactions of oxidation of organic molecules, including lipids, proteins, DNA and RNA. Therefore, the $O_2^{\bullet-}$ radical appears as the toxic substance that triggers the undesirable reactions, the so-called "oxidative stress," in cells and tissues [45]. Hence, from the reliability point of view, the fact that this radical appears is to be considered as the random malfunction of ETC, similarly to "recurrent failures" in engineering. This interpretation of superoxide radicals as the "free-radical failures" was proposed first in [10-13].

In accordance with the above-mentioned theorem, an essential increase in the free-radical failure rate should be expected when the catalytic conditions for the mitochondrial nanoreactors move away from the physiological optimum. Indeed, inadequate supply of oxygen under short-term anoxia/ischemia conditions causes the increase in the reactivity of the mitochondrial ubisemiquinones to oxygen along with the relevant increase in the production of $O_2^{\cdot-}$. It was experimentally proved that heart mitochondria become the intensive generators of $O_2^{\cdot-}$ after transient anoxia/ischaemia conditions [46].

There is the special antioxidant enzyme in mitochondria, the so-called superoxide dismutase (SOD), which catalyzes the reaction of dismutation of $O_2^{\cdot-}$ into hydrogen peroxide (H_2O_2) and oxygen (O_2). This enzyme works in cooperation with other antioxidant enzymes, catalase and glutathione peroxidase, which catalyze the elimination of H_2O_2 [47]. As a matter of fact, the antioxidant enzymes provide the preventive maintenance against the reactive oxygen forms.

Elementary acts of occurrence of the $O_2^{\cdot-}$ radicals, as well as elementary acts of disappearance of these radicals in the dismutation reaction, are the stochastic processes. Since SOD, like all other enzymes, operates with the limited reliability, the radicals can slip through the defense system. We have analyzed the stochastic dynamics of this system by the mathematical "Birth and Death" model, often used in the reliability theory [12, 15, 17, 31]. The calculations, based on the experimental data from the available literature, show that the rate parameter for the free-radical malfunctions in normal mitochondria, $\lambda \approx 0.25$ s^{-1}, about 1 radical every 4 sec. The rate parameter for elimination of $O_2^{\cdot-}$ by mitochondrial SOD, i.e., the probability of elimination of one $O_2^{\cdot-}$ per unit time, is

$$\mu \approx -\Delta n(t)/n(t)\Delta t = k_e[E] \approx 1.3 \cdot 10^4 \text{ s}^{-1},$$

where $\Delta n(t)$ is the number of the radicals eliminated during the time interval Δt, k_e and $[E]$ are the reaction rate constant and the concentration of SOD, $k_e \approx (2-3) \cdot 10^9$ L mol^{-1} s,$^-$ $[E] \approx (0.4-0.5) \cdot 10^{-5}$ M. Then the probability of the slipping of $O_2^{\cdot-}$ through the SOD defense has been estimated to be:

$$z = (\lambda/\mu)/(1+\lambda/\mu) \approx 1.9 \cdot 10^{-5},$$

i.e., about 2 radicals from every hundred thousand may penetrate the defense system. With the intense radical fluxes in cells, the probability of the free-radical damages in biomolecular constructs of cells can be high enough.

RELIABILITY VERSUS MORTALITY

Despite the complexity and the phenotypic variety of living organisms, aging is governed by some common quantitative laws or, more precisely, the "patterns of relationship." First, there is the so-called species-specific maximal life-span potential. Indeed, it is common knowledge that there are no mice nor rats exceeding 3-4 years of age, and that a human life-span does not exceed ≈ 120 years provided we take reliable data into account, not any sensational press reports or legends [48-50]. The limited lifetime of diploid cell strains *in vitro* is also a well-known phenomenon. For example, human fibroblasts *in vitro* die or mutate into cancer cells after performing about 50 doublings. American biologist Hayflick discovered this effect in 1961 and Russian biologist Olovnikov explained the Hayflick's limit suggesting the mechanism of the under-reparation (incomplete copying) of telomere ends of DNA, see Refs. in [49]). According to the Olovnikov's theory of marginotomy, a cell division is accompanied by the reduction of the telomere ends of the cell chromosomes. In essence, it means that the cell division stops as soon as the telomere circumcision runs up to the limit fatal level.

Another "pattern of relationship" is the correlation, for placental mammals, between the life-span potential and the rate of the basal oxygen consumption:

$$T \cdot V_0 = 4.12 \cdot 10^{10} \cdot B^{1.37},$$

where T is the maximal life-span value of the species (in sec), V_0 is the basal oxygen consumption (resting metabolic rate, ml/sec), B is the brain mass (in kilograms). This correlation, first discovered by Rubner in 1883, has been confirmed since then for different mammalian and non-mammalian species as the universal scaling relation (see Refs. in [51]).

Furthermore, the growth of the mortality rate with age obeys to the universal kinetics law. Namely, if $n(t)$ is a number of live persons of the age t, Δn is a number of those who died during the time interval Δt (usually taken to be 1 year), then the mortality rate:

$$h(t) = -\Delta n(t) / n(t) \Delta t = h_0 \exp(\gamma t),$$

where the parameters h_0 and γ are independent of time. The relevant expression for the survival function (the probability of being alive at a moment t) is

$$R(t) = \text{Prob}\{\tau > t\} = \exp\{(h_0 / \gamma)[1 - \exp(\gamma t)]\}.$$

This is the so-called "Gompertz law" of mortality that has been confirmed for people (of age approximately from 35 to 90 years), other mammals, flies, mollusks [48, 49].

Moreover, it has been shown that aging of prokaryote cells, *Acholeplasma laidlawii*, in the stationary phase of growth, namely – the loss of their viability measured as the ability to form macro-colonies, follows the same kinetic pattern [52]. Noteworthy that the cited work [52] has been the first one where it was demonstrated that the cell viability in cellular cultures declines accordingly to the Gompertz law.

Contrastingly to the so-called "robustness," there are many mathematical models in the engineering theory of reliability [1-4]. The Gompertzian mortality function corresponds to the Type 1 asymptotic distribution for the minimum value known from the so-called statistics of extremes [53]. Namely, the hazard function for a complex physical system consisting of a large number of components increases exponentially whenever the components are connected in series and are all subjected to a "wearing-out" process in which the risk of failure increases progressively [53]. This limit theorem of the statistics of extremes makes the Gompertzian mortality law appear as if it is almost universally valid, much like the central-limit theorem makes the normal distribution appear as the very appropriate model in the general theory of errors.

It is generally known that any organism is a hierarchical structure in which a relatively small number of key elements, which manage a large number of executive elements, can be distinguished. The template principle of organization of living systems implies that the information DNA structures are of the first operation importance in the cell hierarchy. A multi-cellular organism is governed by genes of a special anatomically isolated group of cells like the specialized neurons of hypothalamus in animals. Furthermore, from the mathematical theory of reliability, it is known that the effectiveness of operation of a complex system is determined mainly by the reliability of the system's governing elements, "the power structure."

Following this line, the systems reliability approach to the problems of mortality and longevity was developed in our papers [6, 12, 13, 15, 17-21, 30-33]. This approach is based on the simple general principles. The 1st one is the template principle of organization of living systems implying that the information structures rank first in the cell hierarchy ("original idiotype" of the molecular design or, in other words, the template principle of organization of living systems). Any organism works like a system of biomolecular constructs designed in accordance with the genetic program (*information plan*) in order to perform the preset programmed functions (*purpose*). The 2nd principle is that all biomolecular constructs operate with the limited reliability, namely, for each and every biological device starting from enzymes, normal operation acts alternate with accidental malfunctions. The 3rd principle states that the preventive maintenance replacement of functional elements in cells and tissues is the main line of assuring the high systems reliability, just as in engineering. Following the preset genome pattern, unreliable elements should be timely replaced for novel ones ahead the phase of their wear-out begins. In essence, it is the metabolic turnover. The 4th principle states that there is a finite number of critical elements which perform the supervisory functions over the organism's repair and renewal processes, i.e., – over the metabolic turnover. Since these critical elements of the highest hierarchic level exert the control over the systems reliability, they can be called "supervisors" or "longevity-assurance structures" (LAS). The 5th principle states that the supervisors also operate with the limited (genetically preset) reliability so that the stochastic damages are accumulated with time in "the power structure" up to the preset threshold dysfunction level. As a result, each organism has the limited life-span.

Following this reliability-theory approach, the simple mathematical model of aging was suggested first in our papers [12, 13]. It was taken that LAS accumulate the stochastic flaws resulting in the disarray of their functions. Account was also taken of another widespread peculiarity of living systems, i.e., – the existence of the threshold values for the most important functional parameters. According to this general idea, there is to be an upper limit value, m_c, at which LAS fails. The set of initial flaws, m_j ($j = 1, 2, ..., N$), represents a random sample of the exponential, though truncated, distribution with the density function:

$$ f(m) = \alpha \exp(-\alpha m)/[1 - \exp(-\alpha m_c)], $$

where $\alpha > 0$ is the parameter of this distribution, and $0 \leq m \leq m_c$. To underlay this hypothetical density function, some simple arguments were brought into account. As the flaws to LAS occur as rare events, the probability of getting an extensive flaw should obviously be less than the probability of getting a smaller one. Then, the exponent was used as the simplest asymmetric distribution known from mathematical statistics. The similar truncated exponential distributions have been known for many years ago as the simplest asymmetrical distributions in physics of linear polymer chains [54]. The organism has been assumed to perish the moment that any of the LAS develops the threshold dysfunction, i.e., the expected life-span:

$$ \tau = \min \tau_j $$

Here $\tau_j = b(m_c - m_j)$, where $b > 0$ is the reciprocal of the dysfunction growth rate in LAS with time. As a matter of fact, the life-span of the organism is determined by the weakest link's longevity. Then, the survival function is given by the smallest value of the random sample of size N:

$$ R(t) = \{1 - [exp(\gamma t) - 1]/[exp(\gamma T) - 1]\}^{N}. $$

where N is a number of LAS, $T = bm_c$ and $\gamma = \alpha/b$. For not very high values of time, the following approximation can easily be derived:

$$R(t) \approx \exp\{(h_0/\gamma)[1-\exp(\gamma t)]\}$$

with the relevant expression for mortality rate being:

$$h(t) = h_0\exp(\gamma t), \text{ where } h_0 = \gamma N/[\exp(\gamma T)-1].$$

Here is the Gompertz law of mortality. Hence, this law gets its explanation in the context of the reliability-theory approach stated above. The limit life-span T has appeared as the direct result of existence of the limit dysfunction, m_c, for the LAS. Formally, this limit is the life-span of an "ideal" organism with no flaws at $t = 0$.

All the hypothetical LAS are differently fallible since they are initially flawed at statistically varying degrees. However, they were postulated to have the same values for the reliability characteristics (α, b, m_c). This was certainly assumed for the sake of mathematical simplicity. However, an evolutionary mechanism could be proposed to support this assumption. The arrangement of the appropriate level of reliability for these structures falls into the basic cell maintenance processes of defense, restore and renewal because each of them is vitally important. All processes of this kind are metabolically expensive. Meanwhile, the energy budget of a cell is limited. If the organism perishes the moment that any one of LAS fails, there is no use in natural selection making some of them more reliable than others. The acquisition of the greater maintenance for any one, than is necessary for others, should obviously require an excess cost.

If we take that the maximum life-span for human populations, on the average, is about 95 years, the magnitude of γ varies from 0.0612 to 0.119 years^{-1} and the magnitude of h_0 varies from $0.820 \cdot 10^{-3}$ to $0.022 \cdot 10^{-3}$ years^{-1} [48], then, using the expression for h_0, we find that $N \approx 5-15$. It is worthy to note that this estimation corresponds, by the order of magnitude, to the number of the so-called "longevity-assurance genes" which have been recently discovered in nematodes, yeasts, drosophilae, mice, and other organisms (see, for example, [55, 56] and Refs. therein). It has been assumed that "the power structure," other words the supervisors or LAS in the organisms of humans and animals are the longevity-assurance genes located in the special cells of, most probably, suprachiasmatic nucleus of hypothalamus [15, 17, 18].

There are reports on deceleration of the mortality-rate functions in cohorts of *Drosophila* flies at the advanced age. The similar findings for humans were taken up in the literature, notwithstanding the facts that the statistical data on the mortality at the geriatric ages are poor (see, for example, [56-57]). A qualitative attempt to highlight this limitation of the classical Gompertzian approach was undertaken by assuming a simple mixture of a few homogeneous populations [15]. The first quantitative stochastic model of mortality and aging for heterogeneous populations was suggested in [56]. In succeeding years, the question of how the inhomogeneity, i.e., a genetic or phenotypic variability of populations, may affect the behavior of the reliability model was examined quantitatively in [17-20]. Namely, the parameters T and γ were averaged over the ensemble assuming the normal distributions for these parameters with the respective probability density functions. At the advanced time values, the mortality rate function, generated from the heterogeneous model, may accelerate its run, slow it down, display a maximum or level it off depending upon the extent of heterogeneity of the parameters, thereby behaving in the quantitative agreement with the mortality rate curves of the real populations [17, 19, 31, 32]. At this, the quantitative estimations of N, obtained from the death statistics of the heterogeneous populations, exceed the previous estimation obtained for the case of the homogenous population. The origin of this diversity is quite obvious. Individuals of a homogeneous population, being alike, die from a limited number of similar pathological reasons. However, it is not the case for heterogeneous populations. In this case, on the "tails" of the distribution function there are different individuals, from a centenarian who dies in the age of older than 100 years to a short-lived person who carries a mutant fatal gene in one of his 46 chromosomes. In part, the life-tables of the 1969-1973 calendar periods for Swedish men in the age range 35-105 years have been computed and the set of the fitting parameters, T_0 ($\pm \sigma_T$) = 120 ($\pm$0.3) years, γ_0 ($\pm \sigma_\gamma$) = 0.095 ($\pm$ 0.001) years^{-1} and N = 46, have given the agreement between the reliability model and the overall mortality data (saving the infant mortality range) with the accuracy of 13% [19].

Basing on this reliability-theory approach, one can formulate a more complex mathematical model to take into account the preset pattern of the longevity-assurance genes, their functional interrelations (feedbacks) and other non-linear effects. It is to be hoped that a non-linear reliability-theory model will explain even so sophisticated cases as the ridiculous demographic profiles of *Drosophila melanogaster* strains [57] and justify the Gompertz curves of mortality of human populations via the generalized Polya process of shocks [58].

FREE-RADICAL TIMER OF AGING: RELIABILITY-THEORY STANDPOINT

In the case of damages in LAS due to the superoxide radicals ($O_2^{\cdot-}$), the following equation was derived for the maximum lifespan [13, 15]:

$$T = bm_c \approx m_c /[(qV/E)u + D]$$

In this equation q is probability of the malfunction in mitochondrial nanoreactors leading to the superoxide occurrence, V is respiration rate, E is activity of the mitochondrial SOD in LAS, u is probability for the free-radical failures to provoke functional violations. In part, the parameter u takes into account that the deleterious effects of $O_2^{\cdot-}$, which slipped through the antioxidant defense, are of no concern if the preventive replacement of the damaged biological constructs is properly maintained in cells and tissues. D is index to incorporate other damage factors that are not associated with the oxygen free radicals. As a matter of fact, the latter equation explains the universal quantitative law of aging, the so-called "Rubner scaling relation." Besides, this equation predicts that it should be a linear correlation between the reciprocal of the species-specific maximum lifespan ($1/T$) and the ratio of the respiration rate to the SOD activity (V/E). Tolmasoff et al. have measured the SOD activity in brain, liver and heart tissues of men and animals of 13 species [59]. Using their data on the SOD activity (E) and the literature data on the species-specific oxygen consumption rates (V) from the same paper, we have plotted graphs between the reciprocal maximum lifespan potential ($1/T$) versus the ratio of V/E. Figure 3 demonstrates the graph for brain.

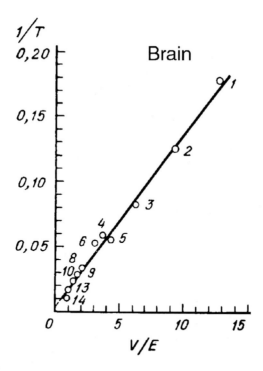

Figure 3. The correlation graph between the reciprocal maximum life-span potential ($1/T$) of different mammalian species and the ratio of the species-specific metabolic rate to the superoxide dismutase activity (V/E) for brain. 1 – house mouse (*Mus musculus*), 2 – deer mouse (*Peromyscus maniculatus*), 3 – common tree shrew (*Tupaii glis*), 4 – squirrel monkey (*Saimarii scuireus*), 5 – bush baby (*Galago crassicaudatus*), 6 – moustache tamarin (*Saguinus mystak*), 7 – lemur (*Lemur macaca fulvus*), 8 – African green monkey (*Cercopithecus aethiops*), 9 – rhesus monkey (*Macaca mulatta*), 10 – olive baboon (*Papio anubis*), 11 – gorilla (*Gorilla gorilla*), 12 – chimpanzee (*Pan troglodytes*), 13 – orangutan (*Pongo pygmaeus*), 14 – man (*Homo sapiens*). From [18, 31].

The straight linear correlations have been obtained, in accordance with the prediction of our reliability-theory model:

Brain $(r = 0.997)$; $1/T = (0.0132 \pm 0.0002)(V/E) + (0.004 \pm 0.002)$

Liver $(r = 0.997)$; $1/T = (0.0144 \pm 0.0003)(V/E) + (0.005 \pm 0.002)$

Heart $(r = 0.981)$; $1/T = (0.0110 \pm 0.0009)(V/E) + (0.011 \pm 0.006)$

By using the free coefficient D, it has been estimated that the longevity of human brain could reach 250 years, should the reliability of the antioxidant enzymes be absolutely perfect. With the values of D from the correlation equations for heart and liver, the limit longevity values have been estimated to be 100 and 200 years, respectively. Although these estimations are illustrative, it should be emphasized from these estimations that the "reactive oxygen species" do play a role in pathogenesis of cardiovascular system. Thus, the theory of reliability essentially lends credence to the free radical theory of aging that was put forward by Denham Harman 60 years ago [60].

In the free radical theory of aging it has been originally suggested that the free radicals initiate oxidative damages of DNA, proteins and lipids in cells and tissues [61]). The radical $O_2^{\cdot-}$ is, however, not the oxidant. On the contrary, this radical is the reductant (see Refs. in [28, 34]). In this regard, of great importance are the recent discoveries that identified the sirtuins, a new family of nicotine adenine dinucleotide (NAD^+)-dependent enzymes. It has been experimentally proved that these NAD^+-dependent deacetylases are the key regulators of epigenetic DNA modifications, i.e., the changes in the gene activity through the chemical modifications to DNA and histone proteins without the changes in the DNA sequence. These epigenome modifications include DNA methylation, noncoding RNA interference and modifications of the histone proteins and, thus, the sirtuins regulate many cellular functions including the glucose metabolism, the secretion of insulin, the adaptations to oxidative stress and to hypoxia, as well as the cell cycle and apoptosis (see Refs. in [62-64]). Meanwhile, the expression of the sirtuin genes depends on the redox state of their environment [62-64]. With these facts in mind, it can be assumed that $O_2^{\cdot-}$, as the reducing agent, may essentially affect the ratio of $NAD(P)H/NAD(P)^+$. As a matter of fact, the radicals are targeted onto the NAD^+-dependent sirtuin system that performs, in its turn, the function of the biological amplifier of the $O_2^{\cdot-}$ impact [28, 33, 34].

Furthermore, one can assume that the radicals impact on the epigenetic sirtuin regulators of the "longevity-assurance genes" in the "the power structure", thereby triggering the delay in the metabolic repair and renewal processes. As the consequence, the oxidative-stress products and other metabolic slag accumulate in peripheral cells and tissues with resulting impetus to the autophagic or apoptotic cell death and, thereby, the age-associated clinical disorders.

The living organisms are designed in accordance with the genetic programs, and the genetic program sets the limit to the lifespan. However, the stochastic free radical failures crucially modulate the programmed "melody" filed in the longevity-assurance genes. Thus, the free-radical redox timer, located presumably in the special cells of the suprachiasmatic nucleus of hypothalamus, serves as the effective stochastic mechanism of realization of the genetically preset deficiency in reliability ("robustness") of the organism as the biosystem taken in its entirety.

ANTIOXIDANTS: SYSTEMS RELIABILITY STANDPOINT

In chemistry, by definition, antioxidants represent a broad class of compounds, both synthetic and natural, molecules of which are capable to react with active free radicals with formation of inactive radicals of the antioxidant and, thereby, terminate free radical chain reactions (see Refs. in [28, 30, 34, 65]). Some of the phenolic inhibitors of the chain free radical peroxidation, when regularly introduced into diet or water of experimental animals, reveal the beneficial effects and prolong the animal's lifespan. Denham Harman was first who successfully tested antioxidants in experiments with laboratory animals. It was discovered that the antioxidant radiation protector 2-mercaptoethylamine prolongs life spans of C3H female mice and of AKR male mice [61]. Since then, the beneficial effects of the antioxidant therapy were experimentally proved over and over again (see Refs. in [27, 28, 33, 34, 65]). However, the free-radical chemical mechanism of action of antioxidants in living systems (*in vivo*) does not currently seem as unambiguous as half a century ago.

In 1968, the enzyme SOD was discovered by J. M. McCord and I. Fridovich (see Refs. in [47]). It has since become clear that neither natural nor synthetic antioxidants are able to compete for the reactive oxygen species with the specialized anti-oxidative enzyme systems of cells and tissues. Contrary to the popular opinion, neither natural antioxidants, like vitamin E, ascorbic acid or flavonoids, nor synthetic antioxidants, like 4-methyl-2,6-ditretbutylphenol (butylated hydroxytoluene, BHT, insoluble in water) or 2-ethyl-3-hydroxy-6-methylpyridine hydrochloride (soluble in water) are able to operate *in vivo* in the same way as *in vitro*, i.e., – as the simple chemical scavengers of free radicals. It should be taken into account that the rate constants (k) and the real concentrations of the antioxidants are negligibly low to compete for the reactive oxygen species with the specialized anti-oxidative enzymes. SOD catalyzes the reaction of dismutation of $O_2^{\cdot-}$ into H_2O_2 and oxygen, thereby scavenging $O_2^{\cdot-}$, with $k \approx 10^9$ L mol^{-1} s^{-1} [47]. Meanwhile, the k values for the reactions of ascorbic acid and other antioxidants with $O_2^{\cdot-}$ do not exceed 10^4 L mol^{-1} s^{-1}. The rate constant for the reaction of the antioxidant α-tocopherol with $OH^\bullet$ radical can be as high as $8 \cdot 10^{10}$ L mol^{-1} s^{-1}. Meanwhile, the $OH^\bullet$ radical is known to react with any organic molecules as the strong oxidant with the rate constants close to the diffusion limit, $>10^{10}-10^{11}$ L mol^{-1} s^{-1} (see Refs. in [28, 34]). Therefore, none of the antioxidants can compete for the hydroxyl radical *in vivo* with other organic molecules which are obviously present around this radical in considerably greater numbers than the molecules of any antioxidants. Of course the peroxyl radicals $RO_2^\bullet$ can appear in the reactions of $OH^\bullet$ radicals with lipids. *In vivo*, however, $RO_2^\bullet$ and other products of peroxidation arise mainly as the secondary products in the reactions that accompany cell death at apoptosis or autophagocytosis during utilization of the cellular waste by lyzosomes and peroxysomes. The rate constants for the reactions of the synthetic and natural antioxidants with $RO_2^\bullet$ in the model reactions may range up to about 10^6 L mol^{-1} s^{-1}. However, the antioxidants are unlikely to be highly necessary for scavenging the active radicals in the catabolic processes. Thus, the manifold effects of antioxidants *in vivo* can hardly be interpreted on the basis of the simple chemical analogy with the action of the same antioxidants as the radical scavengers *in vitro*. Over the years, more and more experimental results indicate that the true mechanisms of the "antioxidant prophylaxis" are to be studied on the ways of systems biology instead of the free-radical chemistry [17, 27, 28, 30, 34, 66-68].

As stated above, the most efficient way to increase the systems reliability, be it a technical system or a biological system, is the well-timed prevention of malfunctions (failures) of functional elements. Following this reliability-theory guide-line, it was proposed [10, 15, 17] that the antioxidants provide the preventive protection against free radicals *in vivo*. At this, the particular protection mechanisms may be different for antioxidants of different types.

For BHT, it was found that this antioxidant prevents the generation of $O_2^{\bullet-}$ radicals as the by-products of the mitochondrial electron transport. In the studies of the low-temperature ESR (electron spin resonance) signals of the rat tissues, we found that BHT increases the myocardium oxygenation [66]. It is known that hypoxia results in the structural damage in the mitochondrial membranes resulting in the considerable decrease in the reliability of electron transport, so that the mitochondria become generators of the intense $O_2^{\bullet-}$ fluxes [46]. It stands to reason that BHT prevents the development of hypoxia by increasing the degree of myocardium oxygenation thereby preventing the transformation of the electron-transport nanoreactors of the myocardial mitochondria into the intensive generators of $O_2^{\bullet-}$. Furthermore, it has been proved that BHT produces the dramatic hormonal changes in the animal's blood, the increase of corticotropin and corticosteroids along with the decrease of thyrotropin and triiodothyronine in blood plasma of rats after the BHT administration [67, 68]. Hence, BHT induces the substantial shift in the activity of adenohypophysis gland which is the source of corticotropin and thyrotropin hormones and this is accompanied with the relevant shifts in the activity of peripheral endocrine glands, the adrenal cortex (the source of corticosteroids) and the thyroid gland (the source of triiodothyronine). It is common knowledge that the release of corticotropin into blood, followed by the increase in synthesis of corticosteroids and the decrease in synthesis of thyroid hormones, is the significant phase of the systems adaptation to stress. It seems that, with regular introduction into animals' food, BHT as a mild stress factor trains the neuro-hormonal system and, thus, increases the systems reliability, i.e., – adaptive capabilities of the organism [27, 67, 68]. Hence, BHT is actually able to decrease the level of the active oxygen species in myocardial cells and, probably, other cells too. However, the beneficial effect of this antioxidant is manifested not through the direct elimination (scavenge) of the free radicals but in the preventive manner, namely, through the decrease in the probability of generation of the radicals.

Another example of the synthetic antioxidants is 2-ethyl-3-hydroxy-6-methylpyridine hydrochloride ("Emoxipine"). This water soluble antioxidant was first introduced in biomedicine as the anti-radiation protector in 1980 [11]. Now the antioxidants of this type are used to treat brain circulation disorders, in ophthalmology, etc (see Refs. in [28, 34]). The mechanism of the antioxidant prophylaxis in this case differs from that for BHT. The antioxidants based on hydroxypyridines are the analogs of pyridoxine and pyridoxal phosphate which are the vitamins of the B_6 group. Meanwhile, pyridoxal phosphate is the cofactor of glutamate aspartate aminotransferase, RNA polymerase, and of some other enzymes of biosynthesis of the nitrogen-containing compounds [45]. This implies that hydroxypyridine antioxidants are the anti-metabolites of vitamin B_6 and, as such, they inhibit the key enzymes of synthesis of amino acids and nucleotides. In particular, this allows understanding of the efficiency of 2-ethyl-3-hydroxy-6-methylpyridine as the anti-radiation protector. The inhibition of biosynthesis retards the cell division and thus provides the cells with the additional time for restoring the genetic structures damaged by ionizing radiation [11, 28, 34].

The so-called mitochondria-targeted antioxidants, MitoVit-E (vitamin E derivative [69]) and SkQ (ubiquinone derivative [70]) can also act in a preventive manner. As the phenolic compounds, MitoVit-E and SkQ have weakly acidic properties and, as such, they can serve as protonophore uncouplers of oxidative phosphorylation, i.e., they can uncouple electron transport and ATP synthesis in mitochondria like, for example, 2,4-dinitrophenol. Besides, as the hydrophobic cations, they can transfer counter-ions through the mitochondrial lipid membrane and, thereby, they can decrease the transmembrane potential. Meanwhile, it is generally known that the electron transport in mitochondria experiences a "back pressure" of the transmembrane potential [45]. Therefore, as the transmembrane transfer agents of protons and anions, MitoVit-E and SkQ decrease the transmembrane potential thereby decreasing the generation of $O_2^{\cdot-}$ and its active products in mitochondria. This provides grounds for believing that the mitochondria-targeted antioxidants not so much scavenge directly the $O_2^{\cdot-}$ radical (or its protonated form $HO_2^{\cdot}$) but prevent the formation of these radicals in mitochondria.

Mathematical Theory of Reliability and Biological Robustness 69

Mechanisms of antioxidant activity of natural antioxidants are being revised too. For example, glutathione (GSH), the physiological antioxidant and second messenger in cells, is considered now as the post-translational modifier that control over the epigenetic mechanisms at different levels, including the substrate availability and enzymatic activity for DNA methylation, expression of microRNAs, and participation in the histone code [71].

Furthermore, there is a wide class of natural antioxidants called flavonoids, among them – querticin, flavones, and resveratrol (the last one is especially abundant in grapes and red wine). These antioxidants can provide the preventive protection from oxygen radicals by induction of the specific antioxidant enzymes. Indeed, the induction of the synthesis of SOD and catalase was detected in blood erythrocytes of humans who received the food additive *Protandim* (extracts from five medical plants) [72]. The authors concluded that the modest induction of the antioxidant enzymes, SOD and catalase, may be a much more effective approach to the problem of defense from free radicals than supplementation with antioxidants "that can, at best, stoichiometrically scavenge a very small fraction of total oxidant production" [72]. Noteworthy, that resveratrol activates expression of the sirtuin proteins thereby providing, in part, the increase in expression of mitochondrial SOD *in vivo* (see Refs. in [28, 62]).

Inasmuch as the expression of SOD and other antioxidant enzymes in humans and animals is under the hormonal control, flavonoids also seem to make their preventive maintenance defense through the hormonal regulation mechanisms. Indeed, in the experiments with *Macaca mulatta* monkeys it was found that the diurnal changes (circadian rhythms) in the SOD activity in erythrocytes tightly and positively correlate with the diurnal changes in the levels of cortisol and dehydroepiandrosterone sulfate (DHEAS) in blood plasma [73]. For young animals, the values of correlation coefficient were 0.92 ± 0.09 (cortisol *versus* SOD) and 0.99 ± 0.02 (DHEAS *versus* SOD). With aging, the circadian rhythms of SOD, cortisol and DHEAS are smoothed out although the correlation between the diurnal changes in cortisol and in SOD still maintains even for old animals. These results, like the above-mentioned experiments with BHT, testify that corticosteroid hormones play the essential role in regulation of SOD activity.

Quite a lot of data have now been accumulated demonstrating that even vitamin E (α-tocopherol), a "key antioxidant," can hardly serve as a free radical inhibitor *in vivo* and, hence, this issue in handbooks should be revised too. There are four tocopherol isomers: α-, β-, γ-, and δ-tocopherol. All four isomers react *in vitro* with the $RO_2{}^{\bullet}$ radical with approximately the same rate constants of about 10^6 L mol^{-1} s^{-1}. In the living nature, however, mainly α-tocopherol is encountered. As shown in the experiments on the cell cultures and the isolated enzymes, this form of vitamin E inhibits a key regulator enzyme of biosynthesis, protein kinase C. Besides, it inhibits 5-lipoxygenase and phospholipase A_2 and activates protein phosphatase 2A and diacylglycerol kinase. It was proved that α-tocopherol modulates the expression of the genes encoding synthesis of a number of the protective proteins including α-TTP, α-tropomyosin and collagenase. Moreover, α-tocophenyl phosphate, rather than the antioxidant phenolic form of vitamin E, serves as the bioregulator. It has been suggested that α-tocopherol acts as a ligand for yet unidentified specific proteins regulating the signal transduction and gene expression (see Refs. in [74]).

Furthermore, there are more and more data indicating that the therapeutic effects of many pharmaceutical drugs are due to their beneficial action not only on the cells and tissues of the host organism but also on the gastric and intestinal microbiota. The number of microbiota cells in the gastrointestinal tract, on the skin, in some other organs and tissues nearly exceeds the number of cells of the host organism. Of even greater importance is that the microbial cells produce the physiologically active substances that markedly affect all organs and tissues including immune system. Moreover, there are the data that the microbial metabolites promote metabolic benefits in the brain cells via the gut-brain neural circuits. As a matter of fact, a new synthetic biomedical concept has being emerged that the human microbiota is a source of therapeutic drug targets (see Refs. in [28, 34, 75, 76]).

In view of the advances in systems biology, one can suggest that the so-called antioxidants, both natural and synthetic ones, attack the organism's microbial population. In high doses, these substances are toxic, as implied, because of their deleterious effects on the microbiota. In low doses, however, the same compounds produce the favorable effects on the organism's microbiota, in a hormetic-like fashion, and, thereby, increase the system reliability and the organism's lifespan. One can further assume that the so-called "mitochondria-targeted" compounds like MitoVit-E and SkQ actually affect the microbiotic cells. Thus, in this century, which is the century of systems biology, the theory which was put forward in the early 20th century by Metchnikoff about the considerable effects of the microbial population on the body health and aging [77], is actually revived. One can say with reasonable confidence that "Metchnikoff arises."

In closing, such terms as "polyphenols", instead of antioxidants", and "redox regulation/redox signaling pathways", instead of "oxidative stress", came into use at last [78]. Moreover, the Society for Free Radical Biology and Medicine has been recently renamed in the Society for Redox Biology and Medicine. Yet, the paradigm that the antioxidants directly intercept free radicals *in vivo* as well as they do it *in vitro* had a very long-lived existence. As said in [79], "it is harder to overcome old ideas, rather than create the new ones."

CONCLUSION

Reliability ("robustness") of biological systems as a research field of systems biology is based on the mathematical theory of reliability. The systems reliability approach, which was developed in our papers, is based on the simple general principles. First, it is the template principle of organization of living systems implying that the information structures rank first in the cell hierarchy. An organism works like a system of the biomolecular constructs designed in keeping with the genetic program in order to perform the preset programmed functions. Second, the biomolecular constructs operate with the limited reliability, namely, for each and every bio-device the normal operation acts alternate with the failures or accidental malfunctions. Third, the preventive maintenance is the main line of assuring the high systems reliability. Following the preset genome pattern, unreliable elements should be timely replaced for novel ones ahead the phase of their wear-out begins, just as in engineering. Forth, there is the finite number of the critical elements which perform the supervisory functions over the preventive maintenance. Fifth, the supervisors also operate with the genetically preset reliability, so that the stochastic damages are accumulated with time in the supervisors up to the preset threshold dysfunction level. As a result, the life-span of the organism as the system is limited. The reliability systems approach integrates both general concepts of aging, the concept of aging program and the free-radical theory of aging, in the unified pattern. On this basis, the universal features of aging, such as the exponential growth of mortality rate with time and the correlation of longevity with the species-specific resting metabolism, are naturally explained. The systems theory of reliability testifies that aging is the stochastic consequence of the genetically limited reliability of the biomolecular constructs at all functional levels, from nanoreactors to the organism as a whole. The malfunctions of the mitochondrial electron transport nanoreactors, which produce oxygen anion-radicals ($O_2^{\cdot-}$, "superoxide radicals") as the by-products of respiration, seem to be of first importance. The free-radical redox-timer, located presumably in the specialized neurons of central nervous system, serves as the effective stochastic mechanism of realization of the preset deficiency of bioreliability. As the reducing agent, $O_2^{\cdot-}$ affects the ratio of $NADH/NAD^+$ and, by changing the activity of sirtuins, slows down the renewal of biomolecular constructs. As the consequence, the oxidative-stress products and other metabolic slag accumulate with the resulting impetus to autophagic or apoptotic cell death accompanied with the age-associated clinical disorders. Furthermore, the systems reliability approach serves as the heuristic methodology in biomedicine, in part, in searching the realistic mechanisms of the therapeutic effects of antioxidants.

ACKNOWLEDGMENT

This work was realized with support from Federal Agency for Scientific Organizations (FASO, Russia), project no. 0089-2014-0042.

The mathematicians consider theory of reliability as a part of probability theory. Boris V. Gnedenko, outstanding mathematician from Kiev, Ukraine, was one of

Vitaly K. Koltover

Founding Fathers of the mathematical theory of reliability. The problem of reliability of biological systems has been first put forward by D. M. Grodzinsky and his collaborators [5, 6]. The first conference on reliability of biological systems was held in Kiev in 1975. The first books on biological reliability were published in Kiev by "Naukova Dumka," the publishing office of Ukrainian Academy of Sciences [5-10]. The first dissertation on reliability of biological systems was defended in Kiev, the A. Bogomolets Institute of Physiology [17]. Thus, located at the cross-roads of Western Europe and the Orient, Kiev has spurred the studies on reliability ("robustness") of biological systems. It confirms the old saying of the Middle Ages that "Teaching comes from Kiev."

REFERENCES

[1] Bazovsky, I. *Reliability. Theory and Practice*. London: Prentice-Hall; 1961.

[2] Lloyd, DK.; Lipov, M. *Reliability: Management, Methods and Mathematics*. New Jersey: Prentice Hall, Inc.; 1962.

[3] Gnedenko, BV; Belyaev, YuK; Soloviev, AD. *Mathematical Methods in Theory of Reliability*. Moscow: Nauka; 1965 (in Russian).

[4] Barlow, RE; Proschan F. *Statistical Theory of Reliability and Life Testing: Probability Models*. New York: Holt, Reinhart & Wiston, Inc.; 1975.

[5] Grodzinsky, DM. *Models of living matter and mathematician bionics*. Kiev (fSU): Naukova Dumka; 1966 (in Russian).

[6] Grodzinsky, DM; Vojtenko, VP; Kutlakhmedov, YA; Koltover, VK. *Reliability and Aging of Biological Systems*. Kiev (fSU): Naukova Dumka; 1987 (in Russian).

[7] Grodzinsky, DM (ed). *Systems of Reliability of Cell (Proceedings of the 1st all-union conference "Systems of Reliability of Cell," Kiev, 1975)*. (fSU): Naukova Dumka; 1977 (in Russian).

[8] Grodzinsky, DM (ed) *Reliability of Cells and Tissues (Proceedings of the 2nd all-union conference "Reliability of Cells and Tissues," Kiev, 1977)*. (fSU): Naukova Dumka; 1980 (in Russian).

[9] Grodzinsky, DM; Kutlakhmedov, YA; Gudkov, IN (eds.) *Reliability of Biological Systems (Proceedings of the 3rd all-union conference "Reliability of Biological Systems," Kiev, 1980)*. Kiev (fSU): Naukova Dumka; 1985 (in Russian).

[10] Koltover, VK; Kutlakhmedov, YA. Free radical mechanisms of failures and reliability of the cell defense systems. In: Grodzinsky DM (ed.) *Reliability of Cells and Tissues (Proceedings of the 2nd all-union conference "Reliability of Cells and Tissues," Kiev, 1977)*, Kiev (fSU): Naukova Dumka; 1980, pp. 41-51 (in Russian).

[11] Koltover, VK; Kutlakhmedov, YA; Afanaseva, EL. Recovery of cells from radiation-induced damages in the presence of antioxidants and the reliability of

biological systems. *Doklady Biophysics (Doklady Akad Nauk SSSR)*, 1980, 254, 3, 159-161.

[12] Koltover, VK. Reliability of enzymatic protection of a cell against superoxide radicals and the aging. *Doklady Biophysics (Doklady Akad Nauk SSSR)*, 1981, 256, 1, 3-5.

[13] Koltover, VK. Reliability of enzyme systems and molecular mechanisms of ageing. *Biophysics (Moscow)*, 1982, 27, 4, 635-639.

[14] Doubal, S. Theory of reliability, biological systems and aging. *Mech. Ageing. Develop.*, 1982, 18, 4, 339-353.

[15] (a) Koltover, V. K. *Theory of Reliability, Superoxide Radicals and Aging.* Chernogolovka: ICPH, USSR Acad. Sci.; 1983, 42 P. (b) Koltover, VK. Theory of reliability, superoxide radicals and aging. *Uspekhi Sovremennoj Biologii (Advances in Modern. Biology)*, 1983, 96, 4, 85-100 (in Russian).

[16] Witten, M. A return to time, cells, systems and aging: Rethinking the concept of senescence in mammalian organisms. *Mech. Ageing and Develop.*, 1983, 21, 69-81.

[17] Koltover, VK. *Reliability of Electron-Transport Membranes and the Role of Oxygen Anion-Radicals in Aging (Doctoral Dissertation in Biophysics).* Kiev (fSU): A. Bogomolets Institute of Physiology, Acad. Sci. of Ukraine SSR; Moscow: N. Semenov Institute of Chemical Physics, Acad. Sci. of USSR, Moscow, 1988, 351 p. (in Russian).

[18] Koltover, VK. Free radical theory of aging: View against the reliability theory. In: Emerit I, Chance B (eds.) *Free Radicals and Aging.* Basel: Birkhauser; 1992, pp. 11-19.

[19] Koltover, VK; Andrianova, ZS; Ivanova, AN. Simulation of survival and mortality curves of human populations based on the theory of reliability. *Russ. Biology Bulletin (Izv. Akad. Nauk Biol.)*, 1993, 20, 1, 95-101.

[20] Koltover, VK. Reliability concept as a trend in biophysics of aging. *J. Theor. Biol.*, 1997, 184, 2, 157-163.

[21] Koltover, VK. Reliability concept as a trend in biophysics. *J. Biosciences*, 1999, 24, Suppl. 1 (13th Inter. Biophys. Congress, September 18-26, 1999, New Dehli), 193.

[22] Gavrilov, LA; Gavrilova, NS. The reliability theory of aging and longevity. *J. Theor. Biol.*, 2001, 213, 527-545.

[23] Kutlakhmedov, YA; Korogodin, VI; Koltover, VK. *Foundations of Radiation Ecology.* Kiev (Ukraine): Vyshcha shkola, 2003, 320 p. (in Ukrainian).

[24] Finkelstein, M. On some reliability approaches to human aging. *Int. J. Reliability, Quality Safety Eng.*, 2005, 12, 337-346.

[25] Steinsaltz, D; Goldwasser, L. Ageing and total quality management: Extending the reliability metaphor for longevity. *Evolutionary Ecology Res.*, 2006, 8, 1445-1459.

[26] Kutlakhmedov, Yu; Korogodin, V; Rodina, V; Pchelovskaya, S. Radiocapacity: characteristic of stability and reliability of biota in ecosystems. In: Cigna AA,

Durante M (eds.) *Radiation Risk Estimates in Normal and Emergency Situations.* Dordrecht: Springer, NATO Security Trough Science Series B: Physics and Biophysics; 2006, Vol. 9, pp. 185-195.

[27] Koltover, VK. Bioantioxidants: The systems reliability standpoint. *Toxicology and Industrial Health*, 2009, 25, 4-5, 295-299.

[28] Koltover, VK. Antioxidant biomedicine: from free radical chemistry to systems biology mechanisms. *Russ. Chemical Bull.*, 2010, 59, 1, 37-42.

[29] Dimitrov, B. Ages in reliability and biosystems: interpretations, control, and applications. In: Rykov VV, Balakrishnan N., Nikulin MS (eds.) *Mathematical and Statistical Models and Methods in Reliability Statistics for Industry and Technology*. Dordrecht: Springer; 2010, part 3, pp. 317-334.

[30] Koltover, VK. Reliability of electron-transport membranes and the role of oxygen radical anions in aging: stochastic modulation of the genetic program, *Biophysics (Moscow)*, 2011, 56, 1, 125-28.

[31] Koltover, VK. Theory of reliability in systems biology: aging versus reliability. In: Valente AX, Sarkar A, Gao Y (eds). *Recent Advances in Systems Biology Research*. New York: Nova Science Publishers, Inc.; 2014, pp. 109-130.

[32] Koltover, VK. Mathematical theory of reliability and aging: Teaching comes from Kiev. In: Frenkel I, Lisnianski A (eds.) *Proceedings of the Second International Symposium on Stochastic Models in Reliability Engineering, Life Science and Operations Management*. New York: IEEE CPS (The Institute of Electrical and Electronics Engineers Inc., Conference Publishing Services); 2016, pp. 386-392.

[33] Koltover, VK. Free radical timer of aging: from chemistry of free radicals to systems theory of reliability. *Current Aging Sci.*, 2017, 10, 1, 12-17.

[34] Koltover, VK. Antioxidant therapy of aging: from free radical chemistry to systems theory of reliability. In: Vaiserman AM (ed.) *Anti–Aging Drugs: from Basic Research to Clinical Practice*. Cambridge (UK): Royal Society of Chemistry Publishing; 2017, pp. 183-204.

[35] Kitano, H. Biological robustness. *Nat. Rev. Genet.*, 2004, 5, 826–837.

[36] Lehar, J; Krueger, A; Zimmermann, G; Borisy, A. High-order combination effects and biological robustness. *Mol. Systems Biol.*, 2008, 4, 215. DOI: 10.1038/msb.2008.51.

[37] Kaltenbach, HM; Dimopoulos, S; Stelling, J. Systems analysis of cellular networks under uncertainty. *FEBS Lett.*, 2009, 583, 3923-3930.

[38] Larhlimi, A; Blachon, S; Selbig, J; Nikoloski, Z. Robustness of metabolic networks: A review of existing definitions. *Biosystems*, 2011, 106, 1, 1-8.

[39] Kriete, A. Robustness and aging - a systems-level perspective. *Biosystems*, 2013, 112, 1, 37-48.

Mathematical Theory of Reliability and Biological Robustness

[40] Gong, M; Wang, Y; Wang, Sh; Liu, W. Enhancing robustness of interdependent network under recovery based on a two-layer-protection strategy. *Sci. Reports*, 2017, 7, 12753, DOI:10.1038/s41598-017-13063-2.

[41] Van Valen, L. A new evolutionary law. *Evolutionary Theory*, 1973, 1, 1-30.

[42] Kirkwood, TBL; Rose, MR. Evolution of senescence: late survival sacrificed for reproduction. *Phil. Trans. R. Soc. London B*, 1991, 332, 15-24.

[43] Kafri, R; Springer, M; Pilpel, Y. Genetic redundancy: new tricks for old genes. *Cell*, 2009, 136, 3, 389-392.

[44] Blumenfel'd, LA; Kol'tover, VK. Energy transformation and conformational transitions in mitochondrial membranes as relaxation processes. *Mol. Biol.* (Moscow), 1972, 6, 1, 130-133.

[45] Nelson, DL; Cox, MM. *Lehninger Principles of Biochemistry*. New York: Freeman; 2008.

[46] Nohl, H; Koltover, V; Stolze, K. Ischemia/reperfusion impairs mitochondrial energy conservation and triggers $O_2^{\cdot-}$ release as a byproduct of respiration. *Free Radical Res. Com.*, 1993, 18, 3, 127-137.

[47] McCord, JM; Fridovich, I. Superoxide dismutases: you've come a long way, baby. *Antioxidants and Redox Signaling*, 2014, 20. 10, 1548-1549.

[48] Sacher, GA. Life table modification and life prolongation. In: Finch G; Hayflick L. (eds.) *Handbook of the Biology of Aging*. New York: Van Nostrand Reinhold; 1977, pp. 82-638.

[49] Anisimov, V. N. *Molecular and Physiological Mechanisms of Aging*, 2nd ed. St. Petersburg: Nauka; 2008 (in Russian).

[50] Dong, X; Milholland, B; Vijg, J. Evidence for a limit to human lifespan. *Nature*, 2016, 538, 257-259.

[51] Schmidt-Nielsen, K. *Scaling. Why Is Animal Size So Important?* Cambridge: Cambridge Univ. Press; 1984.

[52] Kapitanov, AB.; Aksenov, MY.; Tatishchev, OS.; Koltover, VK. Cell-culture of *Acholeplasma laidlawii* as an object for the investigation of the age-variation of biological membranes. *Doklady Biophysics (Doklady Akad Nauk SSSR)*, 1985, 281, 1, 186-189.

[53] Gumbel, E. J. *Statistics of Extremes*. New York: Columbia University; 1962.

[54] Flory, PJ. *Principles of Polymer Chemistry*. Ithaka: Cornell Univ.; 1953.

[55] Longo, VD; Shadel, GS; Kaeberlein, M; Kennedy, B. Replicative and chronological aging in *Saccharomyces cerevisiae*. *Cell Metabolism*, 2012, 16, 18-31.

[56] Yashin, AI; Manton, KG; Vaupel JW. Mortality and aging in a heterogeneous population: A stochastic process model with observed and unobserved variables. *Theor. Population Biol.*, 1985, 27, 154-175.

[57] Smith, ED; Tsuchiya, M; Fox, LA; Dang, N; Hu, D; Kerr, EO; Johnston, ED; Tchao, BN; Pak, DN; Welton, KL; Promislow, DE; Thomas, JH; Kaeberlein, M;

Kennedy, BK. Quantitative evidence for conserved longevity pathways between divergent eukaryotic species. *Genome Research*, 2008, 18, 564-570.

[58] Cha, JH; Finkelstein, M. Justifying the Gompertz curves of mortality of human populations via the generalized Polya process of shocks. *Theor. Population Biol.*, 2016, 109, 54-62.

[59] Tolmasoff, J; Ono, T; Cutler, RG. Superoxide dismutase: correlation with life span and specific metabolic rate in primate species. *Proc. Nat. Acad. Sci. USA*, 1980, 77, 5, 2777-2781.

[60] Harman, D. Aging: A theory based on free radicals and radiation chemistry. *J. Gerontol.*, 1956, 11, 298-300.

[61] Harman, D. Free radical theory of aging: History. In: Emerit I., Chance B. (eds.) *Free Radicals and Aging*. Basel, Birkhauser; 1992, pp. 1-10.

[62] Houtkooper, RH; Pirinen, E; Auwerx, J. Sirtuins as regulators of metabolism and health span. *Nature Reviews*. 2012, 13, 225-238.

[63] Watroba, M; Dudek, I; Skoda, M; Stangret, A; Rzodkiewicz, P; Szukiewicz, D. Sirtuins, epigenetics and longevity. *Ageing Res. Reviews*, 2017, 40, 11-19.

[64] Satoh, A; Imai, Sh; Guarente, L. The brain, sirtuins, and ageing. *Nature Reviews Neurosci.*. 2017, 18, 362-374.

[65] Obukhova, LK; Emanuel, NM. Role of free radical chain reactions of oxidation in molecular mechanisms of aging of living organisms. *Russ. Advances in Chemistry*, 1983, 52, 3, 353-372.

[66] Koltover, VK; Gorban, EN; Maior, PS. Mechanism of prolongation of life by dibunol (butylated hydroxytoluene). *Dokl. Biophys. (Dokl. Akad. Nauk SSSR)*, 1984, 277, 130-133.

[67] Frol'kis, VV; Gorban, EN; Kol'tover, VK. Effect of the antioxidant butylated hydroxytoluene (dibunol) on hormonal regulation in rats of various ages. *Dokl. Biophys. (Dokl. Akad. Nauk SSSR)*, 1985, 284, 210-213.

[68] Frolkis, VV; Gorban, EN; Koltover, VK. Effects of antioxidant butylated hydroxytoluene (BHT) on hormonal regulation and ESR signals in adult and old rats. *AGE (J. Am. Aging Assoc.)*, 1990, 13, 5-8.

[69] Murphy, MP. Targeting lipophilic cations to mitochondria. *Biochim. Biophys. Acta*, 2008, 1777, 1028-1031.

[70] Skulachev, VP. Mitochondria-targeted antioxidants as promising drugs for treatment of age-related brain diseases. *J. Alzheimer's Disease*, 2012, 28, 2, 283-289.

[71] García-Giménez, JL; Romá-Mateo, C; Pérez-Machado, G; Peiró-Chova, L; Pallardó, FV. Role of glutathione in the regulation of epigenetic mechanisms in disease. *Free Radic. Biol. Med.*, 2017, 112, 36-48.

[72] Nelson, SK; Bose, GK; Grunwald, PM; McCord, JM. The induction of human superoxide dismutase and catalase in vivo: a fundamentally new approach to antioxidant therapy. *Free Radic. Biol. Med.*, 2006, 40, 2, 341-347.

[73] Goncharova, ND; Shmaliy, AV; Bogatyrenko, TN; Koltover, VK. Correlation between the activity of antioxidant enzymes and circadian rhythms of corticosteroids in *Macaca mulatta* monkeys of different age. *Exp. Gerontol.*, 2006, 41, 778-783.

[74] Galli F; Azzi, A; Birringerc, M; Cook-Mills, JM; Eggersdorfer, M; Frank, J; Cruciani, G; Lorkowski, S; Özerj, NK. Vitamin E: Emerging aspects and new directions. *Free Radicals Biol. Med.*, 2017, 102, 16-36.

[75] Heintz, C; Mair, W. You are what you host: microbiome modulation of the aging process. *Cell*, 2014, 156, 408-411.

[76] Espin, JC; González-Sarrías, A; Tomás-Barberán, FA. The gut microbiota: A key factor in the therapeutic effects of (poly)phenols. *Biochem. Pharmacology*, 2017, 139, 82-93.

[77] Metchnikoff, E. *The Prolongation of Life. Optimistic Studies*. London: Heinemann; 1907.

[78] Davies, KJA. The oxygen paradox, oxidative stress, and ageing. *Arch. Biochem. Biophys.*, 2016, 595, 28-32.

[79] Keynes, JM. *The General Theory of Employment, Interest and Money*. New York: Palgrave Macmillan; 2007.

BIOGRAPHICAL SKETCH

Vitaly K. Koltover
ScD (Biology – Biological Physics)
PhD (Physics & Mathematics – Chemical Physics)

Affiliation:

Chief Researcher (Principal Investigator),

Institute of Problems of Chemical Physics, Russian Academy of Sciences.

http://www.icp.ac.ru

Education:

1966: National Taras Shevchenko University, Kiev, Ukraine (fSU), Department of Physics. Master Degree - Physics (Diploma with Honor).

1971: PhD (Candidate of Physical and Mathematical Sciences – Chemical Physics), Institute of Chemical Physics, USSR Academy of Sciences, Moscow. Dissertation: "Studies of the electron-transport biological membranes by the method of the molecular probes", advisor: Prof. Lev A. Blumenfeld.

1988: Sc. D. (Doctor of Biological Sciences – Biological Physics), A. Bogomolets Institute of Physiology, Ukrainian Academy of Sciences, Kiev; N. Semenov Institute of Chemical Physics, USSR Academy of Sciences, Moscow. Dissertation: "Reliability of electron-transport membranes and the role of oxygen anion-radicals in aging". Diploma of the Highest Attestation Committee, Moscow.

Business Address:

Institute of Problems of Chemical Physics, RAS, Chernogolovka, Moscow Region, 142432, Russia. E-mail: koltover@icp.ac.ru

Research and Professional Experience:

Currently main research interests are: systems theory research, reliability ("robustness") of biological systems, magnetic isotopes and nuclear spin catalysis, chemical nano-bionics,

Lecturing and Research Abroad:

2011 (December): Shamoon College of Engineering, Beer Sheva (Israel)l;

2011 (August): Institute for Physical Chemistry, Albert-Ludwig University, Freiburg (Germany);

2004 (November): Max-Planck Institute for Demographic Research, Rostock (Germany);

2002 (June): National Lawrence Berkeley Laboratory, University of California, Berkeley, (USA);

2002 (January-February): Indian Institute of Technology, Chennai (Madras), Bhabha Atomic Center, Mumbai (India);

2001 (July): Department of Chemistry, Northwestern University, Evanston (USA);

1991 (July) – 1992 (June): Institute of Pharmacology and Toxicology, University of Veterinary Medicine, Vienna (Austria);

1990 (November-December): Department for Biochemistry and Biophysics, head prof. Britton Chance), University of Pennsylvania, Philadelphia (USA);

1989 (February): National Lawrence Berkeley Laboratory, University of California, Berkeley, (USA).

Plenary and oral presentations at international scientific meetings in Russia (1972-present), Austria (1992, 1994), Canada (2001), China (2007, 2011), France (1991, 1998, 2003, 2005), Greece (2006), India (2002), Israel (2010, 2016), Italy (1992, 2014), Japan (1998), USA (1990, 1994, 2001, 2009, 2010), Ukraine (1992-present).

Professional Appointments:

Committee on Reliability of Biological Systems at the Scientific Council on the Problems of Biophysics, USSR Academy of Sciences (vice-chairman, 1978-1992).

Russian Biophysical Society, Russian Gerontological Society.

Inter. journal "Advances in Gerontology", Saint-Petersburg, Russia (editor council); inter. journal "Problems of Aging and Longevity", Kiev, Ukraine (editor board); inter. journal "Research in Medical & Engineering Sciences", New York, USA, Crimson Publ. (editor board); inter. journal "Gerontology & Geriatrics Studies, New York, USA, Crimson Publ. (editor board).

Russian Foundation for Basic Research, Moscow, Russia, expert council member; Russian Scientific Foundation, Moscow, Russia, expert.

Honors:

Never been a member of Communistic party of SU.

Publications from the Last 3 Years:

1. Koltover, V.K., Labyntseva, R.D., Kosterin, S.O. Stable magnetic isotopes as modulators of ATPase activity of smooth muscle myosin. In: Broadbent D. (ed) *Myosin: Biosynthesis, Classes and Function*. New York: Nova Science Publishers Inc.; 2018, pp. 135-158.

2. Smirnova, D.V., Koltover, V.K., Nosenko, S.V., Strizhova, I.A., Ugarova, N.N. Firefly luciferase bioluminescence as a tool for searching magnetic isotope effects in ATP-dependent enzyme reactions. *Moscow University Chemistry Bull.*, 2018, 73, 4, 158-165.

3. Koltover, V.K. Antioxidant biomedicine: from chemistry of free-radicals to reliability of biological systems. *Res. Med. Eng. Sci.*, 2018, 3, 3, 1-6.

4. Koltover, V.K. Mathematical theory of reliability and aging: a little bit of history and the state of art. *Gerontol. & Geriatric Stud.*, 2018, 4, 2, 1-2.

5. Koltover, V.K. Nuclear spin catalysis: from physics of liquid matter to medical physics. *J. Mol. Liquids*, 2017, 235, 44-48.

6. Koltover, V.K. Free radical timer of aging: from chemistry of free radicals to systems theory of reliability. *Current Aging Sci.*, 2017, 10, 1, 12-17.

7. Koltover, V.K. Antioxidant therapy of aging: from free radical chemistry to systems theory of reliability. In: Vaiserman A.M (ed.) *Anti–Aging Drugs: from Basic Research to Clinical Practice*. Cambridge (UK): Royal Society of Chemistry Publishing; 2017, pp. 183-204.

8. Avdeeva, L.V., Koltover, V.K. Nuclear spin catalysis in living nature. *Moscow University Chem. Bull.*, 2016, 71, 3, 160-166.

9. Koltover, V.K., Labyntseva, R.D., Karandashev, V.K., Kosterin, S.A. Magnetic isotope of magnesium accelerates the ATP hydrolysis catalyzed by myosin. *Biophysics*, 2016, 61, 2, 200-206.

10. Koltover, V.K. Mathematical theory of reliability and aging: Teaching comes from Kiev. In: Frenkel I., Lisnianski A. (eds.) *Proceedings of the Second International Symposium on Stochastic Models in Reliability Engineering, Life Science and Operations Management.* New York: IEEE CPS (The Institute of Electrical and Electronics Engineers Inc., Conference Publishing Services); 2016, pp. 386-392.

In: Focus on Systems Theory Research
Editors: Manuel F. Casanova and Ioan Opris

ISBN: 978-1-53614-561-8
© 2019 Nova Science Publishers, Inc.

Chapter 3

QUANTUM MODELS OF COMPLEX SYSTEMS

*Miroslav Svítek**

Faculty of Natural Sciences, Matej Bell University,
Bánská Bystrica, Slovak Republic
Faculty of Transportation Sciences,
Czech Technical University in Prague, Czech Republic

ABSTRACT

This chapter summarizes the theory of complex systems that comes basically from physical - information analogies. The information components and gates are defined in a similar way as components in electrical circuits. Such an approach enables the creation of complex networks through their serial, parallel or feedback ordering. Taking into account wave probabilistic functions (the mathematical instrument of quantum physics), we can enrich the complex system theory with features such as entanglement, parallelism, interference, etc. It is shown on illustrative examples that such approach can explain emergencies or self-organization properties of complex systems.

Keywords: quantum system theory, complex systems, quantum informatics, physical-information analogies, electrical-information analogies, magnetic – information analogies, entanglement, interference, wave probabilistic functions, information power, information action, information memelement, emergencies, self-organization

---

* Corresponding Author: Czech Technical University in Prague, Faculty of Transportation Sciences, 110 00 Konviktska 20, Prague 1, Czech Republic; Email: svitek@fd.cvut.cz.

INTRODUCTION

Analogies among electrical and information circuits seem to be efficient attempts for problems solving within system's sciences [9, 13, 23]. Let us introduce a unit for the current of information and call it *information flow* Φ, which is measured in bits per second and which describes the input or output of information per unit of time.

We can analogously define a quantity of potential, which we would call *information content* I, which determines the quantity of work per bit (Joules per bit). Information content for information systems (IT/ICT) can be defined as the number of 'success events' in the system per bit of information, and one may expect that if received information is significant, in information system a sequence of 'success events' is activated that orders the system. This also means that in order to obtain any concrete information content, we would already have to have done work, such as studying, searching for documentation, preparation, etc. On the other hand, it could be the other way around: the given information content might enable us to obtain a certain quantity of energy or (nowadays) funding in a real physical environment.

From knowledge of information flow and information content, one can define other information physics quantities. One of the important quantities can be *information power* PI, defined as the product of information flow and information content [22, 23]. Analysis easily reveals that the unit of information power is work per second realized thanks to the received bit of information. For information systems (IT/ICT), information power is defined as the number of "success events" per second caused by the receipt of one bit of information.

By introducing the quantity of information power, one can demonstrate that the impact of information is maximized if the received information flow is appropriately processed by the recipient and transformed into the best possible information content (interpretation). If there is a flow of valuable information that the recipient is incapable of processing, the information power level is low. On the other hand, if the recipient is able to make good use of the information flow, but the flow does not carry needed information, the result is likewise a low level of information power.

INFORMATION CIRCUITS

Information Gate

For the sake of simplicity, let us imagine an information subsystem as an input-output information gate given in Figure 1 that issues from a matrix representation in the following form:

$$\begin{pmatrix} I_2 \\ \phi_2 \end{pmatrix} = \begin{pmatrix} t_a & t_b \\ t_c & t_d \end{pmatrix} \cdot \begin{pmatrix} I_1 \\ \phi_1 \end{pmatrix} = T \cdot \begin{pmatrix} I_1 \\ \phi_1 \end{pmatrix} \qquad (1)$$

where the matrix T is called the transmission matrix.

Between the input ports, input information content is available, and input information flow enters the system. Between the output ports, it is possible to obtain output information content, and output information flow leaves the system.

Let us now examine the input-output information gate we have created. Input quantities can describe purely intellectual operations. Input information content includes our existing knowledge, and input information flow describes the change to the environment in which our gate operates and the tasks we want carried out (target behavior). All of the valuable, long-term information gained in this way can be used for the targeted release of energy, where at the output of the input-output gate, there may be information content on the order of millions of Joules per bit (or profits in millions of dollars). The output information flow serves as a model of the providing of such services or knowledge.

The basis of information systems is the ability to interconnect individual information subsystems, or in our case, input-output information gates. It is very easy to imagine the serial or parallel ordering of these subsystems into higher units. A very interesting model is feedback of information subsystems, because it leads to non-linear characteristics, to information systems defined at the limit of stability and other interesting properties. In this manner one may define information filters, which are able to select, remove or strengthen a component of information.

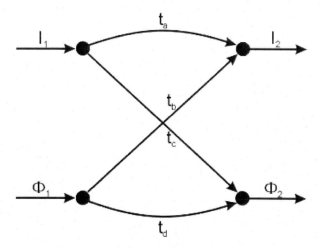

Figure 1. Information gate (Φ - information flow of data measured in bits per second, I - information content measured in Joule per bits).

Professor-Student Information Model

In the context of information model, it is appropriate to deal with the problem of teaching, because the information subsystem called a teacher may be regarded as a source of information content. The teacher has prepared this information content for years with respect to both the content as such (optimizing the information content) and its didactic presentation (optimizing the information flow), so that the knowledge can be passed on to a subsystem known as a student.

If we assume that the teacher subsystem has greater information content than the student subsystem, after their interconnection, the information flow will lead from the teacher to the student, so that the information content of the two subsystems will gradually balance out.

The students receive the information flow and increase their information content. If the students are not in a good mood, or if the information flow from the teacher is confused, the students are unable to understand the information received and to process it, so as to increase their information content.

The individual components and subsystems of complex system can behave in different ways, and their behavior can be compared to everyday situations in our lives. A characteristic of politicians is their ability to use even a small input of information content to create a large output information flow. They have the ability to take a small amount of superficially understood content and to interpret and explain it to the broadest masses of people. On the other hand, a typical professor might spend years receiving input information flow and input information content, and within her/his field, he/she may serve as a medium for transmitting a large quantity of output information content. The professor, however, might not spread the content very far, sharing it perhaps only with a handful of enthusiastic students.

It is hard to find an appropriate system to combine the characteristics of the different information subsystems described above, but it is possible to create a group of subsystems - system alliance [22], where these characteristics can be combined appropriately. In this way, one can model a company or a society of people who together create information output that is very effective and varied, leading to improved chances for the survival and subsequent evolution of the given group.

Through an appropriate combination of its internal properties, the alliance can react and adapt to the changing conditions of its surroundings. Survival in alliances thus defined seems more logical and natural than trying for a combination of all necessary processes within the framework of one universal complex system.

Information Dynamic

It is evident that a relation between the information flow $\Phi(t)$ and the information content $I(t)$ can have a lot of time dependent forms. In accordance to electrical analogies, we can define the *information impedance* $Z(t)$ expressing the acceptance of the information flow $\Phi(t)$ in the studied system:

$$I(t) = Z(t) \cdot \Phi(t) \tag{2}$$

Considering a time dependence we can expect three types of impedances.

First of them, the *information resistance R* yields into linear dependency between $I(t)$ and $\Phi(t)$:

$$I(t) = R \cdot \Phi(t) \tag{3}$$

It gives an information that the transmitted information flow $\Phi(t)$ has a direct impact on the studied system – the number of bits per second is linearly dependent on the number of events in the studied system.

The *information inductance L* has the form:

$$I(t) = L \cdot \frac{d\Phi(t)}{dt} \tag{4}$$

It says that the time change of information flow $\Phi(t)$ (acceleration/deceleration of transmitted bits per second) is linearly proportional to the number of events in the system.

And, the *information capacitance C* can be given as:

$$\Phi(t) = C \cdot \frac{dI(t)}{dt} \tag{5}$$

It means that the time change of information content $I(t)$ (increase/decrease of events number per bit in the system) is proportional to the information flow $\Phi(t)$.

Due to time dependence of all the above mentioned quantities $I(t), Z(t), \Phi(t)$ we can use mathematical instruments known in a theory of electrical circuits – Laplace, Fourier or z-transform – and rewrite these quantities, for example, in $j\omega$-domain as follows [9]:

$$\tilde{I}(j\omega) = F\{I(t)\}$$
$$\tilde{Z}(j\omega) = F\{Z(t)\} \tag{6}$$
$$\tilde{\varphi}(j\omega) = F\{\varphi(t)\}$$

where $F\{.\}$ means Fourier transform and $\tilde{I}(j\omega), \tilde{Z}(j\omega), \tilde{\varphi}(j\omega)$ are Fourier's functions assigned to the information content, to the information impedance and to the information flow, respectively.

Then, the equations (2-5) could be expressed in $j\omega$-domain:

$$\tilde{I}(j\omega) = \tilde{Z}(j\omega) \cdot \tilde{\varphi}(j\omega)$$
$$\tilde{I}(j\omega) = R \cdot \tilde{\varphi}(j\omega)$$
$$\tilde{I}(j\omega) = j\omega \cdot L \cdot \tilde{\varphi}(j\omega) \tag{7}$$
$$\tilde{\varphi}(j\omega) = j\omega \cdot C \cdot \tilde{I}(j\omega)$$

All mathematical instruments developed in the past for dynamic electric circuits can be applied with success for modeling of dynamic information circuits.

QUANTUM MODELS

Wave Probabilities

Bracket or Dirac notation [2, 14] is a standard notation for describing quantum states in the theory of quantum mechanics composed of angle brackets and vertical bars. This name is used because the inner product of two quantum states is denoted by a bracket $\langle \Phi | \Psi \rangle$, consisting of a left part $\langle \Phi |$, called the bra, and a right part, called the ket $| \Psi \rangle$.

Let us define N discrete events A_i, $i \in \{1, 2, .., N\}$ of a sample space S, with defined time-dependent probabilities $P(A_i, t), i \in \{1, 2, ..., N\}$.

The quantum state $|\psi, t\rangle_\eta$ represents the description of the quantum object given by superposition of N discrete events at location η and time instant t:

$$|\psi, t\rangle_\eta = \psi(A_1, t) \cdot |A_1\rangle_\eta + \psi(A_2, t) \cdot |A_2\rangle_\eta + ... + \psi(A_N, t) \cdot |A_N\rangle_\eta \tag{8}$$

with N *wave probabilistic functions* defined as [6]:

$$\psi(A_i,t) = \alpha_i(t) \cdot e^{j \cdot v_i(t)}, i \in \{1,2,...,N\},\tag{9}$$

where $\alpha_i(t) = \sqrt{P(A_i,t)}$ is the modulus, and $v_i(t)$ is the phase of a wave probabilistic function. We suppose the reference phase assigned to event A_1 at time t = 0 is typically chosen as $v_1(0) = 0$.

If we take into consideration k quantum objects, the corresponding wave function $|\tilde{\psi},t\rangle_\eta$ is given by the *Kronecker product* defined [14]:

$$|\tilde{\psi},t\rangle_\eta = |\psi,t\rangle_{\eta+1} \otimes |\psi,t\rangle_{\eta+2} \otimes .. \otimes |\psi,t\rangle_{\eta+k},\tag{10}$$

where the modulus of weighting complex parameters gives probabilities that measurements on the set of k quantum objects at time t will yield into a sequence of predefined events. Their phases represent possible correlations between all events [4].

The quantity of information in bits can be measured e.g., by *von Neumann entropy* [14]:

$$S(\rho) = -tr\left(\rho \cdot \log_2(\rho)\right)\tag{11}$$

where $tr(.)$ means trace operator and ρ density operator:

$$\rho(x,t) = |\psi(x,t)|^2\tag{12}$$

It measures an amount of uncertainty contained within the density operator taking into account wave probabilistic features like entanglement, quantization, etc.

Quantum Information Gate

Let us define a time-dependent wave probabilistic function which describes the *wave information flow:*

$$\psi_\phi(x,t) = |\psi_\phi(x,t)| \cdot e^{j \cdot v_\phi(x,t)}\tag{13}$$

measured e.g., by von Neuman entropy in [bits per second]:

$$S\left(\rho_\phi\right) = -tr\left(\rho_\phi \cdot \log_2\left(\rho_\phi\right)\right) \tag{14}$$

$$\rho_\phi\left(x,t\right) = \left|\psi_\phi\left(x,t\right)\right|^2 \tag{15}$$

The term the *wave information content* can be represented as well by:

$$\psi_I\left(x,t\right) = \left|\psi_I\left(x,t\right)\right| \cdot e^{j \cdot v_I\left(x,t\right)} \tag{16}$$

The number of "success events" in the studied system can be likewise measured by von Neumann entropy [number of success events per bit of received information]:

$$S\left(\rho_I\right) = -tr\left(\rho_I \cdot \log_2\left(\rho_I\right)\right) \tag{17}$$

$$\rho_I\left(x,t\right) = \left|\psi_I\left(x,t\right)\right|^2 \tag{18}$$

From the above analysis it is apparent that von Neumann entropy is just an information measure that plays the same role in the theory of wave probabilistic functions as *Shannon entropy* measure in a classical theory of probability [14].

Wave Information Dynamic

We can define in the same manner the *wave information impedance* $\psi_Z\left(Z,t\right)$ expressing an acceptance of the information flow $\Phi\left(t\right)$ by the system:

$$\psi_I\left(I,t\right) = \psi_Z\left(Z,t\right) \cdot \psi_\phi\left(\Phi,t\right) \tag{19}$$

The *wave information resistance* R_ψ yields into:

$$\psi_I\left(I,t\right) = R_\psi \cdot \psi_\phi\left(\Phi,t\right) \tag{20}$$

The *wave information inductance* L_ψ is defined:

$$\psi_I\left(I,t\right) = L_\psi \cdot \frac{d\psi_\phi\left(\Phi,t\right)}{dt} \tag{21}$$

And the *wave information capacitance* C_ψ is given:

$$\psi_\phi(\Phi, t) = C_\psi \cdot \frac{d\psi_I(I, t)}{dt} \qquad (22)$$

All quantities $\psi_I(I, t), \psi_Z(Z, t), \psi_\varphi(\Phi, t)$ can be transformed with help of Fourier transform $F\{.\}$ into $j\omega$-domain:

$$\tilde{\psi}_I(I, j\omega) = F\{\psi_I(I, t)\}$$
$$\tilde{\psi}_Z(Z, j\omega) = F\{\psi_Z(Z, t)\} \qquad (23)$$
$$\tilde{\psi}_\varphi(\Phi, j\omega) = F\{\psi_\varphi(\Phi, t)\}$$

and the equations (18-21) then rewritten as:

$$\tilde{\psi}_I(I, j\omega) = \tilde{\psi}_Z(Z, j\omega) \cdot \tilde{\psi}_\varphi(\Phi, j\omega)$$
$$\tilde{\psi}_I(I, j\omega) = R_\psi \cdot \tilde{\psi}_\varphi(\Phi, j\omega)$$
$$\tilde{\psi}_I(I, j\omega) = j\omega \cdot L_\psi \cdot \tilde{\psi}_\varphi(\Phi, j\omega) \qquad (24)$$
$$\tilde{\psi}_\varphi(\Phi, j\omega) = j\omega \cdot C_\psi \cdot \tilde{\psi}_I(I, j\omega)$$

Due to serial, parallel or feedback ordering of quantum information gates represented by dynamic wave probabilities or by their Fourier's functions the very specific features of complex systems could be modelled.

FEATURES OF QUANTUM MODELS

Interference

Let us define two quantities of quantum gate in following way (for the sake of simplicity we suppose that all quantities are time independent and they acquire only N finite values):

$$\psi_\Phi = \alpha_{\Phi,1} \cdot |\Phi_1\rangle + \alpha_{\Phi,2} \cdot |\Phi_2\rangle + ... + \alpha_{\Phi,N} \cdot |\Phi_N\rangle \qquad (25)$$

$$\psi_I = \alpha_{I,1} \cdot |I_1\rangle + \alpha_{I,2} \cdot |I_2\rangle + ... + \alpha_{I,N} \cdot |I_N\rangle \qquad (26)$$

where $\Phi_1,..,\Phi_N$ and $I_1,...,I_N$ are possible values of information flow and information content, respectively. Complex parameters $\alpha_{\Phi,1},..,\alpha_{\Phi,N}$ and $\alpha_{I,1},..,\alpha_{I,N}$ represent wave probabilities taking into account both probability of falling relevance value of flow or content together with their mutual dependences [10].

The *wave information power* PI can be expressed using wave probabilistic functions (25, 26) as follows:

$$\psi_{PI} = \psi_\Phi \otimes \psi_I = \alpha_{\Phi,1} \cdot \alpha_{I,1} \cdot |\Phi_1, I_1\rangle + ... + \alpha_{\Phi,1} \cdot \alpha_{I,N} \cdot |\Phi_1, I_N\rangle + .. + $$
$$+ \alpha_{\Phi,N} \cdot \alpha_{I,1} \cdot |\Phi_N, I_1\rangle + ... + \alpha_{\Phi,N} \cdot \alpha_{I,N} \cdot |\Phi_N, I_N\rangle \tag{27}$$

where symbol $\otimes$ means Kronecker multiplication [14].

Each i,j-th component $|\Phi_i, I_j\rangle$ represents particular value of information power that characterizes the falling/measuring of information flow Φ_i and information content I_j.

Both values Φ_i and I_j could be either positive (the information is given into the system), or negative (information is withdrawn out of the system).

It is evident that possible different combinations of information flows and contents $|\Phi_i, I_j\rangle$, $|\Phi_k, I_l\rangle$ can achieve the same (similar) information power:

$$\Phi_i \cdot I_j \approx \Phi_k \cdot I_l \approx K_r \tag{28}$$

We can unite these two components into one value of information power:

$$\left(\alpha_{\Phi,i} \cdot \alpha_{I,j} + \alpha_{\Phi,k} \cdot \alpha_{I,l}\right) \cdot |\Phi_i, I_j\rangle = \beta_r \cdot |K_r\rangle \tag{29}$$

It could be seen that the interferences of wave probabilities could emerge and the wave resonances among wave parameters are possible as well.

Finally, the wave information power in renormalized form can be expressed:

$$\psi_{PI} = \beta_1 \cdot |K_1\rangle + \beta_2 \cdot |K_2\rangle + ... + \beta_r \cdot |K_r\rangle + ... \tag{30}$$

where we can use von Neumann entropy for its assessment:

$$S(\rho_{PI}) = -tr(\rho_{PI} \cdot \log_2(\rho_{PI})) \tag{31}$$

$$\rho_{PI} = |\psi_{PI}|^2 \tag{32}$$

It is supposed that each element of information circuit has its input/output information flow Φ_i and input/output information content I_j. With respect to this statement we can, therefore, define the input/output information power PI_{in}, PI_{out} assigned into this element and find the optimized ordering of quantum gates to achieve the best possible information power at the output of the whole complex information circuit.

Mass-Parallelism

Let us imagine that thanks to wave probability functions, a situation may arise when we shall be monitoring the probability of the union of several phenomena, e.g., that either the first phenomenon will occur, OR the second will occur, OR the third will not occur, etc., and that this probability works out to equal zero. Naturally, this situation cannot arise under the classical theory of probability, because their probabilities are merely added together, and at the most, repeating overlaps of phenomena are subtracted.

In the newly introduced area of complex wave probability functions (quantum systems), it can also occur, through the influence of the existence phases, the subtracting of probabilities, and under certain conditions it is possible to find such a constellation of phenomena, that their union works out to zero probability [13].

This, however, automatically means that the inversion phenomenon (intersection) for the given union (in our case, this inversion phenomenon would mean that the first phenomenon does not occur, AND at the same time the second phenomenon does not occur, AND the third phenomenon does occur) will occur with 100% probability, regardless of how the phenomena are arranged spatially.

Such feature is called *quantum entanglement* and it is caused by the resonance of complex wave functions. Among the ways this resonance manifests itself is that thanks to it we arrive from a purely probabilistic world to a completely deterministic world, where there is a disruption of the probabilistic characteristics of various phenomena, and the links between the entangled phenomena become purely deterministic events that even show up in different places (generally even at different times), and for that reason they are also often designated as spatial (or generally temporo-spatial) distributed system states. Similarly, one may arrive at the conclusion that thanks to the principle of resonance, selected (temporo-spatial) distributed states absolutely cannot occur in parallel, and this leads to an analogy with the *Pauli exclusion principle*.

The selection of a group entangled states can, of course, have a probabilistic character, as long as the entanglement is not one hundred percent. This means that parallel behavior occurs only with a certain probability, and this leads to the idea of the selection of one variant according to the given probability function.

In reference [14], we read that the behavior of entangled states is very odd. Firstly, it spreads rapidly among various phenomena, where for this spreading it makes use of a property known as *entanglement swapping*. Here is a simple example of this behavior. If we have four phenomena, the first and second being entangled, the third and fourth phenomenon being entangled as well, then as soon as it comes to an entanglement between the first and third phenomenon, the second and fourth are also entangled, without any information being exchanged between them. Not- withstanding that those phenomena can be spatially quite remote from each other.

Complexity Reduction

Many complex systems are typically characterized by a high level of redundancies. The surrounding complex reality can be modelled either by very complicated model or approximated by a set of many different and often overlapping easier models which represent different pieces of knowledge.

Wave probabilities could be used to set up final behavior of complex system. Phase parameters can compensate overlapping information among models as it was presented in [5, 6, 11, 12]. Feynman rule [24] says that all paths (in our case each of the models) contributes to a final amplitude (in our case to a final model) by its amplitude with different phase.

In classical examples the more models the more possible trajectories of the future complex system behavior. This problem is mentioned in literature as *"the curse of dimensionality"*. But for wave probabilistic models some trajectories could be due to phase parameters mutually canceled up and others, by contrast, strengthened.

If we take a sum of all trajectories assigned to all wave models this sum can converge into "right" trajectory of the complex system. With respect to *Feynman path diagram* [25], the more available models could not note the complexity increase.

Information Resonance

We can continue in our way of thinking and define basic principles of information resonance. For example, we can imagine two hemispheres of our brain. The left hemisphere plays the role of the information inductor – the source of information flow $\Phi_i(t)$ based on identified knowledge. On the contrary, the right hemisphere could be described as the information capacitor – the source of information content $I_i(t)$ based on the observed data - analytical part that attempts to interpret the available data. The resonance principle can be modeled by the means of co-operation between both hemispheres. The bigger data flow $\Phi_i(t)$ is generated by the left hemisphere the higher knowledge $I_i\ t$ can be extracted by the right hemisphere. The higher knowledge $I_i\ t$ then encourages higher data flow $\Phi_i(t)$ and so on.

We can assume that the information flow $\Phi_i(t)$ represents a number of different evolution variants/stories/conclusions that are afterwards analyzed/interpreted/modeled as the information content $I_i\ t$. The result of the resonance principle is maximizing the link between the two hemispheres and achieving the best balance between the syntactical and semantical part of the information.

ADVANCED PHYSICAL-INFORMATION ANALOGIES

Information Memelements

The circuit theoretician Chua [15] introduced the basic concept of electrical components together with the links between them as it is shown in Figure 2.

There are six different mathematical relations connecting pairs of the four fundamental electrical circuit variables:

$q(t)$ - charge,

$\varphi(t)$ - magnetic flux,

$i(t)$ - electric current,

$v(t)$ - voltage.

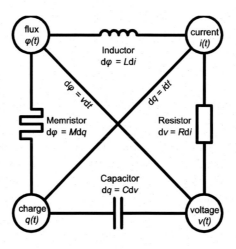

Figure 2. Chua's concept of electrical quantities.

94   *Miroslav Svítek*

From electrical variables definition we know that the charge is the time integral of the current. Faraday's law tells us that the flux is the time integral of the electromotive force, or voltage. There should be four basic circuit elements described by relations between variables: resistor, inductor, capacitor and memristor. Chua's concept is famous due to an envisioned new electrical component named "memristor" that provides a functional relation between charge $q(t)$ and flux $\varphi(t)$.

The equations for memelement (memristor, memcapacitor, meminductor) can be generalized [17]:

$$y(t) = g\big(w(t)\big) \cdot x(t) \tag{33}$$

$$\frac{dw(t)}{dt} = x(t) \tag{34}$$

where y(t) and x(t) are the terminal memelement's variables and w(t) is the internal state variable.

We can describe basic memelements as follows:

- *Information Memristor:* y(t) represents the information content $I_i\ t$, x(t) the information flow $\Phi_i(t)$ and w(t) the information in bits,
- *Information Meminductor:* y(t) represents the information flow $\Phi_i(t)$, x(t) the information content $I_i\ t$ and w(t) the information action in Joule-second per bit,
- *Information Memcapacitor:* y(t) represents the information content $I_i\ t$, x(t) the information flow $\Phi_i(t)$ and w(t) the time-domain integral of information in bits.

The butterfly-shaped hysteresis loop is expected to occur at a sufficiently large input of $q(t)$ or $\varphi(t)$ [18]. Information memelements as a part of information circuit can cause the hysteresis that were introduced e.g., in the *theory of catastrophes* [21].

Electric – Information Analogies

In the current state of *information analogies*, an electric circuit with its electric current [coulomb per second] and voltage [Joule per coulomb] represents the analogy of an *information model* with quantities:

- *Information content - I* [Joule per bit] defines the model of a real system together with its appropriate features and suitable control strategies (extracted uncertainty of data flow, data interpretation, model structure identification, model parameters' estimation, mixture of multi-models, model's verification and validation and model-based control)
- *Information flow - Φ* [bits per second] describes the syntax strings of data flow assigned to a real system (data collection and signals transmission to/from a real system).

The information model only works with available knowledge and creates a suitable representation of a real system. In the electric analogy, Joule per bit means the energy required for finding the most suitable model for a real system.

Magnetic – Information Analogies

The *magnetic circuit* with the magnetic flux φ [Joule-second per coulomb] and with the magneto motive force (mmf) F [Joule-second per coulomb] represents the action assigned to one coulomb. *Action* is an attribute of dynamics of a physical system from which the equation of real motion can be derived. In this text we will rather use the "rate of magnetic flux" $\frac{d\varphi}{dt}$ in [Joule per coulomb] which is related to the energy flow (energy transmission) carried by a coulomb.

In information analogies it means the changes of a real system to achieve more energy. Such approach is like the Kauffman's principle of self-organized agents [6] continuously looking for more and more sophisticated ways of obtaining energy.

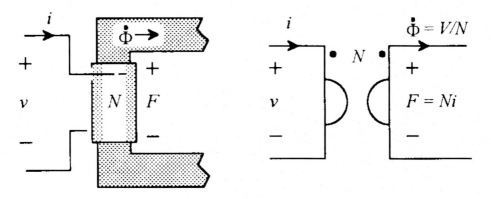

Figure 3. Gyrator model of electric/magnetic transformer [20].

The electric - magnetic transformation can be modeled by a gyrator[1] as it is shown in Figure 3. On the left side there are electrical parameters: v – electric voltage, i – electric current and on the right site there are magnetic parameters: F – magneto motive force (mmf) and $d\Phi/dt$ - rate of magnetic flux.

For a winding of N turns we can write:

$$v = N \cdot \frac{d\Phi}{dt}$$

(35)

$$i = \frac{F}{N}$$

(36)

The magnetic circuit (right side of Figure 3) represents in an information analogy a modification of a physical system based on the available information (left side of Figure 3). With respect to this it is possible to define two new information parameters assigned to a real physical system (to distinguish the right side of Figure 3 we use the term 'knowledge-based'):

- *Knowledge-based action A* [Joule-second per bit] – Magneto motive force (mmf) can be interpreted in magnetic-information analogy as an action that describes the amount of energy[2] that could be obtained from a real system based on one-bit of information during one second. Different changes of a real system yield to different values of physical actions[3]. Information flow Φ from an information model identifies actions in the real world. On the other hand, new actions (in the real system) can generate new information flows or, in other words, a new modification of the information model.

- *Knowledge-based energy flow E* – the rate of magnetic flux $d\Phi/dt$ in the magnetic-information analogy can be interpreted as knowledge-based resources extraction. The information content I, represented by the information model, enables us to realize changes of the real physical system (changes in structure,

---

[1] According to Wikipedia, a gyrator is a passive, linear, lossless, two-port electrical network element proposed in 1948 by Bernard D. H. Tellegen as a hypothetical fifth linear element after the resistor, capacitor, inductor and ideal transformer. An important property of a gyrator is that it inverts the current-voltage characteristic of an electrical component or network. In the case of linear elements, the impedance is also inverted. In other words, a gyrator can make a capacitive circuit behave inductively: a series LC circuit behaves like a parallel LC circuit, and so on. It is primarily used in active filter design and miniaturization.

[2] The new source of energy that can be exploited using available information.

[3] The principle of least "knowledge-based action" can be applied to obtain the optimized behavior of a complex system. The solution requires finding the path that has the least value. This principle remains the central point in modern physics, being applied in thermodynamics, the theory of relativity, quantum mechanics, particle physics and we propose to be a focus of complex system theory for an explanation of features like self-organization, etc.

organization, processes, etc.) in such a way that new resources of identified energy could be extracted. Parameter E describes the speed of flow of the extracted energy in [Joules per second].

The presented approach of electrical- and magnetic-information analogies allows for the connection of the real physical world with its information model and describes the benefit of the available information.

We can go further on and create *complex network* with both real (analogy to magnetic part) and virtual (analogy to electric part) components including their serial, parallel or feedback ordering. Such approach can be extended also to *quantum complex networks* similarly as it was done in previous parts. In this case the model can be enriched by features like interference, entanglement, etc. among all the real and virtual components.

DISCUSSION

The presented approach to quantum models of complex systems can be shown on some illustrative examples. One already discussed is the *co-operation of two brain hemispheres* – the left hemisphere with more rational abilities and the right hemisphere with more emotional abilities. In this approach, the left hemisphere can be newly modelled as electric circuit that collects and processes data and builds the information model. On the other hand, the right hemisphere is responsible for feeling/visualization of different stories or triggering emotions, e.g., working with physical parts of our body.

Memelements included to an information circuit can represent historical experiences because the integral part of variables contains a memory. The circuits with these features are much richer and can model more sophisticated situations.

Other extension could be studied in information- or knowledge-based variables. Historically, information power PI [22, 23] in [joule per second] was defined as multiplication of information flow Φ and information content I on the left side of Figure 3. In a similar way we can define *physical action AP* in [Joule-second] (right side of Figure 3) as multiplication of knowledge-based action A in [Joule-second per bit] and available information in [bits].

Physical energy EP in [Joule] (right side of Figure 3) can be obtained by multiplication of knowledge-based action A in [Joule-second per bit] and information flow Φ in [bits per second]. Similarly, the *information energy EI* (energy necessary to create the model) in [Joule] (left side of Figure 3) can be defined by multiplication of available information in [bits] and information content I in [joule per bit].

The all above discussed physical-information analogies can be easily changed into the wave representation. Considering the wave representations of different information parameters, the quantum model of complex system should explain e.g., the emergent behavior, catastrophic phenomena. The inner resonances could surprisingly arrive to the features such as self-organization or, by other words, to unexpected jump reduction of complexity.

We can then ask the following questions: Is the resonance principle a fundamental rule of self-organization? Are different components organized (structured) through the links so that the knowledge in each of them is maximized? Are such rules of self-organization compatible to minimal energy principle known in physics? If only a minimum of energy is spent in the system, can we define the *Law of minimal information* as the basic principle of complex systems?

The conclusion of the discussion remains still open but let us finish by quote of Albert Einstein: "If at first the idea is not absurd, then there is no hope for it".

CONCLUSION

In this chapter the quantum models of complex systems were introduced based on physical-information analogies. The mathematical comparison between usually used probabilistic models and wave probabilistic models was presented. With the help of mathematical theory we derived the features of quantum models. The mathematical theory points out on the applicability of quantum models and their special features in the area of complex systems.

From the examples given above, we can see the possibility for linking the physical world with the world of information, because every information flow must have its transmission medium, which is typically a physical object (e.g., physical particles) or a certain property of such an object [17]. The case is again similar to an information content, which also must be connected to a real, physical system. The operations defined above the information model can then likewise be depicted in a concrete physical environment and vice versa. Such approach yields to finding and extracting better energy resources in the area of a real system.

We believe that the capturing of processes in the world around us with the help of information subsystems organized into various interconnections (modeled by wave probabilities), especially with feedbacks, can lead to the controlled dissemination of macroscopic work in real system as described by Stuart Kauffman [19], and after the overcoming of certain difficulties, even to the description of the behavior of living organisms or our brain [22].

Wave probabilistic approach can capture Soft Systems Models (SSM) which can bring new quality of understanding the complex systems. Such approach can enrich our learning and we can then speak about quantum cybernetics [11] or quantum system theory [5, 7].

The inspiration for the above defined problems came from physical-information analogies. The link with quantum mechanics [1, 2, 3, 14] could be seen as very interesting and is likely to bring a lot of inspiration for the future work within the complex systems modelling by wave probabilistic functions.

The presented results should not be treated as a finished work, but rather the beginning of a journey. It is easy to understand that a lot of mentioned theoretical approaches should continue to be tested in practical applications.

ACKNOWLEDGMENT

This work was supported by the Project AI & Reasoning CZ.02.1.01/0.0/0.0/ 15_003/0000466 and the European Regional Development Fund.

REFERENCES

[1] Deutsch, D. Quantum theory, the Church-Turing principle and the universal quantum computer, *Proceedings of the Royal Society of London Series A*, 400, 97-117, 1985.

[2] Derek, F. Lawden: *The Mathematical Principles of Quantum Mechanics*, Dover Publication, Inc., Mineola, New York, 1995, ISBN 0-486-44223-3.

[3] Gold, JF. *Knocking on the Devil's Door - A Naive Introduction to Quantum Mechanics*, Tachyon Publishing Company, 1995.

[4] Khrennikov, A. Reconstruction of Quantum Theory on the Basis of the Formula of Total Probability, Proc. of Conf. of Probability and Physics -3, *American Inst. of Physics, Ser. Conf. Proc.*, 750, pp. 187-219, 2005.

[5] Svítek, M. *Dynamical Systems with Reduced Dimensionality, Monograph NNW* No. 6, Czech Academy of Science, 161 pages, 2006, ISBN 80-903298-6-1.

[6] Svítek, M. Wave probabilistic models, *Neural Network World*, 5/2007, pp. 469-481, 2007.

[7] Svítek, M. Quantum System Modelling, *International Journal on General Systems*, Vol. 37, No. 5, pp. 603-626, 2008.

[8] Svítek, M. Wave probabilities and quantum entanglement, In: *Neural Network World*, 5/2008, pp. 401-406, 2008.

[9] Svítek, M; Votruba, Z; Moos, P. Towards Information Circuits, In: *Neural Network World*, 2010, vol. 20, no. 2, p. 241-247. ISSN 1210-0552.

[10] Svítek, M. Wave probabilistic information power, In: *Neural Network World*, 2011, vol. 21, no. 3, p. 269-276, ISSN 1210-0552.

[11] Svítek, M. Wave probabilistic functions for quantum cybernetics, 2012, *IEEE Transactions on Systems Man and Cybernetics, Part C-Applications and Reviews*, Volume 42, Issue 2, pp. 233-240, 2012.

[12] Svítek, M. Applying Wave Probabilistic Functions for Dynamic System Modeling, *IEEE Transactions on Systems Man and Cybernetics, Part C-Applications and Reviews*, Volume 41, Issue 5, pp. 674-681, 2011.

[13] Svítek, M. Towards to complex system theory, *NNW*, 1/15, 2015.

[14] Vedral, V. *Introduction to Quantum Information Science*, Oxford University Press, 2006.

[15] Chua, LO. Memristor – The Missing Circuit Element, *IEEE Transactions on Circuit Theory*, 1971, 18/5.

[16] Mohamed, MGA; HyungWon, Kim; Tae-Won, Cho. Modeling of Memristive and Memcapacitive Behaviors in metal-Oxide Junctions, Hindawi Publishing Corporation, *Scientific World Journal*, Volume 2015, Article ID 910126, 16 pages, http://dx.doi.org/10.1155/2015/910126.

[17] Marszalek, W. On the action parameter and one-period loops of oscillatory memristive circuits, *Nonlinear Dyn*, (2015), Springer, 82, 619-628, DOI 10.1007/s11071-015-2182-2.

[18] Shen, Shi-Peng; Shang, Da-Shan; Chai, Yi-Sheng; Sun, Young. Realization of a flux-driven memtranstor at room temperature. *Chinese Physics B*, 2016, 25(2), 027703.

[19] Kauffman, Stuart. *At Home in the Universe: The Search for Laws of Self-Organization and Complexity*. Oxford University Press. ISBN 0195111303.

[20] Hamill, DC. Gyrator-Capacitor Modelling: A better Way of Understanding Magnetic Components, Applied Power Electronics Conference and Exposition, 1994. APEC '94. *Conference Proceedings*, 1994, Pages 326 – 332, vol. 1.

[21] Thom, René. *Structural Stability and Morphogenesis: An Outline of a General Theory of Models*. Reading, MA: Addison-Wesley, 1989. ISBN 0-201-09419-3.

[22] Novák, M; Votruba, Z. *Theory of System Complexes Reliability*, Aracne edit., Roma, 2017.

[23] Vlček, J. Systems Engineering (in Czech: Systémové inženýrství), *CTU in Prague*, 1999, ISBN 80-01-01905-5.

[24] Feynman, R; Leighton, R; Sands, M. *Feynman lectures of physics*, Addison Wesley Longman, Inc., USA, 1966.

[25] Feynman, R. *QED: The Strange Theory of Light and Matter by Richard Feynman*, Addison Wesley Longman, Inc., USA, 1966.

In: Focus on Systems Theory Research
Editors: Manuel F. Casanova and Ioan Opris

ISBN: 978-1-53614-561-8
© 2019 Nova Science Publishers, Inc.

Chapter 4

MODEL-ORDER REDUCTION WITH H_2/H_∞ PERFORMANCE

Salim Ibrir[*]
Department of Electrical Engineering
King Fahd University of Petroleum and Minerals
Dhahran, Kingdom of Saudi Arabia

Abstract

Model Order Reduction (MoR) has demonstrated its usefulness and tremendous applicability in simulation and control of large-scale mathematical models that appear in engineering, medicine, biology, and other sciences. Recently, the interest in developing more accurate reduced-order models has increased due to the nature of integrated dynamical systems and the need of the synergistic integration of electronics, mechanics, control theory, internet of things, and computer science within product design and manufacturing. This chapter discusses a new approach to model-order reduction with H_2/H_∞ performance measure. The developed MoR approach is seen as a combination of Petrov-Galerkin projection with H_2/H_∞ error-norm minimization. The proposed numerical algorithm is stated as a solution of set of Linear Matrix Inequalities (LMIs). The algorithm is compared to classical MoR methods and the main features are clearly demonstrated.

1. Introduction

Simulation and control of feedback control systems necessitate the design of accurate models that best describe the true behaviors of the systems' dynamics. However, accurate models may involve a huge number of states with high complexity of computation. Examples of those systems are encountered in many engineering fields where the system dynamics is originally described by a set of partial-differential equations (PDEs). After spatial discretization, the number of the discrete states is usually very high. It is therefore, very time

---

[*]Email: sibrir@kfupm.edu.sa

consuming to simulate or control such large-scale systems. To overcome this inherent difficulty, a reduced-order model can be built to preserve the most important characteristics of the original system with some expense of inaccuracy.

Historically, the fundamental problem of model-order reduction has received a prominent attention in the literature and quite successful methods have been proposed for both continuous time and discrete time systems (Benner, Hinze, & Maten, 2011), (Tan & He, 2007), (Antoulas, 2005), (Antoulas, Sorensen, & Gugercin, 2001), (Desrochers, 1981). The balanced-truncation algorithms (Heinkenschloss, Reis, & Antoulas, 2011), moment matching techniques (Antoulas, 2005), projection-based procedures, optimal and convex-optimization techniques (Grigoriadis, 1995), (Geromel, Kawaoka, & Egas, 2004), (Ibrir, 2018), (Ibrir & Bettayeb, 2014), (Ibrir & Bettayeb, 2015), (Ibrir, 2017) are examples of computational techniques that have been extensively used for a variety of dynamical systems. Combination of these techniques has also led to more accurate algorithms with a priori quantification of approximation errors. Further details on available techniques for model-order reduction are discussed in the survey paper (Antoulas et al., 2001) and the references therein.

The approximation error, induced by the reduced-order system, depends essentially upon the relevance of the imposed optimization criteria and the feasibility of the solutions under multiple constraints. Referring to the literature in this area of research, it is found that the minimization of H_∞ norm of the difference of two transfer functions leads to satisfactory approximation error, see e.g., (Kavranoglu & Bettayeb, 1993). In particular, H_2-based algorithms (Gugercin, Antoulas, & Beattie, 2008), (Yan & Lam, 1999), (Ibrir, 2018), convex-optimization-based procedures (Geromel et al., 2004), (Grigoriadis, 1995), (Zhang, Huang, & Lam, 2003), (Zhang et al., 2003), and Hankel-based algorithms (Safonov, Chiang, & Limebeer, 1990) have ever demonstrated satisfactory performances for linear dynamical systems. Other variant algorithms may be traced in the references (Moore, 1981), (Al-Saggaf & Franklin, 1987), (Glover, 1984), (Antoulas, 2005), (Penzl, 2006), (Heinkenschloss et al., 2011), (Sou & Rantzer, 2012), (Luitel & Venayagamoorthy, 2010).

To the best of our knowledge, the MoR problem with mixed H_2/H_∞ performance has not been considered in the literature as a projection method. In this paper, a convex-optimization procedure is proposed for the solution of the mixed H_2/H_∞ model-order reduction for linear-time-invariant (LTI) continuous-time systems. The matrices of the reduced-order model are given in terms of the entries of a positive definite matrix that plays the role of an estimate of the observability Gramian. Numerical simulations showed that the proposed approach gives better results when compared to the classical balanced-truncation method and the MoR Hankel algorithm.

2. Problem Statement and Preliminary Results

Throughout this chapter, we note by $\mathbb{R}$, $\mathbb{N}$, and $\mathbb{Z}_{\geq 0}$ the set of real numbers, the set of natural numbers, and the set of positive integer numbers, respectively. The notation $A > 0$ (resp. $A < 0$) means that the matrix A is positive definite (resp. negative definite). A' is the matrix transpose of A. We note by $\| \cdot \|$ the usual Euclidean norm. The notation $\mathbf{0}$ and I stand for the null matrix and the identity matrix of appropriate dimensions while $I_{n,n}$ and

$0_{n,n}$ stand for the identity matrix of dimensions $n \times n$ and the null matrix of dimensions $n \times n$, respectively. The symbol "$\star$" as a matrix entry stands for any element that is induced by transposition. If A is a matrix, $\mathrm{He}(A) = A + A'$. The following technical Lemmas will thoroughly used in the proofs of the main results. Therefore, for sake of clarity, the statements of these Lemmas are recalled.

Lemma 1 (The Schur complement lemma (Boyd, Ghaoui, Feron, & Balakrishnan, 1994)). *Given constant matrices M, N, Q of appropriate dimensions where M and Q are symmetric, then $Q > 0$ and $M + N'Q^{-1}N < 0$ if and only if*

$$\begin{bmatrix} M & N' \\ N & -Q \end{bmatrix} < 0, \text{ or equivalently } \begin{bmatrix} -Q & N \\ N' & M \end{bmatrix} < 0.$$

Lemma 2 (Elimination procedure (Boyd et al., 1994)). *Given matrices G, U, V of appropriate dimensions, there exists a matrix X such that*

$$G + UXV' + VX'U' > 0, \tag{1}$$

if and only if

$$\tilde{U}'G\tilde{U} > 0, \quad \tilde{V}'G\tilde{V} > 0 \tag{2}$$

holds, where $\tilde{U}$ and $\tilde{V}$ are the orthogonal complements of U and V respectively.

Consider the stable LTI system described by the state-space formulation:

$$\begin{aligned} \dot{x} &= A\,x + B\,u, \\ y &= C\,x, \end{aligned} \tag{3}$$

where $x = x(t) \in \mathbb{R}^n$ denotes the state vector, $u = u(t) \in \mathbb{R}^m$ is the control input, and $y = y(t) \in \mathbb{R}^p$ is the system measured output. The matrices A, B and C are real-valued known matrices of appropriate dimensions. Our ultimate objective is to set up a reduced-order system of dimension r; $r < n$ whose state-space realization is given by:

$$\begin{aligned} \dot{x}_r &= A_r\,x_r + B_r\,u, \\ y_r &= C_r\,x_r, \end{aligned} \tag{4}$$

where $A_r \in \mathbb{R}^{r \times r}$, $B_r \in \mathbb{R}^{r \times m}$ and $C_r \in \mathbb{R}^{p \times r}$ are the state, the input, and the output matrices, respectively. Additionally, the following specifications are required to be fulfilled simultaneously.

i) The matrix A_r is Hurwitz;

ii) Find the minimum value of $\gamma > 0$ such that the H_2 norm of the transfer function $G(s) - G_r(s) = C(s\,I - A)^{-1}B - C_r(s\,I - A_r)^{-1}B_r$ is less than γ;

iii) Find the minimum value of $\gamma_\infty > 0$ such that the H_∞ norm of the transfer function $G(s) - G_r(s) = C(s\,I - A)^{-1}B - C_r(s\,I - A_r)^{-1}B_r$ is less than γ_∞.

The transfer function $\tilde{G}(s) = G(s) - G_r(s)$ is seen as the transfer function of the following system:

$$\begin{pmatrix} \dot{x} \\ \dot{x}_r \end{pmatrix} = \begin{pmatrix} A & 0 \\ 0 & A_r \end{pmatrix} \begin{pmatrix} x \\ x_r \end{pmatrix} + \begin{pmatrix} B \\ B_r \end{pmatrix} u,$$

$$\tilde{y} = \begin{pmatrix} C & -C_r \end{pmatrix} \begin{pmatrix} x \\ x_r \end{pmatrix} \tag{5}$$

where $u = u(t)$ and $\tilde{y} = \tilde{y}(t)$ are seen as the input and the output of (5), respectively. Let

$$A_\Delta = \begin{pmatrix} A & 0 \\ 0 & A_r \end{pmatrix}, B_\Delta = \begin{pmatrix} B \\ B_r \end{pmatrix}, C_\Delta = \begin{pmatrix} C & -C_r \end{pmatrix}. \tag{6}$$

Then, for the null-initial condition $x(0) = 0$ and $x_r(0) = 0$, the H_2 norm of $\tilde{G}(s)$; noted $\|\tilde{G}\|_{H_2}$, is equal to $\sqrt{\mathrm{trace}(B'_\Delta Q B_\Delta)}$ where $Q \in \mathbb{R}^{(n+r) \times (n+r)}$ is the observability Gramian defined as the solution of the Lyapunov equation:

$$A'_\Delta Q + Q A_\Delta + C'_\Delta C_\Delta = 0. \tag{7}$$

The H_∞ norm of the transfer function $\tilde{G}(s)$ is defined as

$$\|\tilde{G}\|_{H_\infty} = \mathrm{ess} \sup_{\|u(t)\|_{\mathscr{L}_2} \neq 0} \frac{\|\tilde{y}(t)\|_{\mathscr{L}_2}}{\|u(t)\|_{\mathscr{L}_2}} = \sup_\omega \bar{\sigma}(\tilde{G}(j\omega)), \tag{8}$$

where $\bar{\sigma}$ stands for the maximum singular value. The H_2/H_∞ model-order reduction problem can be stated as follows. Find $\hat{Q} > 0$, A_r, B_r and C_r that solve the following optimization problem:

$$\min_{\hat{Q}, A_r, B_r, C_r} \gamma^2 + \gamma_\infty^2 \tag{9a}$$

s.t.

$$\hat{Q} > 0, \quad \mathrm{trace}(B'_\Delta \hat{Q} B_\Delta) < \gamma^2, \tag{9b}$$

$$A'_\Delta \hat{Q} + \hat{Q} A_\Delta + \frac{1}{\gamma_\infty^2} \hat{Q} B_\Delta B'_\Delta \hat{Q} + C'_\Delta C_\Delta < 0. \tag{9c}$$

Conditions (9a)-(9c) are sufficient conditions to ensure $\|\tilde{G}\|_{H_2} < \gamma$ and $\|\tilde{G}\|_{H_\infty} < \gamma_\infty$. This comes from the fact that, if condition (9c) is satisfied, then $A'_\Delta \hat{Q} + \hat{Q} A_\Delta + C'_\Delta C_\Delta < 0$, and consequently, $\hat{Q}$, that solves (9c), verifies $\hat{Q} > Q$. As a result, $\mathrm{trace}(B'_\Delta Q B_\Delta) < \mathrm{trace}(B'_\Delta \hat{Q} B_\Delta) < \gamma^2$. Actually, condition (9c) is a sufficient condition to make the condition: $\|\tilde{y}(t)\|^2_{\mathscr{L}_2} \leq \gamma_\infty^2 \|u(t)\|^2_{\mathscr{L}_2}$ satisfied. To prove this result, let $\xi = \begin{pmatrix} x' & x'_r \end{pmatrix}'$ be the augmented state vector of dimension $n + r$ and let $\mathscr{W}(\xi) = \xi' \hat{Q} \xi$ be the Lyapunov function associated with the dynamics (5). If the following condition:

$$\int_0^t \tilde{y}'(s)\tilde{y}(s)ds - \gamma_\infty^2 \int_0^t u'(s)u(s)\, ds < -\mathscr{W}(\xi(t)) \tag{10}$$

Model-Order Reduction with H_2/H_∞ Performance 105

is satisfied for the null-intial conditions then, inequality $\|\tilde{y}(t)\|^2_{\mathscr{L}_2} \le \gamma^2_\infty \|u(t)\|^2_{\mathscr{L}_2}$ is satisfied. If (10) holds true; the following integral inequality:

$$\int_0^t \left(\tilde{y}'(s)\tilde{y}(s)ds - \gamma^2_\infty u'(s)u(s) + \dot{\mathscr{W}}(\xi(s)) \right) ds < 0 \tag{11}$$

holds true as well. After straightforward development, the last integral inequality is explicitly reduced to the following inequality:

$$\int_0^t \left(\begin{array}{c} \xi(s) \\ u(s) \end{array} \right)' \left(\begin{array}{cc} A'_\Delta \hat{Q} + \hat{Q} A_\Delta + C'_\Delta C_\Delta & \hat{Q} B_\Delta \\ B'_\Delta \hat{Q} & -\gamma^2_\infty I \end{array} \right) \left(\begin{array}{c} \xi(s) \\ u(s) \end{array} \right) ds < 0. \tag{12}$$

From the last inequality, it can be inferred, by the Schur complemet Lemma that, condition (9c) is a sufficient and a necessary condition to fulfill (12). Notice that the optimization problem, as stated in (9a)-(9c), is not convex which makes the numerical search of one possible solution a very difficult task because of the high number of the matrix variables to be determined. For instance, the matrices A_r, B_r, C_r and $\hat{Q}$ are all unknown, and therefore, the reduction of the number of matrix variables is quite necessary to diminush the degree of the problem complexity. As a first step, necessary and sufficient conditions to make the optimization problem (9a)-(9c) solvable are summarized in the following statement.

Theorem 3. *The optimization problem (9a)-(9c) has a solution if and only if there exit a positive definite matrix $\hat{Q}_1 \in \mathbb{R}^{n \times n}$ and a positive semidefinite matrix $Z \in \mathbb{R}^{n \times n}$ such that the following optimization problem:*

$$\min_{\hat{Q}_1 > 0, \, Z \ge 0} \gamma^2 + \gamma^2_\infty \tag{13a}$$

s.t.

$$\hat{Q}_1 - Z > 0; \quad rank(Z) \le r, \tag{13b}$$

$$trace\left(B'(\hat{Q}_1 - Z)B \right) \le \gamma^2, \tag{13c}$$

$$A'\hat{Q}_1 + \hat{Q}_1 A + C'C < 0, \tag{13d}$$

$$\left(\begin{array}{cc} A'(\hat{Q}_1 - Z) + (\hat{Q}_1 - Z)A & (\hat{Q}_1 - Z)B \\ B'(\hat{Q}_1 - Z) & -\gamma^2_\infty I \end{array} \right) < 0 \tag{13e}$$

is solvable.

Proof. Let us take the partition of $\hat{Q}$ as follows:

$$\hat{Q} = \left(\begin{array}{cc} \hat{Q}_1 & \hat{Q}_2 \\ \star & \hat{Q}_3 \end{array} \right), \quad \hat{Q}_1 \in \mathbb{R}^{n \times n}, \hat{Q}_2 \in \mathbb{R}^{n \times r}, \hat{Q}_3 \in \mathbb{R}^{r \times r}. \tag{14}$$

Using the result of the Schur complement Lemma, conditions (9b) and (9c) are equivalent to the following:

$$trace(B'_\Delta \hat{Q} B_\Delta) < \gamma^2,$$

$$\left(\begin{array}{ccc} A'_\Delta \hat{Q} + \hat{Q} A_\Delta & C'_\Delta & \hat{Q} B_\Delta \\ \star & -I & 0 \\ \star & \star & -\gamma^2_\infty I \end{array} \right) < 0. \tag{15}$$

Using the partition of $\hat{Q}$, the last inequality is rewritten as

$$
\begin{pmatrix}
A'\hat{Q}_1 + \hat{Q}_1 A & A'\hat{Q}_2 + \hat{Q}_2 A_r & C' & \hat{Q}_1 B + \hat{Q}_2 B_r \\
\star & A'_r \hat{Q}_3 + \hat{Q}_3 A_r & -C'_r & \hat{Q}'_2 B + \hat{Q}_3 B_r \\
\star & \star & -I & 0 \\
\star & \star & \star & -\gamma_\infty^2 I
\end{pmatrix} < 0. \tag{16}
$$

Inequality (16) is expanded as

$$
\underbrace{\begin{pmatrix}
A'\hat{Q}_1 + \hat{Q}_1 A & A'\hat{Q}_2 & C' & \hat{Q}_1 B \\
\star & 0 & 0 & \hat{Q}'_2 B \\
\star & \star & -I & 0 \\
\star & \star & \star & -\gamma_\infty^2 I
\end{pmatrix}}_{G}
$$

$$
+ \underbrace{\begin{pmatrix}
0 & 0 \\
I & 0 \\
0 & 0 \\
0 & I
\end{pmatrix}}_{U} \underbrace{\begin{pmatrix}
A'_r & -C'_r \\
B'_r & 0
\end{pmatrix}}_{X'} \underbrace{\begin{pmatrix}
\hat{Q}'_2 & \hat{Q}_3 & 0 & 0 \\
0 & 0 & I & 0
\end{pmatrix}}_{V'} \tag{17}
$$

$$
+ \begin{pmatrix}
\hat{Q}'_2 & \hat{Q}_3 & 0 & 0 \\
0 & 0 & I & 0
\end{pmatrix}' \begin{pmatrix}
A'_r & -C'_r \\
B'_r & 0
\end{pmatrix}' \begin{pmatrix}
0 & 0 \\
I & 0 \\
0 & 0 \\
0 & I
\end{pmatrix}' < 0.
$$

The orthogonal complement of U verifies the following:

$$
U'_\perp = \begin{pmatrix}
I & 0 & 0 & 0 \\
0 & 0 & I & 0
\end{pmatrix}, \quad U'_\perp U = 0, U'_\perp U_\perp > 0. \tag{18}
$$

Similarly,

$$
V'_\perp = \begin{pmatrix}
I & -\hat{Q}_2 \hat{Q}_3^{-1} & 0 & 0 \\
0 & 0 & 0 & I
\end{pmatrix}, \quad V'_\perp V = 0, V'_\perp V_\perp > 0. \tag{19}
$$

Using the result of the Elimination Lemma, inequality (17) holds if and only if the following

$$
U'_\perp G U_\perp < 0, \quad V'_\perp G V_\perp < 0 \tag{20}
$$

holds. Inequality $U'_\perp G U_\perp < 0$ leads to the following condition:

$$
\begin{pmatrix}
A'\hat{Q}_1 + \hat{Q}_1 A & C' \\
\star & -I
\end{pmatrix} < 0; \tag{21}
$$

which is equivalent to: $A'\hat{Q}_1 + \hat{Q}_1 A + C'C < 0$. The necessary and the sufficient condition: $V'_\perp G V_\perp < 0$ gives:

$$
\begin{pmatrix}
\mathrm{He}\left((\hat{Q}_1 - \hat{Q}_2 \hat{Q}_3^{-1} \hat{Q}'_2)A\right) & (\hat{Q}_1 - \hat{Q}_2 \hat{Q}_3^{-1} \hat{Q}'_2)B \\
\star & -\gamma_\infty^2 I
\end{pmatrix} < 0. \tag{22}
$$

Model-Order Reduction with H_2/H_∞ Performance 107

By setting $Z = \hat{Q}_2\hat{Q}_3^{-1}\hat{Q}_2'$, the last inequality takes the new compact form:

$$\begin{pmatrix} A'(\hat{Q}_1 - Z) + (\hat{Q}_1 - Z)A & (\hat{Q}_1 - Z)B \\ \star & -\gamma_\infty^2 I \end{pmatrix} < 0. \tag{23}$$

Now, let us deal with the trace condition: $\text{trace}(B_\Delta'\hat{Q}B_\Delta) < \gamma^2$. Let $W > 0$ be a positive definite matrix verifying $W - B_\Delta'\hat{Q}B_\Delta > 0$, or equivalently,

$$\begin{pmatrix} W & B'\hat{Q}_1 + B_r'\hat{Q}_2' & B'\hat{Q}_2 + B_r'\hat{Q}_3 \\ \star & \hat{Q}_1 & \hat{Q}_2 \\ \star & \star & \hat{Q}_3 \end{pmatrix} > 0. \tag{24}$$

Inequality (24) is expanded as

$$\underbrace{\begin{pmatrix} W & B'\hat{Q}_1 & B'\hat{Q}_2 \\ \star & \hat{Q}_1 & \hat{Q}_2 \\ \star & \star & \hat{Q}_3 \end{pmatrix}}_{\Omega} + \underbrace{\begin{pmatrix} I \\ 0 \\ 0 \end{pmatrix}}_{\Phi} B_r' \underbrace{\begin{pmatrix} 0 & \hat{Q}_2' & \hat{Q}_3 \end{pmatrix}}_{\Psi'}$$

$$+ \begin{pmatrix} 0 & \hat{Q}_2' & \hat{Q}_3 \end{pmatrix}' B_r \begin{pmatrix} I \\ 0 \\ 0 \end{pmatrix}' > 0. \tag{25}$$

Using again the result of the Elimination Lemma, the necessary and the sufficient conditions guaranteeing $\text{trace}(B_\Delta'\hat{Q}B_\Delta) < \gamma^2$ are:

$$\Phi_\perp'\Omega\Phi_\perp > 0, \quad \Psi_\perp'\Omega\Psi_\perp > 0, \quad \Phi_\perp' = \begin{pmatrix} 0 & I & 0 \\ 0 & 0 & I \end{pmatrix}, \quad \Psi_\perp' = \begin{pmatrix} I & 0 & 0 \\ 0 & I & -\hat{Q}_2\hat{Q}_3^{-1} \end{pmatrix}. \tag{26}$$

With the condition $\Phi_\perp'\Omega\Phi_\perp > 0$, one recovers the condition $\hat{Q} > 0$ while condition $\Psi_\perp'\Omega\Psi_\perp > 0$ leads to:

$$\begin{pmatrix} W & B'(\hat{Q}_1 - \hat{Q}_2\hat{Q}_3^{-1}\hat{Q}_2') \\ \star & \hat{Q}_1 - \hat{Q}_2\hat{Q}_3^{-1}\hat{Q}_2' \end{pmatrix} > 0. \tag{27}$$

Inequality (27) implies $W > 0$, $W > B'(\hat{Q}_1 - Z)B$ and $\hat{Q}_1 - Z > 0$. If $\text{trace}(W) < \gamma^2$; then, $\text{trace}(B'(\hat{Q}_1 - Z)B) < \gamma^2$. This ends the proof. $\qquad\square$

3. H_2/H_∞ Model-Order Reduction

In this section the problem of H_2/H_∞ model-order reduction is considered. Before presenting the main result of this Section, the link between the optimal value of the input matrix B_r and the entries of the observability gramian is highlighted. The optimal selection of the input matrix B_r will subsequently help in defining the structure of the remaining matrices, namely, the state and the output matrices A_r and C_r. In the following statement, it will be shown that the optimal value of the input matrix B_r, that minimizes the H_2 norm of $G(s) - G_r(s)$ could be determined from the entries of the observability gramian that depends in turn upon A_r and C_r.

108   *Salim Ibrir*

Theorem 4. *Consider the stable LTI system (3) of dimension n and let (4) be the reduced-order system of dimension r; $r < n$. Assume that there exist a positive definite matrix $Q \in \mathbb{R}^{(n+r)\times(n+r)}$, and two real-valued non-null matrices $A_r \in \mathbb{R}^{r\times r}$ and $C_r \in \mathbb{R}^{p\times r}$ such that the following optimization problem:*

$$\min_{Q>0} \ trace\left(B'(Q_1 - Q_2 Q_3^{-1} Q_2')B\right),$$

s.t.   (28)

$$A_\Delta' Q + Q A_\Delta + C_\Delta' C_\Delta = 0, \quad Q = \begin{pmatrix} Q_1 & Q_2 \\ \star & Q_3 \end{pmatrix} > 0,$$

has a solution then, the optimal value of the input matrix B_r, that minimizes the H_2 norm of $G(s) - G_r(s)$, is $B_r = -Q_3^{-1} Q_2' B$ where A_Δ and C_Δ are defined as in (6), $G(s)$ and $G_r(s)$ are the transfer functions of system (3) and (4), respectively.

Proof. Let $B_r = W'B$ where $W \in \mathbb{R}^{n\times r}$ is a real-valued matrix to be determined. The matrix $Q \in \mathbb{R}^{(n+r)\times(n+r)}$ is the observability gramian of system (5), and hence, it is positive definite once A and A_r are Hurwitz and the pair (A_Δ, C_Δ) is observable. By definition, the square of the H_2 norm of $G(s) - G_r(s)$ is equal to trace$(B_\Delta' Q B_\Delta)$. We have,

$$Q = \begin{pmatrix} Q_1 & Q_2 \\ \star & Q_3 \end{pmatrix}, Q_1 \in \mathbb{R}^{n\times n}, Q_2 \in \mathbb{R}^{n\times r}, Q_3 \in \mathbb{R}^{r\times r}. \tag{29}$$

where Q_1 and Q_3 are positive definite matrices. Since

$$\frac{d}{dW}\text{trace}(B_\Delta' Q B_\Delta) = 2\frac{d}{dW}\text{trace}\left(B'WQ_2'B\right)$$
$$+ \frac{d}{dW}\text{trace}\left(B'WQ_3W'B\right) \tag{30}$$

Using the following equalities:

$$\frac{\partial}{\partial X}\,\text{trace}\left(AXBX'C\right) = A'C'XB' + CAXB$$
$$\frac{\partial}{\partial X}\,\text{trace}\left(AXB\right) = A'B'. \tag{31}$$

Then,

$$\frac{d}{dW}\text{trace}(B'WQ_2'B) = BB'Q_2,$$
$$\frac{d}{dW}\text{trace}(B'WQ_3W'B) = 2BB'WQ_3. \tag{32}$$

This yields,

$$\frac{d}{dW}\text{trace}(B_\Delta' Q B_\Delta) = 2BB'Q_2 + 2BB'WQ_3. \tag{33}$$

The square of the H_2 norm of the transfer function $G(s) - G_r(s)$ is optimal when $\frac{d}{dW}\text{trace}(B_\Delta' Q B_\Delta) = 0$; that is,

$$2BB'Q_2 + 2BB'WQ_3 = 0, \tag{34}$$

Since Q_3 is positive definite, the optimality condition (34) is equivalent to:

$$2BB'Q_2Q_3^{-1} + 2BB'W = 0 \tag{35}$$

which implies $W = W^\star = -Q_2Q_3^{-1}$. Substituting the optimal solution $W^\star$ in the expression of $\|G(s) - G_r(s)\|_{H_2}^2$ gives

$$\begin{aligned}
\|G(s) - G_r(s)\|_{H_2}^2 &= \text{trace}(B'Q_1B) \\
&\quad + 2\,\text{trace}(B'W^\star Q_2'B) \\
&\quad + \text{trace}(B'W^\star Q_3 W^{\star'}B) \\
&= \text{trace}(B'(Q_1 - Q_2Q_3^{-1}Q_2')B).
\end{aligned} \tag{36}$$

Since $\text{trace}(B'(Q_1 - Q_2Q_3^{-1}Q_2')B)$ is reaching its minimum value, then $W = W^\star$ is the optimal value realizing this objective. This ends the proof. $\qquad\square$

Theorem 5. *Consider the stable LTI system (3). If there exist a positive definite matrix $\hat{Q}_1 \in \mathbb{R}^{n\times n}$ and a positive semidefinite matrix $Z \in \mathbb{R}^{n\times n}$ such that the following optimization problem:*

$$\min_{\hat{Q}_1 > 0,\, Z \geq 0} \gamma^2 + \gamma_\infty^2 \tag{37a}$$

s.t.

$$\hat{Q}_1 - Z > 0; \quad rank(Z) \leq r, \tag{37b}$$

$$trace\left(B'(\hat{Q}_1 - Z)B\right) \leq \gamma^2, \tag{37c}$$

$$\begin{pmatrix}
A'\hat{Q}_1 + \hat{Q}_1 A + C'C & A'\hat{Q}_1 + ZA + C'C & (\hat{Q}_1 - Z)B \\
\star & A'\hat{Q}_1 + \hat{Q}_1 A + C'C & 0 \\
\star & \star & -\gamma_\infty^2 I
\end{pmatrix} < 0, \tag{37d}$$

$$\begin{pmatrix}
A'(\hat{Q}_1 - Z) + (\hat{Q}_1 - Z)A & (\hat{Q}_1 - Z)B \\
B'(\hat{Q}_1 - Z) & -\gamma_\infty^2 I
\end{pmatrix} < 0 \tag{37e}$$

is solvable then, for the following state-space matrices:

$$\begin{cases}
A_r = \hat{Q}_2' A \hat{Q}_1^{-1} \hat{Q}_2 \hat{Q}_3^{-1}, \\
B_r = -\hat{Q}_2' B, \\
C_r = -C\hat{Q}_1^{-1}\hat{Q}_2\hat{Q}_3^{-1}, \\
Z = \hat{Q}_2\hat{Q}_3^{-1}\hat{Q}_2',
\end{cases} \qquad \hat{Q} = \begin{pmatrix} \hat{Q}_1 & \hat{Q}_2\hat{Q}_3^{-1} \\ \star & \hat{Q}_3^{-1} \end{pmatrix} \tag{38}$$

the reduced-order system (4) verifies

$$\begin{aligned}
\|G - G_r\|_{H_2}^2 &\leq \gamma^2 - c^2, \\
\|G - G_r\|_{H_\infty}^2 &\leq \gamma_\infty^2,
\end{aligned} \tag{39}$$

where,

$$c^2 = trace\left(B_\Delta'(\hat{Q} - Q)B_\Delta\right), \quad B_\Delta = \begin{pmatrix} B \\ B_r \end{pmatrix}. \tag{40}$$

110 *Salim Ibrir*

Proof. The proof is omitted for space limitation. □

The conditions of Theorem 5 are stated as linear matrix inequalities except the rank condition that is not numerically tractable. To make the conditions of Theorem 5 free from this rank condition, a predefined structure of the matrix Z could be set to enforce the fulfillment of the rank condition. Actually, there are many possible structures of the matrix Z that make the condition $\text{rank}(Z) \leq r$ and $B_r \neq 0$. Algorithm 1 gives one possible solution to fulfill all the conditions of Theorem 5 including the rank condition.

Algorithm 1 : Galerkin H_2/H_∞ MoR Algorithm

Require: Define the reduced-order r.

Step 1. Solve the following convex optimization problem with respect to $\gamma^2 > 0$, $\gamma_\infty^2 > 0$, $\hat{Q}_1 \in \mathbb{R}^{n \times n}$ and $Z_1 \in \mathbb{R}^{r \times r}$

$$\min_{\hat{Q}_1 > 0, Z \geq 0} \gamma^2 + \gamma_\infty^2$$

s.t.

$$Z = \begin{pmatrix} Z_1 & 0 \\ 0 & 0 \end{pmatrix} \geq 0, Z_1 > 0, \hat{Q}_1 > 0,$$

s.t.

$$\hat{Q}_1 - Z > 0,$$

$$\text{trace}\left(B'(\hat{Q}_1 - Z)B \right) \leq \gamma^2,$$

$$\begin{pmatrix} A'\hat{Q}_1 + \hat{Q}_1 A + C'C & A'\hat{Q}_1 + ZA + C'C & (\hat{Q}_1 - Z)B \\ \star & A'\hat{Q}_1 + \hat{Q}_1 A + C'C & 0 \\ \star & \star & -\gamma_\infty^2 I \end{pmatrix} < 0,$$

$$\begin{pmatrix} A'(\hat{Q}_1 - Z) + (\hat{Q}_1 - Z)A & (\hat{Q}_1 - Z)B \\ B'(\hat{Q}_1 - Z) & -\gamma_\infty^2 I \end{pmatrix} < 0.$$

Step 2. Obtain the Schur decomposition of the matrix Z_1, i.e., finding a quasi-triangular Schur matrix T and a unitary matrix U such that $Z_1 \leftarrow UTU'$.

Step 3. $\hat{Q}_2 \leftarrow \begin{pmatrix} U \\ 0_{n-r,r} \end{pmatrix}$ and $\hat{Q}_3 \leftarrow T^{-1}$. Verify: $Z \leftarrow \hat{Q}_2\hat{Q}_3^{-1}\hat{Q}_2'$.

Step 4. Set the state and the output matrices as
$A_r \leftarrow \hat{Q}_2'A\hat{Q}_1^{-1}\hat{Q}_2\hat{Q}_3^{-1}$;
$B_r \leftarrow -\hat{Q}_2'B$; % The condition $\hat{Q}_2'B \neq 0$ should be satisfied.
$C_r \leftarrow -C\hat{Q}_1^{-1}\hat{Q}_2\hat{Q}_3^{-1}$;
Step 5. Write the dynamics of the reduced-order model as in (4).
End.

---

4. Simulation Results

The proposed model-order reduction design is compared to the balanced truncation and the Hankel procedures by considering the stable linear system given by the state-space equations:

$$\dot{x} = \begin{pmatrix} 0 & 0 & 0 & -2 \\ 1 & 0 & 0 & -4 \\ 0 & 1 & -1 & -5 \\ 0 & 0 & 1 & -2 \end{pmatrix} x + \begin{pmatrix} 1 \\ 0 \\ 0 \\ 0 \end{pmatrix} u, \qquad (41)$$

$$y = \begin{pmatrix} 1 & 0 & 0 & 0 \end{pmatrix} x.$$

In Figures 1, 2, the output of the original system and the outputs of the reduced-order models are represented for $r = 3$ and $r = 2$, respectively. For this example, the methods perform pretty well and give comparable results. As a second assessment of the proposed MoR method, one dimensional continuous-time system is build to approximate the fourth-dimensional system having the following dynamics:

$$\dot{x} = \begin{pmatrix} 0 & 0 & 0 & -8 \\ 1 & -1 & 0 & -4 \\ 0 & 1 & -1 & -6 \\ 0 & 0 & 1 & -6 \end{pmatrix} x + \begin{pmatrix} 1 \\ 0 \\ 0 \\ 0 \end{pmatrix} u, \qquad (42)$$

$$y = \begin{pmatrix} 0 & 0 & 0 & 1 \end{pmatrix} x.$$

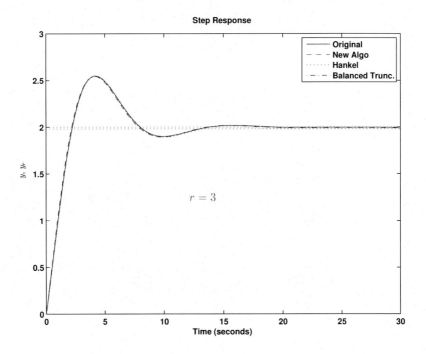

Figure 1. Comparison of different MoR methods for $r = 3$

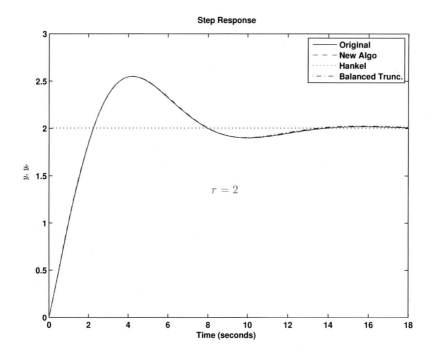

Figure 2. Comparison of different MoR methods for $r = 2$

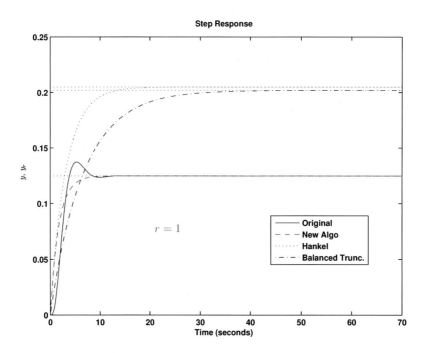

Figure 3. Comparison of different MoR methods for $r = 1$

As seen in Figure 3, the proposed algorithm ensures the convergence of the reduced-order model output to the true steady-state value. The balanced-truncation along with the Hankel MoR procedures exhibit some static errors. Extensive simulations showed that the proposed algorithm gives excellent results when the system is represented in some of the controllable/observable canonical forms. Moreover, it is noticed that the upper bound γ_∞ may not describe a tighter bound for the true norm $\|\tilde{G}\|_{H_\infty}$. However, the value of $\sqrt{\gamma^2 - c^2}$ does provide a good estimate of the true $\|\tilde{G}\|_{H_2}$.

Conclusion

A mixed H_2/H_∞ model-order reduction procedure is proposed for LTI continuous-time systems. The design is accomplished through the solution of a set of linear-matrix inequalities. The number of the optimization variables is reduced by setting a reduced-order model of pre-defined structure. The state-space matrices of the reduced-order system are explicitly given. Simulation results showed that the proposed algorithm provides better results than classical MoR methods like the Hankel and the balanced-truncation methods. Additionally, the H_2 and the H_∞ performances of the reduced-order system are evaluated.

Acknowledgments

The author gratefully acknowledge the support and the constant help of the Deanship of Scientific Research at King Fahd University of Petroleum and Minerals. This work is under the KFUPM DSR grant referenced: IN131043.

References

Al-Saggaf, U. M., & Franklin, G. F. (1987). An error bound for a discrete reduced order model of a linear multivariable system. *IEEE Transactions on Automatic Control*, **32**(9), 815-819.

Antoulas, A. C. (2005). *Advances in design and control: Approximation of large scale dynamical systems*. Society for Industrial and Applied Mathematics (SIAM).

Antoulas, A. C., Sorensen, D. C., & Gugercin, S. (2001). A survey of model reduction methods for large-scale systems. *Contemporary Mathematics*, **280**, 193-219.

Benner, P., Hinze, M., & Maten, E. J. W. ter (Eds.). (2011). *Model reduction for circuit simulation*. Springer.

Boyd, S., Ghaoui, L. E., Feron, E., & Balakrishnan, V. (1994). *Linear matrix inequality in systems and control theory*. SIAM, Philadelphia.

Desrochers, A. A. (1981). On an improved model reduction technique for nonlinear systems. *Automatica*, **17**(2), 407-409.

Geromel, J. C., Kawaoka, F. R., & Egas, R. G. (2004). Model reduction of discrete time systems through linear matrix inequalities. *International Journal of Control*, **77**(10), 978-984.

Glover, K. (1984). All optimal Hankel-norm approximations of linear multivariable systems and their L^∞ error bounds. *International Journal of Control*, **39**(6), 1115-1193.

Grigoriadis, K. M. (1995). Optimal H_∞ model reduction via linear matrix inequalities: Continuous and discrete-time cases. *Systems and Control Letters*, **26**(5), 321-333.

Gugercin, S., Antoulas, A. C., & Beattie, C. A. (2008). H_2 model reduction for large-scale linear dynamical systems. *SIAM Journal on Matrix Analysis and Applications*, **30**(2), 609-638.

Heinkenschloss, M., Reis, T., & Antoulas, A. C. (2011). Balanced truncation model reduction for systems with inhomogeneous initial conditions. *Automatica*, **47**(3), 559-564.

Ibrir, S. (2017, December). $\mathcal{H}_2$-Galerkin projection method for model order reduction of linear and nonlinear systems. In *Proc. 56th IEEE Conference on Decision and Control*. Melbourne, Australia.

Ibrir, S. (2018, July). A projection-based algorithm for model-order reduction with H_2 performance: A convex-optimization setting. *Automatica*, **93**, 510-519.

Ibrir, S., & Bettayeb, M. (2014). Model reduction of a class of nonlinear systems: A convex-optimization approach. *IMA Journal of Mathematical Control and Information*, **31**(4), 519-531.

Ibrir, S., & Bettayeb, M. (2015). Model reduction of a class of discrete-time nonlinear systems. *Applied Mathematics and Computation*, **250**(1), 78-93.

Kavranoglu, D., & Bettayeb, M. (1993). Characterization of the solution to the optimal H_∞ model reduction problem. *Systems and Control Letters*, **20**(2), 99-107.

Luitel, B., & Venayagamoorthy, G. K. (2010). Particle swarm optimization with quantum infusion for system identification. *Engineering Applications of Artificial Intelligence*, **23**(5), 635-649.

Moore, B. C. (1981). Principal component analysis in linear systems: Controllability, observability and model reduction. *IEEE Transactions on Automatic Control*, **26**(1), 17-32.

Penzl, T. (2006). Algorithms for model reduction of large dynamical systems. *Linear Algebra and its Applications*, **415**(2-3), 322-343.

Safonov, M. G., Chiang, R. Y., & Limebeer, D. N. (1990). Optimal Hankel model reduction for nonminimal systems. *IEEE Transactions on Automatic Control*, **35**(4), 496-502.

Sou, K. C., & Rantzer, A. (2012). Controller reduction via minimum rank matrix approximation. *Automatica*, **48**(6), 1069-1076.

Tan, S. X.-D., & He, L. (2007). *Advanced model order reduction techniques in VLSI design*. Cambridge University Press.

Yan, W.-Y., & Lam, J. (1999). An approximate approach to H_2 optimal model reduction. *IEEE Transactions on Automatic Control*, **47**(7), 1341-1358.

Zhang, L., Huang, B., & Lam, J. (2003). H_∞ model reduction of markovian jump linear systems. *Systems and Control Letters*, **50**(2), 103-118.

In: Focus on Systems Theory Research
Editors: Manuel F. Casanova and Ioan Opris

ISBN: 978-1-53614-561-8
© 2019 Nova Science Publishers, Inc.

Chapter 5

SYSTEMS THINKING IN HEALTH CARE: FROM THEORY TO IMPLEMENTATION

Sheuwen Chuang, PhD[1], and Peter P. Howley, PhD[2]*
[1]Graduate Institute of Data Science, Taipei Medical University, Taiwan
[2]School of Mathematical and Physical Sciences/Statistics,
The University of Newcastle, Australia

ABSTRACT

The world's health care systems have experienced varying and ongoing endeavors over recent decades towards improving quality of care and patient outcomes. Fundamentally, the healthcare systems are becoming increasingly complex and dynamic and previous linear thinking needs to be supplanted by systems understanding.

This chapter introduces the reader to the concept of systems thinking, describing key theories underpinning its characteristics, and utilizes the authors' experiences and research to clarify the need for holistic systems thinking and integration. The chapter draws upon the authors' research and demonstrates the implementation of systems thinking in different contexts.

Keywords: systems thinking, holistic health care systems, accreditation and quality measurement systems, integrated systems

---

* Corresponding Author Email: sheuwen@tmu.edu.tw.

INTRODUCTION

Over recent decades, the world's health care systems have experienced varying efforts or approaches to improve their efficiency and effectiveness and ultimately outcomes for patients. The release of the Institute of Medicine's (IOM) landmark report, "To Err Is Human: Building a Safer Health System" in 2000 (IOM, 2000) pushed significant improvements in patient safety and quality worldwide. However, increases in the cost of health services, rapidly growing technology dependence, compliance with the international quality standards, and satisfying patients' needs have continually challenged health care organizations (Al-Shdaifat, 2015). Fifteen years after the IOM's report, the Health Foundation, UK and National Patient Safety Foundation (NPSF) advocated that despite some progress, much more needs to be done to improve health care to ensure it is as safe as it should be for all patients (Illingworth, 2015; NPSF, 2015).

The NPSF highlights a notable accomplishment of the progress in the past 15 years, namely, that much of the language relevant to patient safety and the concepts of the system approach now permeate health care. People are aware of human factors and team training and the need to use checklists, other aids, and technology (NPSF, 2015). However, research has revealed that successful application of quality improvement initiatives or methods is primarily the effect of context not the efficacy of the methods themselves (Kaplan et al., 2012). The context includes characteristics of the organizational setting, the environment, the individuals, and their roles in the everyday clinical work and the relationships among them (Fulop and Robert, 2015).

Further, research has shown that healthcare staff commonly understand that hospital acquired infections (HAIs), for example, are usually a consequence of delayed diagnosis of infected patients and a failure to coordinate notification, education, treatment, and disinfection (Wu et al., 2008; Wolf and Davidovici, 2010). Nevertheless, people within the healthcare system deal with each root cause contributing to a HAI in relative isolation, react to such outcomes rather than have an holistic and integrated plan to ensure their prevention (or proactively seek to ensure the desired outcome), and generally lack the understanding of, and ability to implement, systems thinking. This creates several limiting choices, with splintering, diluting, and confounding root causes analyses (Vincent, 2004; Chuang et al., 2015).

Health care systems are complex and dynamic in nature, with care provided by increasingly specialized individuals and organizations that employ specialized methods and technologies. In such systems, any single process within a system can be influenced by unseen agents or *variables* both internally and externally. The various dimensions of quality care are interconnected and thus interdependent; addressing one may impact another, perhaps positively or negatively, for example, the tradeoffs between faster, better and cheaper care (Cook and Rasmussen, 2005). This context raises the issues of providing a better care that is far more complex than initially understood. Moreover, IT and the internet of things (IoT) technologies create new contributing factors that are far less understood and controlled by healthcare staff and now need attention, such as the potential to introduce errors via electronic health records (IOM, 2012) and alarm fatigue from countless equipment signals (ECRI 2013, Joint Commission, 2013).

As health care is becoming more influenced by advancing technologies, and human-machine interactions are getting interlaced, a conventional linear thinking model is no longer adequate for describing and improving processes and outcomes. Systems thinking has been recognized as being imperative in understanding, studying, and managing complex healthcare systems (Trochim et al., 2006, WHO, 2009; Adam, 2014). A total system approach to deliver a better care was recommended by the NPSF as the future vital strategy (NPSF, 2015).

Despite the growing interest in topics such as systems thinking, complex adaptive systems, and systems science in the published health literature over the past 20 years, the implementation of effective systems approaches remains challenging (Adam, 2014; Trochim et al., 2006). Schyve (2007) believes that systems thinking does not come naturally, especially for health care professionals who have been educated and acculturated to recognize their personal responsibility to master the knowledge and skills. Most of them make decisions for improvement based on their own experiences: hindsight and outcome biases block their ability to see the deeper story of systematic factors that predictably shape human performance (Woods and Cook, 1999).

In order to build the fundamental knowledge and information for implementing systems thinking within people working in health care, the chapter begins by introducing and defining systems and systems thinking, and then provides an overview of general systems theory and complex-adaptive systems that describes healthcare behavior appropriately. The chapter uses examples drawn from current literature and the authors' own research to explain the feasibility of adopting and adapting system theories to implement effective systems thinking in the complex healthcare environment.

SYSTEMS AND SYSTEMS THINKING

Systems

Several definitions for systems exist. The chapter adopts Meadows' definition (2009). She defined a system as "A set of elements or parts that is coherently organized and interconnected in a pattern or structure that produces a characteristic set of behaviors, often classified as its function or purpose." The definition constructs four basic system's principles, namely:

3. a system is more than the sum of its parts;
4. many of the interconnections in systems operate through the flow of information;
5. the least obvious part of the system, its function or purpose, is often the most crucial determinant of the system's behavior;
6. system structure is the source of system behavior, and system behavior reveals itself as a series of events over time.

Based on this definition, to certify systemic fidelity of systems thinking, Arnold and Wade (2015) tested several definitions of systems thinking made by the leaders in system science, and proposed a systems thinking definition that is able to be clearly understood and used (see *Systems Thinking* section below).

Systems may be classified according to the following four categories: natural or human-made systems, physical or conceptual systems, static or dynamic systems, and closed or open systems (Blanchard and Fabrycky, 2006). Health care delivery is a human-made system in which human beings intervene through components or elements, i.e., medical equipment; computer information system; medication, attributes or patient *characteristics*; staff working experiences; space scale; or relationships among staff and machines. It is a dynamic system in which uncertainty, or variation, often occurs in inputs and the distribution of these inputs over time, and is an open system in which information, objects, and matter cross boundaries and interact. Health care systems, as complex systems, exhibit the characteristics of varied system classifications.

Systems Thinking

The term has been defined and redefined in many different ways. One of the more seminal definitions cited popularly has been one made by Senge (1990). "Systems thinking is, more than anything else, a mindset for understanding how things work. It is a perspective for going beyond events, to looking for patterns of behavior, to seeking underlying systemic interrelationships which are responsible for the patterns of behavior and the events." The systemic interrelationships between the elements of the system are the so called systemic structure or system hierarchy. Senge argues that contemporary society focuses predominantly on events, less on patterns of behavior, and very rarely on system structure. He emphasizes that organizations should focus their attention on system structure for learning while applying the problem-solving model. Only the system structure addresses the underlying causes of behavior at a level such that patterns of behavior can be changed.

Based on Meadows' definition of systems, Arnold and Wade (2015) address three things that should be considered in the definition of systems thinking, they are: elements, interconnections, and function or purpose. Senge's definition is interesting and does describe several highly critical elements of systems thinking, but it does not provide a purpose for systems thinking. Natural and designed physical systems that have clear boundary can be easily defined their function(s) or purpose(s). However, human and conceptual social systems do not have clear-cut and agreed upon aims or purposes, and even when agreed upon, these may change over time. Further, human activity systems being composed of individuals tend to have multiple and overlapping purposes. Thus, human-made systems at least can be distinguished as having three levels: the purpose of the system, the purpose of its parts, and the purpose of the system of which it is a part (Laszlo and Krippner, 1998). Whilst such aspects and goals are fundamental, systems thinking embeds these otherwise seldom-addressed parts of the system, and critically draws focus upon the system's functions or purposes collectively.

In summary, systems thinking is characterized by identifying the multiple system goals and elaborating upon both its elements and the interconnections between these elements. A consideration of all concepts of systems thinking defined by various system thinkers indicates that implementation of systems thinking encompasses: recognizing interconnections; identifying and understanding feedback; understanding system structure; differentiating types of stocks, flows, variables; identifying and understanding non-linear relationships; understanding dynamic behavior; reducing complexity by modeling systems conceptually; understanding systems at different scales (Arnold and Wade, 2015).

Systems Theory

Systems thinking is an approach or a methodology to address problems. It encompasses a body of theory, including, general systems theory; Chaos theory, and others, as well as comprising practical application. This body of theory explains the conceptual system models and exhibits the characteristics of varied system classifications, how systems work, and how a system itself to adapt to change, as well as how to model complex entities by abstracting from certain details of structure and component, and concentrating on the dynamics that define the characteristic functions, properties, and relationships internally or externally to the system (Laszlo and Krippner, 1998).

General Systems Theory (GST)

As a response to the fragmentation and duplication of scientific and technological research of systems in various sciences such as natural sciences and social sciences, in the first half of the 20th century, Ludwig von Bertalanffy advanced the general system theory (GST). The GST simply refers to "a general science of 'wholeness'" and Von Bertalanffy defined the aims of the theory as follows:

(1) There is a general tendency toward integration in the various sciences, natural and social.

(2) Such integration seems to be centered in a general theory of systems.

(3) Such theory may be an important means for aiming at exact theory in the nonphysical fields of science.

(4) Developing unifying principles running "vertically" through the universe of the individual sciences, this theory brings us nearer the goal of the unity of science.

(5) This can lead to a much-needed integration in scientific education (Von Bertalanffy, 1968, p. 38.).

The GST aims to integrate and address the metaphysical fields of science in order to identify universal principles applying to systems in general that can be applied to any system, regardless of the properties or elements of the system. There are two different types of systems classified by Bertalanffy: closed systems and open systems. Closed systems are those that are isolated from its environment, whilst open systems are those that interact with its environment. All organisms are generally considered an open system as there is import and export of material (Von Bertalanffy, 1968); a computer software program, such as Microsoft Word® can be an example of a closed system since entering text does not alter the program (Cordon, 2013).

Complex Adaptive Systems (CAS)

Complex adaptive systems are systems that have large numbers of components, often called agents, which interact and adapt or learn (Holland, 2006). Under a changing environment, some systems, for example immune systems, climate; cities; firms; markets; governments, societies, with various levels of hierarchies, networks, and layers of complexities, have the ability to learn and adapt to its changing components and environment (Cordon, 2013). These inhomogeneous, interacting adaptive agents construct emergent properties of a CAS. Each emergent property is a property of the system as a whole which does not exist at the individual element (agent) level. Therefore to understand a complex adaptive system one has to study the system as a whole and not simply decompose it into its constituents. This is analogous to the more well-known synergy concept, where the whole is greater than simply the sum of its parts.

The key characteristics of CAS are holism, indeterminism, dynamic changes, adaptation, relationships among entities, non-linear relationships (Laszlo and Krippner, 1998; McDaniel et al., 2013), and complex adaptive systems exhibit self-organizing behaviors that emerge from the bottom up, (McDaniel et al., 2009). These characteristic distinguish a CAS from complexity theory and a pure multi-agent system. Complex adaptive systems focus on top-level properties and features such as the capacity and ability of the system to change and adapt itself through self-organization, learning, and reasoning, as a response to variations in its conditions or environment over time.

A CAS is dynamically coping with accompanying surprises, challenges and responses both within the system and between the system and its environment. Feedback loops that move information between agents and between systems are the driving force for adaptive behavior over time. Each feedback loop becomes a focal point for observation, measurement, assessment and intervention.

IMPLEMENTATION OF SYSTEMS THINKING

IOM (2001) described the entire health care system as a complex adaptive system. They are made up agents including individuals such as clinicians, patients and administrators; small organizations such as internal medical practices; processes such as nursing and examination; functional units such as nursing, accounting and marketing; and large organizations such as hospitals, regulatory agencies and insurance companies. Their phenomena of interest often are dynamic and unfold in unpredictable ways, and unfolding events are often unique (McDaniel et al., 2009). Systems thinking is an approach or a methodology to address problems. Its implementation in health care may include the simple building of conceptual system models or the cognition and design of interconnections and system boundaries, how interconnections among major components operate in a certain system structure, through to concentrating in detail on the system dynamics that define the characteristic functions and variables, how feedback loops work, and optimizing relationships internally or externally to the system. The following cases introduce how to implement systems thinking in different system situations.

Continuous Quality Improvement through Accreditation and Quality Measurement/Reporting Systems

More recently, continuous Quality improvement efforts have seen the formation of accreditation systems. Besides, the associated, but often separately considered, quality management/reporting systems which collate data and information are often either not integrated with the other key systems or there is a lack of understanding of how best to utilize the data. Research has revealed a variety of findings about the association of the accreditation and measurement/reporting systems to quality in health care. Positive associations between accreditation and quality improvement (Devkaran1and O'Farrell, 2015; Greenfield and Braithwaite, 2008), as well as partial, inconsistent or conflicting results have been discovered (Merkow et al., 2014; VanSuch 2006; Miller 2005). Since the accreditation system and measurement/reporting system are believed to influence quality outcomes, considerable resources are expended by participating hospitals in support of such endeavors. The contributions of these two systems to effective continuous quality improvement, and how they may sustain quality care has often been questioned in health care.

The issue of how to best utilize these systems within healthcare delivery systems necessitates an embedding and integration of the two systems. This requires application of the two pairs of basic concepts of systems theory: emergence and hierarchy; control and communication (Leveson, 2004; Checkland, 1981). Combining the concept of healthcare systems hierarchy and an analysis of control and communication relationships, a basic holistic healthcare systems relationship model is designed as shown in Figure 2 of the paper identified by doi: 10.1186/1472-6963-9-195 (Chuang and Inder, 2009). As both the horizontal and vertical control/communication relationships are potentially relevant to maintaining an acceptable level of quality within the healthcare systems hierarchy, there are in principle four model relationships of direct interest. These are labeled P1 to P4 in that Figure.

The basic healthcare systems holistic relationship model establishes the inputs, processes and outputs for each of three pivotal systems; the accreditation system, the quality measurement and reporting system (QMS) and the healthcare organization (or hospital) level healthcare system. P1 relates to the control relationship between the accreditation and hospital-level health care system through the provision of standards; P2 the communication relationship reporting on the outputs of the QMS (clinical indicator reports) as part of the inputs to the hospital system; P3 the communication relationship providing associations between the accreditation system outcomes and QMS outcomes; and P4 the potential control relationship between the outcomes of the QMS and the inputs of the accreditation system.

The implementation of systems thinking to explore the issue provides an overall systemic picture of how systems work and influence quality care at the macro system level. Stakeholders, researchers and policy makers may then consider a desired direction of system improvement toward sustainable quality care by understanding the status of each relationship. For instance, the authors discovered the fourth implicit relationship (P4), a feedback between quality performance reporting components and choice of accreditation components that is likely to play an important role in health care outcomes. Two studies by the authors triggered by the model were designed to investigate this potential control relationship in two national healthcare system environments (Chuang and Howley, 2017; Chuang et al. 2013). Significantly, this relationship potential remains to be utilized and developed.

This exemplifies the need for considering and thinking holistically, in this case in the macro system level, see Figure 2 of that paper in https://www.ncbi.nlm.nih.gov/pmc/articles/PMC2773779/. Building a conceptual system model, understanding the interactions (relationships) between system components, and identifying the global effect on the end result based on the four relationships would be the first systems thinking practice. Further, an implementation typology of hospital accreditation systems was developed based on the holistic relationship model. This additional study was conducted through an international systems-theoretic comparison of hospital accreditation systems between five countries: United States of America, Canada, Australia, Taiwan and France. The implementation typology of hospital accreditation could serve as a roadmap for refining hospital accreditation systems toward an integrative approach for continuous quality improvement (Chuang et.al, 2018).

This level of implementing systems thinking does not require professional systems thinking skills or technologies, although such may be valuable in guiding; rather it requires broadening of people's mindset and changes of habits from linear to a non-linear way of thinking.

The Cessation of Repeated Scabies Outbreaks in a Respiratory Care Ward

Scabies outbreaks are common in long-term care facilities worldwide (Achtari et al., 2007; Vorou et al., 2007; Buehlmann et al. 2009). Scabies is a major safety concern for both health care providers and the residents in these settings and among elderly or immune compromised patients in hospitals, owing to its highly contagious nature. Considerable management-related and economic burdens, including prolonged hospitalizations, ward closures, a large number of frequent and intensive patient treatments, laundry and environmental disinfection procedures, and the need for extra staffing ensues from such outbreaks, draining resources. However, it is not a notifiable disease in most countries, and thus institutional scabies outbreaks in health care settings are underreported (Vorou et al., 2007; Buehlmann et al., 2009).

The following overview of a case illustrates the value from a practical implementation of systems thinking to ceases repeated scabies outbreaks over a 17-month period in a 60-bed respiratory care ward (RCW) of a Taiwan public hospital (Chuang et al., 2015). The RCW was a controlled area, open daily to patient visitors for limited hours. Patients who required prolonged mechanical ventilation were mostly unconscious and required assistance with bathing, positioning, and other nursing care. In the period of August 2007 and March 2009, the hospital experienced 3 scabies outbreaks, with increasing infection densities of 3.8%, 15.9%, and 20.7%. During the third outbreak, as for the first two outbreaks, a root cause analysis (RCA) was conducted. This time, however, the hospital was concerned with the 2 previous failures to provide sustained interventions to end the scabies outbreaks through traditional guidelines and RCA. The hospital also assessed the third outbreak using a newly developed systems-oriented event analysis (SOEA) method (Chuang and Howley, 2013).

This case demonstrates use of systems thinking to build a detailed system model corresponding to the outbreak based on the concepts of system functions or purposes, to identify the non-linear cause-and-effect relationships which led to the outbreak, to construct a prioritized system hierarchy to direct the resources allocation of relevant interventions, and to smooth and enhance documentation and communications between practitioners for building consensus and redesigned system model of infection prevention for the future. This was accomplished on the bases of the SOEA implementation procedure as shown in Figure 2 of that paper (Chuang and Howley, 2013); see https://onlinelibrary.wiley.com/doi/epdf/10.1002/sys.21246. The SOEA method was developed and designed based on systems theory and is a structured formulated method supporting the implementation of systems thinking. It provides three core functions: establishment of systems concept, hazard management, alignment of control activities across organizational levels, which are guided by a seven step implementation procedure starting from the micro system level, i.e., clinical units, and developing through to the macro system level, i.e., hospital level.

Implementation of systems thinking can simply start from changing individuals' thinking and mindsets, training people how to think and see both the trees and the forest. To foster such a situation, it is better to have a working environment that encourages all participants to contribute to and share responsibility of problem solving. Such was the process for the scabies outbreak case; improvement of infection prevention and control could not be achieved based on individuals' experiences. All stakeholders should not think of such a responsibility as an additional workload burden, but rather an integral aspect of patient safety and quality of care that will foster a more efficient and effective system, and ultimately a 'prevention is better than cure' mindset and situation. This highlights the importance of developing the required mental model for the implementation of systems thinking in organizations (Senge, 1990).

CONCLUSION

In the wake of globalization and the increasingly complex and dynamic world, the importance of systems thinking is increasing. Individuals, groups, organizations, and nations are expected to understand how to cope in the face of growing uncertainty. For successful implementation of systems thinking, eight challenges must be enacted: support dynamic and diverse network; inspire integrative learning; use system measures and models; foster systems planning and evaluation; expand cross-category funding; utilize system incentives; explore system paradigms perspective; show potential of systems approaches (Trochim et al., 2006). The above examples of explaining how to implement systems thinking should be considered as the basic practice in health care. More advanced use of systems thinking, for example system simulation, and the derivation of system strategies to leverage intervention power need to be learned by different disciplines in the increasing collaborative and integrated workforce. The learning of systems thinking itself as well as implementation of systems thinking is a team exercise. Building organizational support to strengthen these activities is an essential core for its success.

REFERENCES

Achtari JL., Erard P., Gueissaz F., Malinverni R. An outbreak of scabies: a forgotten parasitic disease still present in Switzerland. *Swiss Med Wkly* 2007;137:695-9.

Al-Shdaifat EA., Implementation of total quality management in hospitals, J*ournal of Taibah University Medical Sciences,* 2015;10: 461-466.

Arnold RD, Wade JP. A Definition of Systems Thinking: A Systems Approach. *Procedia Computer Science* 2015; 44 669 – 678.

Blanchard BS and Fabrycky WJ. *Systems engineering and analysis.* Fourth edition. Pearson Education Inc., New Jersey, 2006.

Buehlmann M, Beltraminelli H, Strub C, Bircher A, Jordan X, Battegay M, et al. Scabies outbreak in an intensive care unit with 1,659 exposed individuals: key factors for controlling the outbreak. *Infect Control Hosp Epidemiol.* 2009;30:354-60.

Checkland P. Systems Thinking, Systems Practice. New York: John Wiley & Sons; 1981.

Chuang S., Inder K. An effectiveness analysis of healthcare systems using a systems theoretic approach, *BMC Health Serv Res.* 2009; 9: 195.

Chuang S, Howley P. Strategies for integrating clinical indicator and accreditation systems to improve healthcare management, *International Journal of Healthcare Management,* 2017;15:265-274, DOI: 10.1080/20479700.2017.1300396.

Chuang S., Howley PP., Hancock S. Using clinical indicators to facilitate quality improvement via the accreditation process: the control relationship, *Int J Q HealthCare,* 2013,25: 277-283.

Chuang S., Howley PP., Lin SH. Implementing systems thinking for infection prevention: The cessation of repeated scabies outbreaks in a respiratory care ward. *Am J Infect Control.* 2015;43:499-505.

Chuang S., Howley PP. Beyond root cause analysis: an enriched system-oriented event analysis model for wide application. *Syst Engineer,* 2013;16:427-38.

Chuang S., Gonzales SS., Howley PP. An international systems-theoretic comparison of hospital accreditation – developing an implementation typology, *Int J Q HealthCare,* (accepted, July 9,2018)

Cook RI, Rasmussen J. "Going solid": a model of system dynamics and consequences for patient safety. *Qual Saf Health Care,* 2005;14:130-134.

Cordon CP. System Theories: An Overview of Various System Theories and Its Application in Healthcare. *American Journal of Systems Science* 2013, 2(1): 13-22.

Devkaran S., O'Farrell P. The impact of hospital accreditation on quality measures: an interrupted time series analysis. *BMC Health Services Research* 2015, 15:137.

ECRI. 2013. *Healthcare risk, quality, and safety guidance: clinical alarms.* https://www.ecri.org/components/HRC/Pages/CritCare5.aspx . Accessed Nov 12, 2017.

Fulop N., Robert G. *Context for successful quality improvement, The Health Foundation,* London, 2015. Available at https://www.health.org.uk/sites/health/files/ContextForSuccessfulQualityImprovement.pdf. Accessed May 4, 2018.

Glouberman S., Zimmerman B. *Complicated and Complex Systems: What Would Successful Reform of Medicare Look Like?* Toronto, Ontario, Canada: Commission on the Future of Health Care in Canada; 2002.

Goldberger AL. Non-linear dynamics for clinicians: chaos theory, fractals, and complexity at the bedside. *Lancet.* 1996;347:1312–1314.

Greenfield D., Braithwaite J. Health sector accreditation research: a systematic review. *Int J Qual Health Care* 2008, 20:172-183.

Holland JH. Studying Complex Adaptive Systems. *J SYST SCI COMPLEX*2006;19: 1–8.

Illingworth J. *Continuous improvement of patient safety,* the Health Foundation, London, 2015.

Institute of Medicine (IOM). *Crossing the Quality Chasm: A New Health System for the 21st Century.* Washington, DC: National Academies Press; 2001.

Institute of Medicine (IOM). Health IT and Patient Safety: Building Safer Systems for Better Care. Washington, DC: National Academies Press. 2012.

Kaplan HC., Provost LP., Froehle CM., Margolis PA. The Model for Understanding Success in Quality (MUSIQ): building a theory of context in healthcare quality improvement. *BMJ Qual Saf.* 2012; 21:13-20.

Kohn LT., Corrigan JM., Donaldson MS. T*o Err is Human: Building a Safer Health System.* Institute of Medicine Committee on Quality of Health Care in America; Washington: National Academies Press; 2000.

Laszlo A., Krippner S. Systems Theories: Their Origins, Foundations, and Development. In J.S. Jordan (Ed.), *Systems Theories and A Priori Aspects of Perception.* Amsterdam: Elsevier Science, 1998. Ch. 3, pp. 47-74.

Leveson A. NG: Systems-Theoretic Approach to Safety in Software-Intensive Systems, IEEE Trans. *Dependable Secure Comput.* 2004, 1:66-86.

McDaniel RR Jr, Driebe DJ, Lanham HJ. Health care organizations as complex systems: new perspectives on design and management, *Adv Health Care Manag.* 2013;15:3-26.

McDaniel RR, Lanham HJ, Anderson RA. Implications of complex adaptive systems theory for the design of research on health care organizations, *Health Care Manage Rev.,* 2009;34:191-199.

McDaniel R., Driebe D. Complexity Science and Health Care Management. In: J Blair, M Fottler, and G Savage (Eds), *Advances in Health Care Management.* Stamford, Conneticut: JAI Press 2001; 2:11-36.

Meadows DH. *Thinking in systems. A primer.* London, UK: Earthscan, 2009.

Merkow RP, Chung JW, Paruch JL, Bentrem DJ, Bilimoria KY, Relationship between cancer center accreditation and performance on publicly reported quality measures. *Ann Surg.* 2014;259:1091-7. doi: 10.1097/SLA.0000000000000542.

Miller MR, Pronovost P, Donithan M, Zeger S, Zhan C, Morlock L, Meyer GS. Relationship Between Performance Measurement and Accreditation: Implications for Quality of Care and Patient Safety. *Am J Med Qual* 2005, 20:239-252.

Norberg, J and Cumming, G. *Complexity theory for a sustainable future.* New York, NY: Columbia University Press. 2008.

Plsek PE, Greenhalgh T. The challenge of complexity in health care. *BMJ.* 2001;323:625–628.

Schyve PM. System thinking and patient safety. *Advances in Patient Safety: From Research to Implementation.* Volume 2. Agency for Healthcare Research and Quality. http://www.ahrq.gov/downloads/pub/advances/vol2/ Schyve.pdf, 2007.

Senge P. T*he fifth discipline.* New York, NY: Doubleday, 1990.

Senge, P. *The fifth discipline: The art & practice of the learning organization.* (2nd ed.) New York, NY: Double Day, 2006.

The Joint Commission. 2013. Medical device alarm safety in hospitals. *Sentinel Event Alert* 50:1–3. http://www.jointcommission.org/assets/1/18/SEA_50_alarms_4_5_13_FINAL1.PDF. Accessed Nov 20, 2017.

Trochim WM, Cabrera DA, Milstein B, Gallagher RS, Leischow SJ. Practical Challenges of Systems Thinking and Modeling in Public Health. *Am J Public Health.* 2006; 96:538-46.

Vincent CA. Analysis of clinical incidents: a window on the system, not a search for root causes. *Qual Saf Health Care* 2004;13:242-3.

Wolf R, Davidovici B. Treatment of scabies and pediculosis: facts and controversies. *Clin Dermatol* 2010; 28:511-8.

World Health Organization (WHO), Systems Thinking for Health Systems Strengthening, Adam: Advancing the application of systems thinking in health. *Health Research Policy and Systems* 2014 12:50.

Woods DD and Cook R. Perspectives on human error: Hindsight biases and local rationality. In Durso, Nickerson, et al., eds., *Handbook of Applied Cognition.* New York: Willy, 1999, pp.141-171.

Wu AW, Lipshutz AK, Pronovost PJ. Effectiveness and efficiency of root cause analysis in medicine. *J Am Med Assoc* 2008; 299:685-7.

VanSuch M, Naessens JM, Stroebel RJ, Huddleston JM, Williams AR. Effect of discharge instructions on readmission of hospitalised patients with heart failure: Do all of the Joint Commission on Accreditation of healthcare organizations heart failure core measures reflect better care? *Qual Saf Health Care* 2006, 15: 414-417.

von Bertalanffy L. *General system theory: Essays on its foundation and development,* rev. ed. New York: George Braziller, 1968.

von Bertalanffy L. *General system theory.* New York, NY: George Braziller, 1968.

Vorou R, Remoudaki HD, Maltezou HC. Nosocomial scabies. *J Hosp Infect* 2007; 65:9-14.

ABOUT THE AUTHORS

Dr. Sheuwen Chuang
Associate Professor
Graduate Institute of Data Science,
Taipei Medical University,
Taiwan

Dr. Chuang is currently an Associate Professor in the Graduate Institute of Data Science, Taipei Medical University, Taiwan. Her research and specialist skills include system integration and design, risk management, quality and patient safety, resilience engineering in health care. Dr. Chuang's academic background includes a PhD in systems engineering, and Master's degree in computer and information science. She also has more than 20 years industry experience working in electronics, aerospace, and software development companies, and health care across Asia, Oceania and the United States of America. These experiences enable her to bring authentic learning practices her classroom teaching, and support practical research of risk management and resilience engineering on the basis of systems thinking and systems theory.

She has developed several system models and computer systems for risk management, incident analysis and control in health care. She is known for inspiring people to think differently in a system approach to improve safety and risk. Currently, her studies focus on mass casualty incidents' analysis and innovation of emergency medical service system to enhance resilience in disaster risk reduction.

Dr. Peter Howley
Associate Professor
PhD (Statistics), BMath(Hons), A.Stat.
School of Mathematical and Physical Sciences/Statistics
The University of Newcastle, Australia
www.newcastle.edu.au/profile/peter-howley

Peter Howley is nationally and internationally recognized as a leader and award winning academic and practitioner in statistics. Peter is the National Chair of Statistical Education, Statistical Society of Australia (SSA), an invited member on National and International Advisory Boards for Science and Data Science, International Editorial Board member and Executive Board member of Hunter Innovation and Science Hub, Australia. He is an elected member of the International Statistical Institute.

Peter leads and engages in practical and cross-disciplinary research. His publications, grants and consulting surround process and systems improvement across the fields of health care, education, business, management and industry. He has worked collaboratively with the Australian Council on Health Care Standards, Health Services Research Group, Hunter Medical Research Institute, AMPControl, Taipei Medical University, Taiwan Health and other universities.

In: Focus on Systems Theory Research
Editors: Manuel F. Casanova and Ioan Opris

ISBN: 978-1-53614-561-8
© 2019 Nova Science Publishers, Inc.

Chapter 6

APPLICATIONS OF GENOME-SCALE METABOLIC MODELS AND DATA INTEGRATION IN SYSTEMS MEDICINE

Ali Salehzadeh-Yazdi[1,], Markus Wolfien[1] and Olaf Wolkenhauer[1,2]*

[1]Department of Systems Biology and Bioinformatics,
University of Rostock, Rostock, Germany
[2]Stellenbosch University, Stellenbosch Institute for Advanced Study (STIAS),
Wallenberg Research Centre, Stellenbosch, South Africa

ABSTRACT

The ultimate goal of systems medicine is to understand the underlying mechanism of disease development, diagnostic biomarkers, potential drug targets, and prognosis biomarkers. Generating the context-based/tissue-specific genome-scale metabolic models fosters these goals. In the present chapter, we aim to describe the foundational concepts about metabolic modeling with focus on genome-scale metabolic reconstruction, gene expression integration into metabolic models, constraint-based modeling, model formulation, and applications of metabolic modeling in systems medicine.

Keywords: genome-scale metabolic model, systems medicine, data integration, objective function, context-specific model

---

[*] Corresponding Author Email: ali.salehzadeh-yazdi@uni-rostock.de.

INTRODUCTION

The metabolism is a complex network of dynamical biochemical reactions empowering organisms to grow, reproduce, maintain integrity, defend against harmful environments, and facilitate communication among different living organisms. It is tightly linked to particular diseases and syndromes, such as cancer, obesity, and diabetes. The ability of mathematical modeling methods in description, exploration, and prediction of metabolic phenotypes has been studied thoroughly in recent years [1]. These computational models can illustrate the genotype-phenotype relationship of metabolism and provide answers related to metabolic engineering, drug development, and personalized medicine. However, the representation and modeling of metabolic phenotypes have different levels of abstraction, predictive power, advantages, and limitations that are categorized into three main levels: topological [2], constraint-based [3], and kinetic modeling [4].

Topological analysis is a graph-based approach that has been introduced as an emergent method for simplification, reconstruction, and comprehension of the complex behavior in biological systems. Broadly speaking, topological approaches can be used to explore: 1. Collective behaviors (e.g., diameter, small-world and scale-free properties of a network), 2. Subnetwork behaviors (e.g., functional motif discovery), and, 3. Individual behaviors (e.g., prioritization of important nodes by centrality indices) of network components [5].

A constraint-based modeling approach calculates the flow of metabolites through a given metabolic reaction. This method allows the prediction of a production/consumption rate for a metabolite or growth rate of an organism. Based on environmental, physicochemical, regulatory, enzyme capacity, and thermodynamics principles, different constraints can be applied to the reconstructed metabolic network, because it shrinksthe solution space [3].

Table 1. Summary of the main three methods for analyzing metabolic networks

Method	Input	Analysis	Output	Advantages	Disadvantages	Ref
Topological analysis	SBML	Graph analysis	Centrality indices Motifs Clusters	Handling very large networks	Could not consider dynamics	[2]
Constraint-based analysis	SBML	Flux balance analysis	Essential genes Robustes analysis	Finding the flux distribution of GEM	Steady-state approximation	[3]
Kinetic modeling	SBML	deterministic or stochastic approaches	Concentrations versus time	Considering dynamics of a system	Small number of reactions	[4]

Applications of Genome-Scale Metabolic Models and Data Integration ... 133

Kinetic modeling is an ordinary differential equation-based approach, which analyses the behavior of a biochemical reaction over time. This approach usually applies for a single pathway or only a few reactions [4]. The data used for the method comparison is listed in Table 1.

In the light of the holistic properties of metabolic disorders, genome-scale metabolic models (GEMs) have been developed to demonstrate whole cell functions based on the comprehensive reactions of biochemical networks [6]. GEMs integrate biochemical and physiological data and allow studying the relationships between functions, diseases, and patients at a systems level. GEMs are mathematical representations of the cell metabolism with well-established predictive and functional capabilities. Successful applications of GEMs include industrial biotechnology (e.g., metabolic engineering, antibiotic design, and organismal/enzyme evolution [7]), and systems medicine (e.g., finding potential biomarkers, and identifying new drug targets [8]). Systems medicine has the potential to elucidate the clinical complexity by applying systems biology approaches in medical concepts for individualized high-precision disease diagnostics, onset and progression, treatment and remission, treatment responses as well as adverse events [9].

This book chapter will describe the basic concepts of the GEM reconstruction and constraint-based modeling. In addition, we elucidate general principles of the GEM as a main scaffold for metabolic system analyses and data integration. Finally, we provide an overview of their applications in systems medicine.

BASIC CONCEPTS

Metabolic Model Reconstruction Approaches

GEMs are formal and mathematical representations of the metabolism of a given organism depicted as a genome-scale network. The reconstruction procedure usually starts with the functional annotation of known genes and the specification of the stoichiometry for each metabolic reaction. Thus, the model uses gene-protein-reaction connectivity to link the genotype to the metabolic capability. The GEM reconstruction process is a labor-intensive method, which needs a standardized protocol and structured developmental steps that have been already described by Thiele and Palsson [10]. These steps are categorized in five parts (Figure 1):

1. Creation of a GEM draft according to genome annotation databases of the particular organism and biochemical databases (e.g., MetaCyc [11])
2. The draft should be reassessed and refined. Missing data should be circumvented with phylogenetically closed organisms. Heteromeric enzymes, multifunctional enzymes, and isozymes must be determined for verification and refinement.

3. Incorporating the mathematical representation of the given metabolic reconstructing network.
4. Performing network verification, evaluation, and validation.
5. After obtaining the desired capability of the model, it should be used for the simulation of different conditions. Qualitative or quantitative results will be obtained for further interpretation.

To facilitate the process of the GEM reconstruction, several automatic and semi-automatic approaches were developed (e.g., SEED [12], RAVEN toolbox [13], and merlin [14]). Although these methods have accelerated the reconstruction procedure, manual curation is still needed [15]. On the other hand, there are algorithms devised to generate specific subnetworks that reduce GEMs into core models or generate biosynthetic subnetworks, such as redGEM [16] and LumpGEM [17].

Recently, studies have tried to reframe GEMs towards enhancing phenotype prediction and facilitating genetic design in addition to the integration with expression data. In 2015, Zhang et al. presented an algorithm that is able to simplify the gene-reaction associations and allows the integration with other developed methods by introducing intermediate pseudo reactions [18]. An updated version of this algorithm, which introduced fewer pseudo reactions, was released in 2016 [19].

In 2017, Sánchez et al. developed GECKO, which adds enzymes as part of reactions and thereby ensuring that each metabolic flux does not exceed its maximum capacity [20].

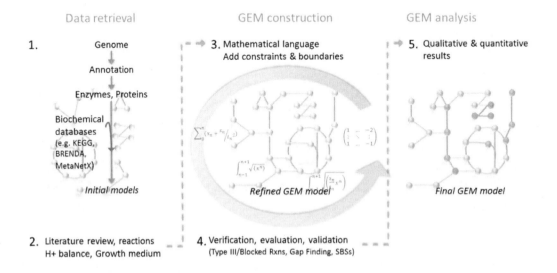

Figure 1. Summary of a GEM reconstruction process.

The History of Publically Available Generic Human Genome-Scale Models

The first high-quality generic human GEMs were released in 2007. Edinburgh Human Metabolic Network (EHMN) [21] and Recon1 [22] were manually reconstructed through assembling biological data from literature, databases, and genome annotation information. The EHMN was updated in 2010 [23] by accumulating the subcellular information for biochemical reactions, transport reactions, and the protein-reaction relationships. In 2012, Agren et al. integrated biological information at the genome, transcriptome, proteome and metabolome level to create iHuman1512 GEM [24]. Recon2 was generated in 2013 by the extension of metabolic information, transport and exchange reactions of Recon1 [25]. In 2016, Recon2.2 improved Recon2 by manual curation and automated error checking [26]. Currently, the latest and most comprehensive human GEM is Recon3D, which was developed by combining large-scale phenotypic data with structural information about proteins and metabolites [27]. The number of reactions, metabolites, and genes of each human GEM is listed in Table 2.

Table 2. Summary statistics for high-quality generic human GEMs

GEM	Number of reactions	Number of metabolites	Number of genes
EHMN (2007)	2823	2671	2322
Recon 1	3843	2712	1496
EHMN (2010)	6216	2634	2699
iHuman1512	5535	4137	1512
Recon 2	7440	5063	2191
Recon2.2	7785	5324	1675
Recon3D	13543	4140	3288

Constraints-Based Modeling Approach

Flux Balance Analysis (FBA) [3] is the most extensively used constraint-based method that was developed about 30 years ago [28]. The main underlying principle of FBA is that under any given environmental condition, the organism will reach a steady-state that satisfies all the physiochemical constraints of the cell, such as the stoichiometric balance of mass and energy [29]. The constraint-based modeling approach exploits biological and chemical constraints to restrict the solution space of a GEM model and finds an optimal solution for a specific condition. In this method, a metabolic network is represented as a stoichiometric set of equations based on an initial matrix. Subsequently, FBA solves underdetermined systems using linear or nonlinear programming and minimizes/maximizes an objective function as follows [30]:

Min/Max: $\sum c_i \cdot |v_i|$

Subject to: $S.v = 0$ $a_i < v_i < b_i$

where S is the stoichiometric matrix, v is the flux matrix, c is the stoichiometric coefficient of metabolite i in a reaction v, and a and b are lower and upper bounds of the given reaction, respectively. Without any constraint, the metabolic flux solutions are underdetermined. Applying constraints, however, would shrink the solution space. Thus, a set of flux vectors corresponding to the metabolic reactions could be calculated based on optimization of a specified objective function [31]. One of the most important steps of the FBA is the definition of a well-chosen objective function. This function could be chosen according to the study perspective or domain expertise. Commonly used objective functions are: the maximal biomass production rate (growth rate), minimum ATP consumption, maximum glucose uptake, minimum oxygen consumption, and maximum production of a given macromolecule [32]. The FBA could be applied to study the metabolic flux distribution and predict metabolic and cellular phenotypes through diverse perturbations in a system [33]. It also explores gene-knockout effects, potential enzyme targets, the robustness of a model, and flux variability analysis [34].

Available Human Objective Function

The computational prediction of human metabolic pathways (HumanCyc), being the first step towards the quantitative modeling of the human metabolism [35], considered no objective function. This also applied to the the EHMN [23] and Reactome, which contains less pathways than former models [36]. For functionality testing of the aforementioned models, the modelers have only examined the synthesis and degradation of different metabolites, such as amino acids, ribonucleotides, deoxyribonucleotides, fatty acids, sterols, glycans, prostaglandins, and heme. When Recon1 was built in 2007, a mouse objective function was used to test its functionality [22]. In 2010, a comprehensive metabolic model for the analysis of the liver physiology called HepatoNet1 was introduced [37]. For validating the models metabolic objectives of human hepatocytes ranging from gluconeogenesis to the degradation of endocytosed plasma, proteins were tested without providing a specific objective reaction. In 2011, the first objective function for a human GEM has been provided by two different groups through analyzing cancer metabolic networks. Folger et al. [38] provided a supplementary file including the biomass composition. Shlomi et al. [39] elaborated more details regarding the biomass reaction. They used the steady-state concentrations of 30 biomass compounds including amino acids (0.78 g/gDW), nucleotides (0.06 g/gDW), lipids (0.16 g/gDW) as well as the growth-associated energy requirement (24 mmol/gDW of ATP). The biomass composition with its corresponding reaction is available in the supplementary file of their manuscript. The first complete description of a human biomass objective function has been presented by Bordbar's et al. study in 2011 [40]. In the supplementary file, they provide details of different compositions based on experimental studies. For hepatocyte cells, free amino acids, lipid, fatty acids, and nucleotides were provided regarding the composition of rat liver cells. For myocyte cells, free amino acids, lipids, phospholipids, fatty acids, and nucleotides were mentioned according to the composition of a human muscle. For adipocyte cells, free amino acids, lipids, phospholipids, and fatty acids were calculated considering the composition of an adipose tissue. In 2012, two research groups (Agren et al. and Wang et al.) generated tissue-specific human metabolic models based on their constructed algorithms called INIT [24] and mCADRE [41], respectively. There is no objective function available in models produced by the INIT algorithm. Agren et al. have mentioned that there is no human biomass equation available in the literature up to the date of their publication. They have thus generated networks allowing for the secretion of all metabolites. In contrast, Wang et al. used a biomass reaction for the validation of one of their models (liver cell). They used a biomass objective function that is very similar to the one used by the Folger group. Finally, in 2013, a new version of the human metabolic model was introduced: Recon2. In its supplementary file, a biomass objective function is provided considering the macromolecular synthesis requirement for proteins (70.6%), DNA (1.4%), RNA (5.8%), lipids (9.7%), carbohydrates (main carbohydrate was assumed to be glucose-6-phosphate) (7.1%), and others (including vitamins, small molecules, ions, cofactors, etc) (5.4%). The cellular weight was estimated as 500×10^{-12} g per cell. The fractional contribution of the different metabolites to the macromolecules was estimated using the nucleotide and amino acid sequence of the ~20,000 annotated ORFs. The energy requirements for translational processes were assumed four ATP per peptidyl bond and an average protein length of 333 amino acids [42, 43].

USING GEMs AS SCAFFOLDS FOR MULTI OMICS DATA INTEGRATION

The availability of high-throughput data, (e.g., genomics, transcriptomics, proteomics, metabolomics, and fluxomics) has allowed a more in-depth study of the metabolism. In particular, integrative data approaches lead to a deeper understanding of the occurrence of certain changes in different conditions and create context-based and tissue-specific models. Following the introduction of a GEM, the integration of gene expression data into the GEM is the subsequent challenge for a better prediction of the metabolic cell fate [44].

The ultimate goal of systems medicine is to understand the underlying mechanism of the disease development, diagnostic biomarkers, potential drug targets, and prognosis biomarkers. The generation of the context-based/tissue-specific GEMs is supporting to achieve these goals. The generic GEM is one of the most prevalent networks that can generate the context-based/tissue-specific GEM by integrating transcriptomics, metabolomics, proteomics, and lipidomics data. These models facilitate the unveiling of the genotype-phenotype relationship and give rise to the extraction of physiologically relevant information from high-quality data [45]. On the other hand, the combination of GEMs with other biological networks (e.g., regulatory [46], signaling, and protein–protein interaction networks [47]) have the potential for further integration of biological knowledge into such mathematical models [48]. There are various studies on the use of GEMs as scaffolds in which high-throughput data can be advantageously combined with. Transcriptome data, however, is the most commonly used omics data for integration into GEMs due to the ease of producing and the fact that they are genome-wide [49]. In the following section, we will focus on the gene expression integration methods into GEMs and their application in systems medicine.

STRATIFICATION OF METHODS TO INTEGRATE TRANSCRIPTOMIC DATA INTO GEMS

From 2002 until now, more than fifty methods have been developed to investigate how gene expression integration into GEMs could affect the model content and predictive accuracy. These methods differ in assumptions and mathematical formulations, using different gene expression datasets (in form of microarray or RNA-sequencing data) and various GEMs of organisms from bacteria to human. These heterogeneous datasets and diverse algorithms are difficult to compare and benchmark. The first study addressing this issue, was published in 2002 by Covert and Palsson [50]. In 2004, Akesson et al. used gene expression data as an additional constraint on the metabolic fluxes in yeast [51]. Afterwards, different algorithms were devised for tackling this challenge: GIMME [52], E-Flux [53], MBA [54], Moxley [55], MADE [56], RELATCH [57], INIT [24], mCADRE [41], tINIT [58], CORDA [59], E-Flux2, SPOT [60], and FASTCORE [61].

These algorithms can be classified in many different ways on the basis of the underlying methodology.

In 2014, Machado and Herrgård classified methods by three main criteria: 1. Regarding their application to the gene expression levels (discrete *vs* continuous, absolute *vs* relative), 2. Their intended functionality regarding flux prediction, or 3. Model building [62].

Kim and Lun (2014) considered four grouping criteria, regarding gene expression and model functionality: 1. Algorithms that require multiple gene expression datasets as input, 2. Requirement for a gene expression threshold to define a gene's high and low expression, 3. Requirement of an appropriate objective function for a given GEM, and 4. Validation of directly predicted fluxes against measured intracellular fluxes [63].

In 2015, Estévez and Nikoloski [64] stratified the methods in three distinct groups: 1. GIMME- and GIM^{3}E-like methods. This group refers to the two-steps approaches with a metabolic functionality (objective function) being optimized through FBA in a first step. Then, the obtained optimal value is employed to minimize the discrepancies between fluxes and data, 2. iMAT-and INIT-like methods. This group of algorithms determines the binary reaction status (i.e., active or inactive), which are in good agreement with the associated data state, 3. MBA-, mCADRE, and fastCORE-like methods. This group defines a core set of active reactions and then finds the minimum essential set of reactions to satisfy the model consistency condition.

Recently, advantages and disadvantages of different approaches of integration of expression data into constraint-based modeling have been systematically evaluated in two comprehensive studies. In the first study, published in 2014, Machado and Herrgård concluded that no method published so far systematically outperforms the others [62]. In the next study, the authors reported that model parameter selection (e.g., gene expression thresholds, metabolic constraints) had the largest impact on the model accuracy [65].

APPLICATION OF GEMs IN SYSTEMS MEDICINE

The human metabolism is altered in many diseases. Therefore, the therapeutic goal is essentially related to the knowledge of the underlying mechanism, diagnostic biomarkers, and drug targets to retrieve the healthy state. GEMs have received considerable attention and many studies have been published about their applications in different aspects of systems medicine.

Inspired by the findings that cancer cells employ aerobic glycolysis, known as the Warburg effect and that such a metabolic modification may lead to cancer, different groups have tailored computational analyses to explore the classical hallmark of cancer metabolism. Despite the fact that the Warburg effect discovery goes back to 1924, its causes still remain poorly understood.

In 2011, Shlomi et al. investigated the metabolic reprogramming of 60 cell lines by employing stoichiometric and enzyme solvent capacity constraints using Recon1 and the gene expression of metabolic genes. Their model successfully predicted a three phase metabolic behavior as well as a glutamine uptake level of cancer cells. They showed that the Warburg effect is a direct consequence of the metabolic adaptation to maximize the growth rate of cancer cells [39].

Folger et al. in 2011 combined microarray data from 59 cancer cell lines with the Recon1 to generate a generic metabolic model of human cancer cells. In addition, the use of integrative approaches demonstrated an improved performance over the independent use of the transcriptomic data or the Recon1 model alone [38].

Wang et al. reconstructed GEMs for 26 human cancer and counterpart normal tissues in 2012. Pathway-level analyses of GEMs revealed the eicosanoid metabolic pathway as a potential selective drug target [41].

Jerby et al. developed a method to interpret metabolic phenotypes of breast cancer patients by integration of transcriptomics and proteomics data into the GEMs [66]. Likewise to an augmented need for ROS detoxification, they discovered a tradeoff linking reduction in the breast cancer tumor cell proliferation rate to evolved metastatic ability.

In 2014, Yizhak et al. explored the role of the Warburg effect in supporting tumor migration by GEMs. Besides the fact that the results were already known and used clinically, they also found metabolic targets inhibiting the cancer migration [67].

Nam et al. (2014) deployed genetic mutation information and transcriptomic data of nine cancer types as well as Recon2 to reconstruct cancer-specific GEMs to predict oncometabolites, which have the potential to dysregulate epigenetic control mechanisms [68].

In 2015, Asgari et al. constructed 13 cancer-specific metabolic models and their corresponding normal models by gene expression integration to Recon1 using the E-Flux method [69]. They compared the flux distribution of normal and cancer reactions in various metabolic subsystems. Their results support the hypothesis that the Warburg effect is a consequence of the metabolic adaptation and is independent of the differential expression of specific metabolic genes.

There are comprehensive reviews covering this topic. For example, the evolution of GEMs of cancer metabolism was published in 2013 [70], in addition a review on the human cell- or tissue-specific GEMs that have been applied in biomedical studies, was published in 2017 [71] and in the same year, Robinson and Nielsen published an anticancer drug discovery study through GEMs [72].

Furthermore, the construction of disease-specific GEMs was used for the identification of biomarkers and drug targets in metabolism-related disorders, including: Type 2 Diabetes (T2D), obesity, Non-Alcoholic Fatty Liver Disease (NAFLD), aging, and Alzheimer Disease (AD).

- T2D is a complex metabolic disease, which is typically accompanied by genome-wide changes in gene expression where dysregulated expression of metabolic genes has a key role. Zelezniak et al. (2010) constructed T2D models according to generic Recon1 and EHMN (2007) and provided a holistic picture of driver metabolic and regulatory nodes that are potentially involved in the pathogenesis of T2D [73].

Väremo et al. (2015) generated a manually curated myocyte-specific GEM by the integration of proteome and transcriptome of six different studies of T2D into the Human Metabolic Reaction database (HMR2) using the tINIT method to identify signatures of a diabetic muscle. They suggested a gene signature, which successfully classified the disease progression of individual samples [74].

- White adipose tissue malfunctions or overload of its lipid storage capacity lead to a range of metabolic diseases such as obesity and its adverse outcomes. In 2011, Bordbar et al. used Recon1 as a starting point to construct adipocytes-, hepatocytes-, and myocytes-specific GEMs. Then, gene expression data from adipose, liver, and skeletal muscle tissue of healthy obese and T2D obese subjects was integrated into this multi-tissue GEM by GIMME. Using this approach, the authors found cysteine dioxygenase, which was reported to be inactive in the adipose of diabetic subjects, as a potential reason for elevated levels of cytotoxic cysteine [40].

  Mardinoglu et al. (2013) reconstructed an adipocyte-specific GEM by integrating proteome, transcriptome, and fluxome from clinical data [75]. iAdipocytes1809 was employed to identify reporter metabolites for the patient stratification and new candidates for potential therapeutic targets of obesity. They showed that the metabolic activity of androsterone and ganglioside GM2 increased in obese subjects and their mitochondrial metabolic activities decreased compared to lean subjects.

- NAFLD is one of the liver disorders resulting from perturbations in the hepatocytic metabolism. In 2013, Mardinoglu et al. identified chondroitin and heparan sulphates as suitable biomarker for the staging of NAFLD by analyzing the reconstructed iHepatocytes2322 [76].

  Hyötyläinen et al. charted liver metabolic activity in NAFLD by integrating the liver gene expression profile (human liver biopsies from subjects with NAFLD and controls) and the metabolic flux data into Recon1 by iMAT. The GEM analysis provided liver functionality scores, reaction activity and pathway enrichment in the context of NAFLD [77].

- New gene expression related research on aging indicated that multiple lowered expression metabolic pathways are involved. Yizhak et al. (2013) developed a new algorithm for the gene expression integration into GEMs called MAT for the identification of drug targets that reverts the metabolism of a diseased cell to a healthy state.

- Scientific evidence showed that the progression of AD links to the cerebral metabolism. Stempler et al. (2014) integrated patients' gene expression with Recon 1 by the iMAT method to predict metabolic biomarkers and drug targets in AD. They demonstrated that the activity of the carnitine shuttle, folate metabolism and mitochondrial transport are significantly decreased. They also predicted several metabolic biomarkers of the AD progression, including succinate and prostaglandin D2 [78].

The availability of omics datasets can also be used to reconstruct personalized patient GEMs to predict metabolic phenotypes and selective drug targets. Agren et al. (2014) used this information to reconstruct personalized GEMs for six HCC patients based on the proteomics data and HMR2 by the tINIT method. These personalized GEMs were successfully employed to identify anticancer drugs [58].

In 2015, Ghaffari et al. generated personalized GEMs for six hepatocellular carcinoma patients from proteomic data and eleven cancer cell-line specific GEMs from RNA-sequencing data. These cancer-specific GEMs were then compared with 83 healthy cell-type GEMs to predict antimetabolites (drugs being structurally similar to metabolites), which would inhibit the cancer growth without perturbing the normal cellular function [79].

One of the most pervasive and ground-breaking pioneer study about personalized GEMs was recently published by Uhlen et al. (2017) [80]. They generated personalized GEMs of 17 types of cancer by integrating the gene expression data into HMR2 using the tINIT method. In addition to predicting driver genes for tumor growth, they demonstrated a widespread metabolic heterogeneity in different patients, highlighting the necessity of personalized medicine for cancer treatments.

Two novel biomedical applications of GEMs are:

- The reconstruction of human pathogen GEMs to unveil the pathogen behavior and mechanism of antibiotic-resistant in bacteria. Carey et al. were pioneers in this research area by working on Malaria [81]. Recently, Dunphy and Papin summarized the latest possibilities in which GEM reconstructions were used to study human pathogens [82].
- The reconstruction of human gut microbiota GEMs. The human gut is colonized with a countless number of microorganisms with extensive interpersonal variation. This complex ecosystem plays a major role in the maintenance of homeostasis. Its dysfunction has been correlated to a broad range of diseases, but the understanding of fundamental mechanisms is hindered by the limited knowledge about interspecies interactions [83]. Therefore, GEMs could provide a well suited framework for the analysis of the human gut microbiota. Recently, a literature-curated interspecies network of the human gut microbiota was developed [84].

All of these studies have increased our understanding of the fundamental mechanisms underlying these diseases and allowed the prediction of drug targets or biomarkers that can be used for designing effective treatment strategies.

DISCUSSION AND CHALLENGES

The generation of generic and context-specific human GEMs has now become a common approach for the prediction of metabolic phenotypes for disorders and health states as well as for the identification of therapeutic targets. With steadily updated generic human GEMs, growing next generation multi-omics approaches, and improvements in integration algorithms, the quality and number of context-specific GEMs will increase accordingly. While there are many advantages about the GEM reconstruction, data integration methods and their applications in system medicine, there are still some challenges to be solved:

- Although there is a standard language for the representation of metabolic models, called the Systems Biology Markup Language (SBML), it seems that different research groups did not consider a unified notation for the representation of their models. For example, a metabolic symbol for the amino acid Alanine was depicted in the human metabolic models by four different character types including underline (ala_L[c]), one dash line (ala-L[c]), three dashed line (ala---L[c]), and DASH (ala-DASH-L[c]). This non-uniform representation hinders readers to easily reproduce results and is very time consuming.
- According to the assumption that transcript or protein levels should provide an accurate snapshot of the metabolism, in almost all data integration algorithms developers use them as surrogates for respective enzyme activity levels. The major obstacle in the integrative analysis of the aforementioned integrative algorithms is the lack of correlation between gene transcription levels, protein levels, enzyme activities and reaction fluxes [62].
- A GEM typically needs a well choosen pre-defined objective function (e.g., a biomass equation), because the model is very sensitive to the definition of the biomass equation, which significantly influences the behavior of the model. Usually, the maximization of the growth rate (biomass equation) is used as an objective function for microorganisms. However, defining an objective function for a human cell is not as straight-forward and the feasibility is very context-specific. Currently, more attention is paid on human model reconstruction precision than on providing biomass-specific functions. Therefore, the human biomass equation needs to be adjusted and defined according to context-specific GEMs [32].

REFERENCES

[1] Mahadevan R. and Palsson, B. O. "Properties of metabolic networks: Structure versus function," *Biophys. J.*, vol. 88, no. 1, 2005.

[2] Asgari, Y., Salehzadeh-Yazdi, A., Schreiber, F. and Masoudi-Nejad, A. "Controllability in cancer metabolic networks according to drug targets as driver nodes," *PLoS One*, vol. 8, no. 11, 2013.

[3] Orth, J. D., Thiele, I. and Palsson, B. Ø. "What is flux balance analysis?," *Nat. Biotechnol.*, vol. 28, no. 3, pp. 245–248, 2010.

[4] Miskovic, L., Tokic, M., Fengos, G. and Hatzimanikatis, V. "Rites of passage: Requirements and standards for building kinetic models of metabolic phenotypes," *Current Opinion in Biotechnology*, vol. 36. pp. 146–153, 2015.

[5] Ma X. and Gao, L. "Biological network analysis: Insights into structure and functions," *Brief. Funct. Genomics*, vol. 11, no. 6, pp. 434–442, 2012.

[6] Palsson, B. "Metabolic systems biology," *FEBS Letters*, vol. 583, no. 24. pp. 3900–3904, 2009.

[7] Mardinoglu A. and Nielsen, J. "Systems medicine and metabolic modelling," in *Journal of Internal Medicine*, 2012, vol. 271, no. 2, pp. 142–154.

[8] O'Brien, E. J., Monk, J. M. and Palsson, B. O. "Using genome-scale models to predict biological capabilities," *Cell*, vol. 161, no. 5, pp. 971–987, 2015.

[9] Wolkenhauer, O., Auffray, C., Jaster, R., Steinhoff, G. and Dammann, O. "The road from systems biology to systems medicine," *Pediatric Research*, vol. 73, no. 4–2. pp. 502–507, 2013.

[10] Thiele I. and Palsson, B. "A protocol for generating a high-quality genome-scale metabolic reconstruction," *Nat. Protoc.*, vol. 5, no. 1, pp. 93–121, 2010.

[11] Caspi, R., Billington, R., Fulcher, C. A., Keseler, I. M., Kothari, A., Krummenacker, M., Latendresse, M., Midford, P. E., Ong, Q., Ong, W. K., Paley, S., Subhraveti, P. and Karp, P. D. "The MetaCyc database of metabolic pathways and enzymes," *Nucleic Acids Res.*, vol. 46, no. D1, pp. D633–D639, 2018.

[12] DeJongh, M., Formsma, K., Boillot, P., Gould, J., Rycenga, M. and Best, A. "Toward the automated generation of genome-scale metabolic networks in the SEED," *BMC Bioinformatics*, vol. 8, 2007.

[13] Agren, R., Liu, L., Shoaie, S., Vongsangnak, W., Nookaew, I. and Nielsen, J. "The RAVEN Toolbox and Its Use for Generating a Genome-scale Metabolic Model for Penicillium chrysogenum," *PLoS Comput. Biol.*, vol. 9, no. 3, 2013.

[14] Dias, O., Rocha, M., Ferreira, E. C. and Rocha, I. "Reconstructing genome-scale metabolic models with merlin," *Nucleic Acids Res.*, vol. 43, no. 8, pp. 3899–3910, 2015.

[15] Notebaart, R. A., van Enckevort, F. H. J., Francke, C., Siezen, R. J. and Teusink, B. "Accelerating the reconstruction of genome-scale metabolic networks," *BMC Bioinformatics*, vol. 7, 2006.

[16] Ataman, M., Hernandez Gardiol, D. F., Fengos, G. and Hatzimanikatis, V. "redGEM: Systematic reduction and analysis of genome-scale metabolic reconstructions for development of consistent core metabolic models," *PLoS Comput. Biol.*, vol. 13, no. 7, 2017.

[17] Ataman M. and Hatzimanikatis, V. "lumpGEM: Systematic generation of subnetworks and elementally balanced lumped reactions for the biosynthesis of target metabolites," *PLoS Comput. Biol.*, vol. 13, no. 7, 2017.

[18] Zhang, C., Ji, B., Mardinoglu, A., Nielsen, J. and Hua, Q. "Logical transformation of genome-scale metabolic models for gene level applications and analysis," *Bioinformatics*, vol. 31, no. 14, pp. 2324–2331, 2015.

[19] Gu, D., Jian, X., Zhang, C. and Hua, Q. "Reframed Genome-Scale Metabolic Model to Facilitate Genetic Design and Integration with Expression Data," *IEEE/ACM Trans. Comput. Biol. Bioinforma.*, pp. 1–1, 2016.

[20] Sánchez, B. J., Zhang, C., Nilsson, A., Lahtvee, P., Kerkhoven, E. J. and Nielsen, J. "Improving the phenotype predictions of a yeast genome-scale metabolic model by incorporating enzymatic constraints," *Mol. Syst. Biol.*, vol. 13, no. 8, p. 935, 2017.

[21] Ma, H., Sorokin, A., Mazein, A., Selkov, A., Selkov, E., Demin, O. and Goryanin, I. "The Edinburgh human metabolic network reconstruction and its functional analysis," *Mol. Syst. Biol.*, vol. 3, 2007.

[22] Duarte, N. C., Becker, S. A., Jamshidi, N., Thiele, I., Mo, M. L., Vo, T. D., Srivas, R. and Palsson, B. O. "Global reconstruction of the human metabolic network based on genomic and bibliomic data," *Proc. Natl. Acad. Sci.*, vol. 104, no. 6, pp. 1777–1782, 2007.

[23] Hao, T., Ma, H. W., Zhao, X. M. and Goryanin, I. "Compartmentalization of the Edinburgh Human Metabolic Network," *BMC Bioinformatics*, vol. 11, 2010.

[24] Agren, R., Bordel, S., Mardinoglu, A., Pornputtapong, N., Nookaew, I. and Nielsen, J. "Reconstruction of genome-scale active metabolic networks for 69 human cell types and 16 cancer types using INIT," *PLoS Comput. Biol.*, vol. 8, no. 5, 2012.

[25] Thiele, I., Swainston, N., Fleming, R. M. T., Hoppe, A., Sahoo, S., Aurich, M. K., Haraldsdottir, H., Mo, M. L., Rolfsson, O., Stobbe, M. D., Thorleifsson, S. G., Agren, R., Bölling, C., Bordel, S., Chavali, A. K., Dobson, P., Dunn, W. B., Endler, L., Hala, D., Hucka, M., Hull, D., Jameson, D., Jamshidi, N., Jonsson, J. J., Juty, N., Keating, S., Nookaew, I., Le Novère, N., Malys, N., Mazein, A., Papin, J. A., Price, N. D., Selkov, E., Sigurdsson, M. I., Simeonidis, E., Sonnenschein, N., Smallbone, K., Sorokin, A., Van Beek, J. H. G. M., Weichart, D., Goryanin, I., Nielsen, J., Westerhoff, H. V., Kell, D. B., Mendes, P. and Palsson, B. O. "A

community-driven global reconstruction of human metabolism," *Nat. Biotechnol.*, vol. 31, no. 5, pp. 419–425, 2013.

[26] Swainston, N., Smallbone, K., Hefzi, H., Dobson, P. D., Brewer, J., Hanscho, M., Zielinski, D. C., Ang, K. S., Gardiner, N. J., Gutierrez, J. M., Kyriakopoulos, S., Lakshmanan, M., Li, S., Liu, J. K., Martínez, V. S., Orellana, C. A., Quek, L. E., Thomas, A., Zanghellini, J., Borth, N., Lee, D. Y., Nielsen, L. K., Kell, D. B., Lewis, N. E. and Mendes, P. "Recon 2.2: from reconstruction to model of human metabolism," *Metabolomics*, vol. 12, no. 7, 2016.

[27] Brunk, E., Sahoo, S., Zielinski, D. C., Altunkaya, A., Dräger, A., Mih, N., Gatto, F., Nilsson, A., Preciat Gonzalez, G. A., Aurich, M. K., Prlić, A., Sastry, A., Danielsdottir, A. D., Heinken, A., Noronha, A., Rose, P. W., Burley, S. K., Fleming, R. M. T., Nielsen, J., Thiele, I. and Palsson, B. O. "Recon3D enables a three-dimensional view of gene variation in human metabolism," *Nat. Biotechnol.*, 2018.

[28] Fell, D. A. and Small, J. R. "Fat synthesis in adipose tissue. An examination of stoichiometric constraints," *Biochem. J.*, vol. 238, no. 3, pp. 781–786, 1986.

[29] Kauffman, J., Prakash, P. and Edwards, J. S. "Advances in flux balance analysis," *Current Opinion in Biotechnology*, vol. 14, no. 5. pp. 491–496, 2003.

[30] Raman, K. and Chandra, N. "Flux balance analysis of biological systems: Applications and challenges," *Briefings in Bioinformatics*, vol. 10, no. 4. pp. 435–449, 2009.

[31] Varma, A. and Palsson, B. O. "Metabolic flux balancing: Basic concepts, scientific and practical use," *Bio/Technology*, vol. 12, no. 10, pp. 994–998, 1994.

[32] Salehzadeh-Yazdi, A. and Asgari, Y. "A Human-Specific Objective Function for Flux Balance Analysis," in *26th International Workshop on Database and Expert Systems Applications*, 2015, pp. 21–25.

[33] Selvarasu, S., Wong, V. V. T., Karimi, I. A. and Lee, D. Y. "Elucidation of metabolism in hybridoma cells grown in fed-batch culture by genome-scale modeling," *Biotechnol. Bioeng.*, vol. 102, no. 5, pp. 1494–1504, 2009.

[34] Lewis, N. E., Nagarajan, H. and Palsson, B. O. "Constraining the metabolic genotype-phenotype relationship using a phylogeny of in silico methods," *Nature Reviews Microbiology*, vol. 10, no. 4. pp. 291–305, 2012.

[35] Romero, P., Wagg, J., Green, M. L., Kaiser, D., Krummenacker, M. and Karp, P. D. "Computational prediction of human metabolic pathways from the complete human genome.," *Genome Biol.*, vol. 6, no. 1, p. R2, 2005.

[36] Matthews, G. Gopinath, M. Gillespie, M. Caudy, D. Croft, B. de Bono, P. Garapati, J. Hemish, H. Hermjakob, B. Jassal, A. Kanapin, S. Lewis, S. Mahajan, B. May, E. Schmidt, I. Vastrik, G. Wu, E. Birney, L. Stein, and P. D'eustachio, "Reactome knowledgebase of human biological pathways and processes," *Nucleic Acids Res.*, vol. 37, no. SUPPL. 1, 2009.

[37] Gille, C., Bölling, C., Hoppe, A., Bulik, S., Hoffmann, S., Hübner, K., Karlstädt, A., Ganeshan, R., König, M., Rother, K., Weidlich, M., Behre, J. and Holzhütter, H. G. "HepatoNet1: A comprehensive metabolic reconstruction of the human hepatocyte for the analysis of liver physiology," *Mol. Syst. Biol.*, vol. 6, 2010.

[38] Folger, O., Jerby, L., Frezza, C., Gottlieb, E., Ruppin, E. and Shlomi, T. "Predicting selective drug targets in cancer through metabolic networks," *Mol. Syst. Biol.*, vol. 7, 2011.

[39] Shlomi, T., T. Benyamini, E. Gottlieb, R. Sharan, and E. Ruppin, "Genome-scale metabolic modeling elucidates the role of proliferative adaptation in causing the warburg effect," *PLoS Comput. Biol.*, vol. 7, no. 3, 2011.

[40] Bordbar, A., Feist, A. M., Usaite-Black, R., Woodcock, B., Palsson, J. O. and Famili, I. "A multi-tissue type genome-scale metabolic network for analysis of whole-body systems physiology," *BMC Syst. Biol.*, vol. 5, 2011.

[41] Wang, Y., Eddy, J. A. and Price, N. D. "Reconstruction of genome-scale metabolic models for 126 human tissues using mCADRE," *BMC Syst. Biol.*, vol. 6, 2012.

[42] Feist M. and Palsson, B. O. "The biomass objective function," *Curr. Opin. Microbiol.*, vol. 13, no. 3, pp. 344–349, 2010.

[43] Dikicioglu, D., Kirdar, B. and Oliver, S. G. "Biomass composition: the 'elephant in the room' of metabolic modelling," *Metabolomics*, vol. 11, no. 6, pp. 1690–1701, 2015.

[44] Nielsen, J. "Systems Biology of Metabolism," *Annu. Rev. Biochem.*, vol. 86, no. 1, pp. 245–275, 2017.

[45] Björnson, E., Borén, J. and Mardinoglu, A. "Personalized cardiovascular disease prediction and treatment-A review of existing strategies and novel systems medicine tools," *Frontiers in Physiology*, vol. 7, no. JAN. 2016.

[46] Vivek-Ananth, R. P. and Samal, A. "Advances in the integration of transcriptional regulatory information into genome-scale metabolic models," *BioSystems*, vol. 147. pp. 1–10, 2016.

[47] Uhlen, M., Hallstro m, B. M., Lindskog, C., Mardinoglu, A., Ponten, F. and Nielsen, J. "Transcriptomics resources of human tissues and organs," *Mol. Syst. Biol.*, vol. 12, no. 4, pp. 862–862, 2016.

[48] Mardinoglu, A. and Nielsen, J. "Editorial: The impact of systems medicine on human health and disease," *Frontiers in Physiology*, vol. 7, no. NOV, 2016.

[49] Sánchez, J. and Nielsen, J. "Genome scale models of yeast: towards standardized evaluation and consistent omic integration," *Integr. Biol.*, vol. 7, no. 8, pp. 846–858, 2015.

[50] Covert, W. and Palsson, B. "Transcriptional regulation in constraints-based metabolic models of Escherichia coli," *J. Biol. Chem.*, vol. 277, no. 31, pp. 28058–28064, 2002.

[51] Åkesson, M., Förster, J. and Nielsen, J. "Integration of gene expression data into genome-scale metabolic models," *Metab. Eng.*, vol. 6, no. 4, pp. 285–293, 2004.

[52] Becker, S. A. and Palsson, B. O. "Context-specific metabolic networks are consistent with experiments," *PLoS Comput. Biol.*, vol. 4, no. 5, 2008.

[53] Colijn, C., Brandes, A., Zucker, J., Lun, D. S., Weiner, B., Farhat, M. R., Cheng, T. Y., Moody, D. B., Murray, M. and Galagan, J. E. "Interpreting expression data with metabolic flux models: Predicting Mycobacterium tuberculosis mycolic acid production," *PLoS Comput. Biol.*, vol. 5, no. 8, 2009.

[54] Jerby, L., Shlomi, T. and Ruppin, E. "Computational reconstruction of tissue-specific metabolic models: Application to human liver metabolism," *Mol. Syst. Biol.*, vol. 6, 2010.

[55] Moxley, J. F., Jewett, M. C., Antoniewicz, M. R., Villas-Boas, S. G., Alper, H., Wheeler, R. T., Tong, L., Hinnebusch, A. G., Ideker, T., Nielsen, J. and Stephanopoulos, G. "Linking high-resolution metabolic flux phenotypes and transcriptional regulation in yeast modulated by the global regulator Gcn4p," *Proc. Natl. Acad. Sci.*, vol. 106, no. 16, pp. 6477–6482, 2009.

[56] Jensen, A. and Papin, J. A. "Functional integration of a metabolic network model and expression data without arbitrary thresholding," *Bioinformatics*, vol. 27, no. 4, pp. 541–547, 2011.

[57] Kim J. and Reed, J. L. "RELATCH: relative optimality in metabolic networks explains robust metabolic and regulatory responses to perturbations," *Genome Biol.*, vol. 13, no. 9, p. R78, 2012.

[58] Agren, R., Mardinoglu, A., Asplund, A., Kampf, C., Uhlen, M. and Nielsen, J. "Identification of anticancer drugs for hepatocellular carcinoma through personalized genome-scale metabolic modeling," *Mol. Syst. Biol.*, vol. 10, no. 3, 2014.

[59] Schultz, A. and Qutub, A. A. "Reconstruction of Tissue-Specific Metabolic Networks Using CORDA," *PLoS Comput. Biol.*, vol. 12, no. 3, 2016.

[60] Kim, K., Lane, A., Kelley, J. J. and Lun, D. S. "E-Flux2 and sPOT: Validated methods for inferring intracellular metabolic flux distributions from transcriptomic data," *PLoS One*, vol. 11, no. 6, 2016.

[61] Pacheco, P. and Sauter, T. "The FASTCORE family: For the fast reconstruction of compact context-specific metabolic networks models," in *Methods in Molecular Biology*, vol. 1716, 2018, pp. 101–110.

[62] Machado, D. and Herrgård, M. "Systematic Evaluation of Methods for Integration of Transcriptomic Data into Constraint-Based Models of Metabolism," *PLoS Comput. Biol.*, vol. 10, no. 4, 2014.

[63] Kim K. and Lun, D. S. "Methods for integration of transcriptomic data in genome-scale metabolic models," *Comput. Struct. Biotechnol. J.*, vol. 11, no. 18, pp. 59–65, 2014.

[64] Estévez, S. R. and Nikoloski, Z. "Context-specific metabolic model extraction based on regularized least squares optimization," *PLoS One*, vol. 10, no. 7, 2015.

[65] Opdam, S., Richelle, A., Kellman, B., Li, S., Zielinski, D. C. and Lewis, N. E. "A Systematic Evaluation of Methods for Tailoring Genome-Scale Metabolic Models," *Cell Syst.*, vol. 4, no. 3, p. 318–329.e6, 2017.

[66] Jerby, L., Wolf, L., Denkert, C., Stein, G. Y., Hilvo, M., Oresic, M., Geiger, T. and Ruppin, E. "Metabolic associations of reduced proliferation and oxidative stress in advanced breast cancer," *Cancer Res.*, vol. 72, no. 22, pp. 5712–5720, 2012.

[67] Yizhak, K., Le Devedec, S. E., Rogkoti, V. M., Baenke, F., de Boer, V. C., Frezza, C., Schulze, A., van de Water, B. and Ruppin, E. "A computational study of the Warburg effect identifies metabolic targets inhibiting cancer migration," *Mol. Syst. Biol.*, vol. 10, no. 8, pp. 744–744, 2014.

[68] Nam, H., Campodonico, M., Bordbar, A., Hyduke, D. R., Kim, S., Zielinski, D. C. and Palsson, B. O. "A Systems Approach to Predict Oncometabolites via Context-Specific Genome-Scale Metabolic Networks," *PLoS Comput. Biol.*, vol. 10, no. 9, 2014.

[69] Asgari, Y., Zabihinpour, Z., Salehzadeh-Yazdi, A., Schreiber, F. and Masoudi-Nejad, A. "Alterations in cancer cell metabolism: The Warburg effect and metabolic adaptation," *Genomics*, vol. 105, no. 5–6, pp. 275–281, 2015.

[70] Lewis, E. and Abdel-Haleem, A. M. "The evolution of genome-scale models of cancer metabolism," *Frontiers in Physiology*, vol. 4 SEP. 2013.

[71] Fouladiha, H. and Marashi, S. A. "Biomedical applications of cell- and tissue-specific metabolic network models.," *J. Biomed. Inform.*, vol. 68, pp. 35–49, 2017.

[72] Robinson, J. L. and Nielsen, J. "Anticancer drug discovery through genome-scale metabolic modeling," *Curr. Opin. Syst. Biol.*, vol. 4, pp. 1–8, 2017.

[73] Zelezniak, A., Pers, T. H., Soares, S., Patti, M. E. and Patil, K. R. "Metabolic network topology reveals transcriptional regulatory signatures of type 2 diabetes," *PLoS Comput. Biol.*, vol. 6, no. 4, 2010.

[74] Väremo, L., Scheele, C., Broholm, C., Mardinoglu, A., Kampf, C., Asplund, A., Nookaew, I., Uhlén, M., Pedersen, B. K. and Nielsen, J. "Proteome- and Transcriptome-Driven Reconstruction of the Human Myocyte Metabolic Network and Its Use for Identification of Markers for Diabetes," *Cell Rep.*, vol. 11, no. 6, pp. 921–933, 2015.

[75] Mardinoglu, A., Agren, R., Kampf, C., Asplund, A., Nookaew, I., Jacobson, P., Walley, A. J., Froguel, P., Carlsson, L. M., Uhlen, M. and Nielsen, J. "Integration of clinical data with a genome-scale metabolic model of the human adipocyte," *Mol. Syst. Biol.*, vol. 9, no. 1, 2013.

[76] Mardinoglu, A., Agren, R., Kampf, C., Asplund, A., Uhlen, M. and Nielsen, J. "Genome-scale metabolic modelling of hepatocytes reveals serine deficiency in patients with non-alcoholic fatty liver disease," *Nat. Commun.*, vol. 5, 2014.

[77] Hyötyläinen, T., Jerby, L., Petäjä, E. M., Mattila, I., Jäntti, S., Auvinen, P., Gastaldelli, A., Yki-Järvinen, H., Ruppin, E. and Orešič, M. "Genome-scale study reveals reduced metabolic adaptability in patients with non-alcoholic fatty liver disease," *Nat. Commun.*, vol. 7, 2016.

[78] Stempler, S., Yizhak, K. and Ruppin, E. "Integrating transcriptomics with metabolic modeling predicts biomarkers and drug targets for Alzheimer's disease," *PLoS One*, vol. 9, no. 8, 2014.

[79] Ghaffari, P., Mardinoglu, A., Asplund, A., Shoaie, S., Kampf, C., Uhlen, M. and Nielsen, J. "Identifying anti-growth factors for human cancer cell lines through genome-scale metabolic modeling," *Sci. Rep.*, vol. 5, 2015.

[80] Uhlen, M., Zhang, C., Lee, S., Sjöstedt, E., Fagerberg, L., Bidkhori, G., Benfeitas, R., Arif, M., Liu, Z., Edfors, F., Sanli, K., Von Feilitzen, K., Oksvold, P., Lundberg, E., Hober, S., Nilsson, P., Mattsson, J., Schwenk, J. M., Brunnström, H., Glimelius, B., Sjöblom, T., Edqvist, P. H., Djureinovic, D., Micke, P., Lindskog, C., Mardinoglu, A. and Ponten, F. "A pathology atlas of the human cancer transcriptome," *Science (80-.).*, vol. 357, no. 6352, 2017.

[81] Carey, M. A., Papin, J. A. and Guler, J. L. "Novel Plasmodium falciparum metabolic network reconstruction identifies shifts associated with clinical antimalarial resistance," *BMC Genomics*, vol. 18, no. 1, 2017.

[82] Dunphy L. J. and Papin, J. A. "Biomedical applications of genome-scale metabolic network reconstructions of human pathogens," *Curr. Opin. Biotechnol.*, vol. 51, pp. 70–79, 2018.

[83] van der Ark, K. C. H., van Heck, R. G. A., Martins Dos Santos, V. A. P., Belzer, C. and de Vos, W. M. "More than just a gut feeling: constraint-based genome-scale metabolic models for predicting functions of human intestinal microbes," *Microbiome*, vol. 5, no. 1. p. 78, 2017.

[84] Sung, J., Kim, S., Cabatbat, J. J. T., Jang, S., Jin, Y. S., Jung, G. Y., Chia, N. and Kim, P. J. "Global metabolic interaction network of the human gut microbiota for context-specific community-scale analysis," *Nat. Commun.*, vol. 8, 2017.

In: Focus on Systems Theory Research
Editors: Manuel F. Casanova and Ioan Opris

ISBN: 978-1-53614-561-8
© 2019 Nova Science Publishers, Inc.

Chapter 7

REALITY IS HIERARCHICALLY ORGANIZED: THE RECURSIVE FOUNDATIONS OF LIVING SYSTEMS AND BEYOND

Patrick Connolly[*]
Department of Counselling and Psychology,
Hong Kong Shue Yan University, Hong Kong, China

ABSTRACT

Hierarchical recursive organization is a fundamental aspect of how the universe works. It forms part of a systems theory picture of reality as a steady emergence of new forms of organization over time, such as the emergence of living organisms from inorganic matter, and the emergence of consciousness, language and culture within the biological world. Each new emergent form of organization comes to change the way systems work, but each is nonetheless founded upon, and constrained by, all that came before. For a long time, living systems presented a challenge to this view, as it had historically been difficult to show how the regulation of living systems were founded upon accepted principles within physics. However, within the last twelve years, this has substantially changed. The free energy principle of Dr. Karl Friston, represents an exciting breakthrough in our understanding of how biological systems are regulated, much as how the laws of thermodynamics and general relativity were considered breakthroughs in our view of how inorganic matter is regulated. This chapter begins with a description of hierarchical recursive organization and how it manifests in some principles of physics, such as loop quantum gravity (Rovelli, 2016) and the slaving principle (Haken, 1983/2004). The nature of living systems is described, first in terms of Maturan and Varela's (1980) concepts of autopoiesis and self-making, and then in terms

---
[*] Email: patrickconnolly@live.com.

Friston's (2010) free energy principle. Specifically, the nature of organizational hierarchies in biological systems and particularly the nervous system is described from the perspective of Dr. Friston's work. The regulatory influence of evolution by natural selection over living systems (and over the free energy principle) is addressed next, including an introduction to the new field of variational neuroethology (Ramstead, Badcock & Friston, 2017). At the end, the final frontier of social and cultural organization, and its regulatory influence over evolution and biological self-organization, is presented. The chapter concludes with the view that future research from a systems theory viewpoint is increasingly likely to use hierarchical computational models that demonstrate recursive organization, and that support a systems theory view of reality.

Keywords: hierarchical recursive organization, free energy principle, markov blankets, variational neuroethology, self-organization, evolution, interpersonal synchrony

INTRODUCTION

Defining Hierarchical Recursive Organization

The concept of recursion in mathematics (and in computer programming) refers to a function that calls itself. However, the usage of the concept of recursion in systems theory has extended beyond this basic definition. It has been used by some systems thinkers (such as Bateson, 1972; Maturana, & Varela, 1980) to describe the stepwise evolution of the principles by which a system is regulated. The description of hierarchical recursive organization (HRO henceforth) to be applied in this chapter is founded on a few assumptions generally held in systems theory.

The first assumption is that systems can be described in terms of hierarchical levels of organization. An example of this might be a cyclone, a spinning vortex of high speed winds around a low-pressure center. At a lower level of organization of the tornado system we might observe that the system is constituted of atoms, bound and interacting with other atoms in the way we understand them to. At a higher level there are air molecules, interacting with one another and with environmental phenomena such as gravity and heat in relatively predictable ways. At the highest level of organization (in this description) is the characteristic organization of the cyclone, the spinning winds around the low-pressure center. In a hierarchical description like this, the highest level of organization is the one which most defines the behavior of the system: we might say that processes at that level control the behavior of the system as a whole.

However, at the same time, we can see that principles operating at the lower levels of organization still hold true. The behavior of individual atoms is still best explained by the principles that govern atoms and their interactions, and the air molecules are still subject to the principles that govern those. Therefore, the overall behavior of the system, while determined by the highest level of organization, cannot violate the principles of the lower levels. In other words, the principles of the lower levels of organization still constrain the overall behavior of the system.

As an aside, we should note that the levels of organization described above are 'selected' in our analysis. The system behaves as a unified whole, and these levels of description are not inevitable or exhaustive. We could extend our description down to subatomic processes, or potentially to even higher-level control processes, potentially such as global patterns of organization of weather systems. Bateson (1972) described a potentially infinite regress of levels of description.

Self-Organization in Systems Theory and Cybernetics

The origin of the field of systems theory (such as in the work of Wiener, 1965 on cybernetics, and of von Bertalanffy, 1969/2009 on general systems theory) began with the question of how those highest levels of organization of systems come to exist, or where their regulatory principles emerge from. One of the central tenets right from this start has been the assumption that they emerge from the activities at the lower levels. Referring to a description found in Wiener and Schade (1965), Grobbelaar (1989) offers a good description of this process with regard to the emergence of a 'pecking order' amongst chickens:

> "... the pecking order [of chickens] which is generated through the interactions of the chickens is spontaneously generated out of the activity of pecking. So that the activity of pecking determines the pattern of dominance, which in turn determines who will peck who." (Grobbelaar, 1989, p. 137)

Grobbelaar suggests that the bigger chickens peck harder, and energetic ones more frequently, leading to a situation where smaller or less energetic ones will steadily peck less and less, until a relatively stable pattern is evident. In other words, the pecking order has emerged from the activities of the existing elements of the system, and the relations between them at this lower order of organization. This has been described as the 'self-organization' of systems, the idea that higher-order regulatory principles of systems emerge from activities at lower-order levels.

This doesn't mean that the activity of pecking is the *only* determinant of the pecking order. In other words, the lower-order principles of organization are not the only determinant of higher-order ones. Other influences play a role, particularly external or environmental influences. For example, Prigogine and Stengers (1984) describe how, when a liquid is heated far enough, characteristic patterns of convection appear in the liquid, which may disappear when the heat reduces. In this way, it is perfectly reasonable to suggest that the patterns of convection are 'caused by' the increase in heat.

However, this is an inadequate description. The convection patterns are a function of the characteristics of the liquid and the atoms and molecules of which it is composed, and the thermodynamic principles which organize their activity.

An analogy might be found in Bateson's (1972) unfortunate example of a man who kicks a dog. The reaction of the dog (e.g., to bite the man, run away or cower and so on) is not determined by the kick, but rather by the way the dog is organized. In other words, the dog's reaction tells you more about the dog than the kick. The kick might be described as an example of 'instigatory' causation in that it influences the system in some way, but the subsequent behavior of the system is more fully determined by the system itself. This is true of the formation of convection patterns in heated liquid as well.

It is this characteristic of systems - that their behavior is largely determined by their own organization rather than just by the external phenomena that influence them - which prompted the emergence of the field of systems theory.

This is also the reason that a hierarchical recursive description of a system is useful. While a cyclone can be said to be formed by the interplay of gravity and the distribution of heat in atmosphere, we cannot explain why a cyclone forms the way that it does without understanding the elements (atoms, molecules) and the relations between them which constitute the cyclone system.

Grobbelaar (1989) describes this interrelationship of hierarchical levels of organization:

> "Although the components and their properties differ from one level to the next, ... a system is constituted by the relations which obtain between the components at the same level as well as between components on different levels which defines the ... [system]... as a unity. Furthermore it is clear that the organization at the lowest level sets the parameters for the recursive ordering of components/elements at the next level, so that the organization at the ... [lowest] ... level will be reflected in a general way at the ... [next highest] ... level, and in an even more indirect way at the ... [highest] ... level." (p. 134-136)

Returning to the self-organizing characteristic of systems (the 'pecking order' example above), this process can be described in dynamic systems theory as the emergence of new dynamic attractor constraining the behavior of the system. In dynamic systems theory, a dynamical attractor specifies a limited set of states that the system can inhabit. It is dynamic in that there is some relative degree of freedom within which the system state can vary relatively unpredictably, but it varies within the specific limits defined by the attractor. Referring to the related field of cybernetics (or regulation of systems) Bateson (1972) suggested that the language of constraint was an appropriate way to understand the behavior of systems:

" ... cybernetic explanation is always negative. We consider what alternative possibilities could conceivably have occurred and then ask why many alternatives were not followed, so that the particular event was one of those few which could, in fact, occur ... In cybernetic language, the course of events is said to be subject to restraints, and it is assumed that, apart from such restraints, the pathways of change would be governed only by equality of probability. In fact, the "restraints" upon which cybernetic explanation depends can in all cases be regarded as factors, which determine inequality of probability. If we find a monkey striking a typewriter apparently at random but in fact writing meaningful prose, we shall look for restraints, either inside the monkey or inside the typewriter. Perhaps the monkey could not strike inappropriate letters; perhaps the type bars could not move improperly struck; perhaps incorrect letters could not survive the paper. Somewhere there must have been a circuit which could identify error and eliminate it." (Bateson 1972, p. 399)

This hypothetical 'circuit' in the last line of the above quote represents that boundary of the dynamic attractor state which constrains the otherwise random (or dynamic) process of the monkey pressing keys.

The emergence of new dynamic attractors in hierarchical levels of organization is step-wise (in other words, organized in discrete levels, and emerging after discrete intervals of time) due to the fact that the system has some relative degree of freedom to move away from its equilibrium state before a new attractor emerges. In other words we might expect that a given system might move between a wide variety of states, but should these changes not obtain stability, there is not a change in regulatory organization as it is defined here.

The stability of this new attractor is often dependent on a feedback loop with the environment. The organization of many physical systems in the universe is dependent on such feedback loops. For example, returning back to the patterns of convection in liquids heated until far from equilibrium described above (Prigogine and Stengers, 1984) the stability of the new attractor state of the convection patterns depends on a relatively stable temperature to be maintained. Should the temperature fall significantly, or should it continue to increase, the patterns of convection may disappear.

Emergent Regulatory Organization

We might understand the emergence of such a new dynamical attractor as the emergence of a new regulatory principle of the system. It essentially represents a new, higher-order organization of the system that most closely describes its overall behavior. As such it means that the system is now doing things that can't be readily predicted from the lower order regulatory principles. In other words, we can't easily predict the

156   *Patrick Connolly*

formation and behavior of cyclones just from knowing the rules by which atoms combine, for example.

Wiener (1965) mentions this problem in different levels of description of weather patterns, where if you were to ask a meteorologist to provide you with a detailed account of the clouds in a weather system, *"... he might laugh in your face, or he might patiently explain that in all the language of meteorology there is no such thing as a cloud, defined as an object with a quasi-permanent identity; and that if there were, he neither possesses the facilities to count them, nor is he in fact interested in counting them. A topologically inclined meteorologist might perhaps define a cloud as a connected region of space in which the density of the part of the water content in the solid or liquid state exceeds a certain amount, but this definition would not be of the slightest value to anyone, and would at most represent an extremely transitory state. What really concerns the meteorologist is some such statistical statement as, "Boston: January 17, 1950: Sky 38% overcast: Cirrocumulus." (p. 30)*

In a similar way, for most practical purposes, the new form of organization that emerges in a system is not predicted by lower order organization, though it can potentially be shown how it is founded upon that lower organization. This phenomenon of HRO, or new emergent self-organization founded upon hierarchical layers of organization, seems pervasive in the natural world, as seen in a number of examples.

Carlo Rovelli's (2016) book 'Reality is not what it seems' addresses a fundamental problem in the field of physics where the laws that govern the activity at a subatomic level of matter (those defined by the field of quantum mechanics) are not compatible with Einstein's laws of general relativity which govern the behavior of matter at a larger scale. He then presents the developing field of loop quantum gravity, which he suggests can offer a means to reconcile these two levels of description. Specifically he states that basic subatomic quanta (that constitute gravitational fields) cluster together in aggregates that interact with one another. At larger and larger scales, these aggregates can be described as occupying different levels of organization. Once aggregates reach a level of scale that begins to 'curve' space-time, profound changes in organization occur that are best described by general relativity.

Hermann Haken's (1983/2004) book 'Synergetics' describes a phenomenon of laser light which shows this emergent organization in a dramatic way. If light is shone onto the rod of a solid state laser at relatively low power, it acts as a lamp, each atom independently emitting a light-wavetrack of 3 meters. However, if the power of light shone on the rod is increased, reaching a level referred to as laser threshold, a completely new phenomenon occurs. The atoms now release a single giant wavetrack with a wavelength of 300,000km. Further increasing the power of the light beyond the laser threshold achieves drastic increases in the output power of the laser. This is represented in Figure 1 below.

The change occurs as the movement of electrons between orbits of the atoms that produce the light wave-tracks becomes synchronized or correlated, producing the coherent wave-track of the laser. Haken (1983/2004) has explained this through what is now known as the slaving principle, which is that slower processes come to slave (the degrees of freedom of) faster microprocesses. This principle has come to be an important foundation of hierarchical organization of systems, that not only defines a temporal relationship between layers of organization, but also often a spatial one, such that activities at larger scale tend to be the slower ones that slave processes at faster, often smaller scale. Haken explains that should one continue to increase the input power, the output goes through a number of additional transitions each reflecting new processes, just as the one described here.

The Problem of Biological Self-Organization

The description of HRO in this chapter presents an image of the universe as an unbroken hierarchical organization, dynamic attractor emerging from dynamic attractor, principles founded upon principles, from the lowest known quanta of space and time as articulated by Rovelli (2016) all the way to human scale physiological and neural activity and beyond. However, for a long time, scientists found great difficulty in linking principles regulating organic life with those regulating its inorganic foundation. Similar to the apparent incompatibility between subatomic physics and general relativity, a key trouble about organic life was the difficulty of reconciling the lower-order laws of thermodynamics with the behavior of organic systems. Where inorganic matter seemed to be invariantly subject to the tendency towards entropy, so organic life seemed to defy entropy, and was characterized by apparent increases in order and complexity, rather than a tendency towards decrease. While work throughout the life sciences was able to successfully model or predict various principles of operation of biological systems, none of these were decisively linked to a foundation of key organizational principles in the inorganic realm, such as those of thermodynamics. The train of hierarchical organization appeared to have derailed.

However, this didn't mean that many scientists didn't believe that such links were possible. Ludwig von Bertalanffy's (1969/2009) influential work on general systems theory began with this premise. Von Bertanlanffy, a biologist, suggested that the principles that regulated biological organisms must emerge from lower-order levels of organization. Though he forwarded ideas about how such linkage could be achieved, he was not able to formulate specific key principles which showed their dependence on lower-order inorganic foundations.

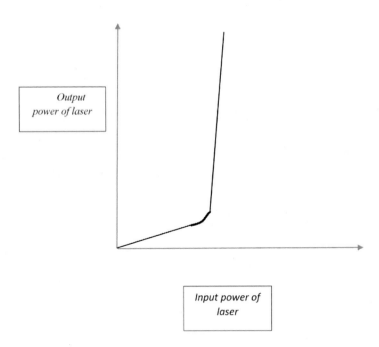

Figure 1. Output power of a laser above and below laser threshold, after Haken, 1983/2004, page 18.

This situation has recently changed. The free energy principle (FEP henceforth) of Dr. Karl Friston (Friston, Kilner & Harrison, 2006; Friston, 2010) represents a critical step forward in describing a fundamental regulatory principle of living systems that can be shown to be founded upon principles regulating lower-order inorganic systems. The remainder of this chapter will be focusing on the describing the revolutionary potential the FEP is having and will have in our understanding of living systems. However, before introducing the FEP, a detour will be taken through the earlier work of Maturana and Varela (1980).

Autopoiesis and Structural Coupling

Humberto Maturana (2002) was asked in 1960 by a student, what could we say happened millions of years ago that means we can say that life began then – the question is really about the fundamental defining characteristic of life. His response to the question was really to identify the circular process whereby organisms constitute themselves:

> "... nucleic acids participate with proteins in the synthesis of proteins, and that proteins participate as enzymes with nucleic acids in the synthesis of nucleic acids, all together constituting a discrete circular dynamics. ... As I was drawing a diagram of this circularity, I exclaimed 'This is it! This is the minimal expression of the circular closed dynamics of molecular productions that makes living systems discrete autonomous molecular systems.'" (Maturana, 2002, p7)

In other words, this formulation suggests that living systems consist of a specific circular relationship with their environment. In this description, the components of the system that are present in the environment build the structures of the system, which themselves act on the environmental components to build the structure. This is a circular, not linear process: it is not one and then the other which occurs, but a single circular process. This defining characteristic of living systems was formalized in the work by Maturana and Varela (1980) with the term 'autopoiesis' or self-making, and it is the first of two preconditions for the existence of life, in their view. The other is a boundary condition that specifies the distinction between the circular, autopoietic system, and its environment. While the boundary condition reflects this distinction, the process of autopoiesis described above specifies a circular process with environment. Maturana and Varela (1980) described this as structural coupling: the continuous recursive structuring of the system in interaction with the environment, where change in one must involve change in the other.

The value of Maturana and Varela's (1980) work is that it provides a model that approximates processes occurring at a specific level of organization, which is roughly at the level of molecular organization and relationships, involving nucleic acids, proteins and enzymes, and their mutual interrelationships. Maturana (2002) took pains to state that it was inappropriate to apply to the concept of autopoiesis to other phenomena and levels of description. In his view, autopoiesis simply describes molecular self-making, not self-organization in general.

Markov Blankets and Living Systems

The work of Friston (2010) introduced below is not just a model approximating a specific process, occurring at a specific level of organization. Rather, we can think of Friston's FEP as a scale-free principle (similar to thermodynamics) which operates at a wide variety of scale in organic life, and specifies that the most fundamental regulatory principle of living systems. The FEP is introduced in the following section, beginning with a description of the basic organization of living systems, that formalizes some aspects of Maturana and Varela's (1980) model.

In a paper entitled 'Life as we know it', Friston (2013) suggests that two preconditions are required for the formation of a living system. One is ergodicity, which is the property that the average amount of time a system spends within a possible or allowed state is proportionate to the probability of the system being in that state. In dynamic systems theory, this is the same as stating that a system has a random dynamical attractor. The second precondition is the existence of a Markov blanket. Since random dynamical attractors characterize virtually all systems (within the present definition), it is this second precondition, the Markov blanket, which is the 'special' one from the perspective of living systems, and deserves closer examination.

Formally a Markov blanket originally described a set of nodes in a Bayesian network, represented below in Figure 2.

In the field of machine learning, a Markov blanket is defined as the set of nodes which contain all the information needed to predict the state inside the blanket. In other words, the state inside the blanket is conditionally independent of the state outside the outside the blanket. Friston (2013) suggests that living systems have the formal properties of a Markov blanket, which is formally very similar to Maturana and Varela's (1980) description of the boundary condition necessary for a living system. As will be seen next, the Markov blanket also has a property similar to structural coupling.

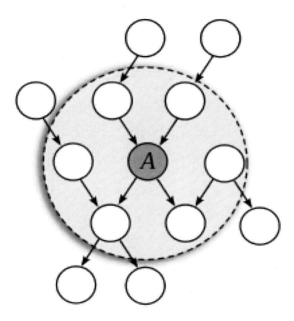

Figure 2. A Markov blanket, a set of nodes surrounding node A. Note in this diagram, higher nodes are called 'parents', ones immediately below are called 'children'. In this diagram, the Markov blanket of node A consists of A's parents, children, and its children's parents. This image was found on https://commons.wikimedia.org/wiki/File%3ADiagram_of_a_Markov_blanket.svg.

In 'Life as we know it', Friston (2013) demonstrates how the existence of the blanket implies that the whole partition (into internal and external states and their Markov blanket) is ergodic. This means that the living system has a tendency to maintain the blanket; if the blanket is penetrated, the system ceases to be a living system. Friston (2013) shows that the maintenance of the Markov blanket requires that internal states are minimizing their FE relative to external states. A detailed discussion of the FE equations can be found in Friston (2010). Here, a simplified, intuitive understanding of the FEP is offered.

Friston's Free Energy Principle (FEP)

The FEP states that a living system's structure specifies a model of its environment, that consists of predictions of its sensory input. This model is referred to as the 'generative' model. At its simplest, the FEP states that the difference between the predictions of the generative model and the actual sensory information (the prediction error) always tends towards a minimum. In other words, the generative model should, over time, become a better and better predictor of environmental stimuli. Sensory input to the system can provoke two responses from the system, both of which achieve the minimization of prediction error. The first response involves 'updating' the generative model to be closer to the sensory information, in the form of Bayesian updating. Alternatively, the system takes an action which changes the sensory information to be closer to that predicted by the generative model. In this way, the FEP specifies a recursive circular process (described as an action-perception cycle) between the system and its environment that is formally very similar to Maturana and Varela's (1980) notion of structural coupling. However, while the concepts of autopoiesis and structural coupling may only specify activities at a specific, molecular level, Friston's (2010) FEP not only demonstrates it foundations on lower order principles of organization, but also specifies a scale-free constraint operating at all higher levels of organization of living systems.

Friston and Stephan (2007) have shown the FEPs foundation on thermodynamics. With regard to the problem of entropy and living systems, they show how, rather than violating the thermodynamic principle of entropy, rather the FEP represents a specific instance of the tendency towards entropy. Fluctuation theorems in statistical mechanics have shown that the level of entropy in the system can increase in open dissipative non-equilibrium systems such as biological ones, which exchange entropy and energy with their environment.

> "The premise here is that the environment unfolds in a thermodynamically structured and lawful way and biological systems embed these laws into their anatomy. ... For example, although disorder always increases, the second law per se is invariant. This invariance is itself a source of order. In short, organisms could maintain configurational order, if they transcribed physical laws governing their environment into their structure." (Friston & Stephan, 2007)

The intriguing implication here is that the tendency towards entropy is encoded in the generative model itself. More than just being far-from-equilibrium, dissipative systems, biological systems are structured to avoid phase changes (perhaps through natural selection, addressed in a later section), indicating why they can endure for long periods in relatively stable environmental conditions.

The power of the FEP lies not only in how it can be linked to lower-order regulatory principles such as thermodynamics, but also how it can be shown to act as a fundamental regulatory constraint in living systems, even though higher-order regulatory principles may emerge that are super-ordinate to the FEP.

Hierarchical Organization in Living Systems

One may have the idea that an organism possesses one Markov blanket. An intuitive example might be a unicellular organism. However, the FEP regulates living systems at all scale, down to the organelles within cells, to individual cells, to tissues, organs, systems, and the whole organism. In fact, the FEP constrains organization beyond the level of the individual organism, such as social systems, but this is returned to later. What this indicates is that Markov blankets are ubiquitous within living systems, and that all these layers, from organelles to the whole organism, have their own Markov blankets. The whole organism nonetheless has a Markov blanket, and the overall free energy state of the organism, is the sum of the free energy of all the components (Connolly & van Deventer, 2017; Friston, personal communication, 13th July 2015; Kirchoff, Parr, Palacios, Friston & Kiverstein, 2018).

Further, this organization is also evidently hierarchical, and also recursively organized. In fact, we could say that the FEP presents a new constraint on HRO. When new regulatory organization emerges in a living system, it does not only mean that the system has a new dynamical attractor: it also has a new Markov blanket. This suggests that living systems are self-organizing at every possible level of their structure (Connolly & van Deventer, 2017; Palacios, Razi, Parr, Kirchoff & Friston, 2017). Kirchoff, et al. (2018) describe hierarchical nested Markov blankets:

> "the assembly of Markov blankets can be understood to occur in a nested and hierarchical fashion, where a Markov blanket and its internal states at the macroscopic scale consist of smaller Markov blankets and their internal states at microscopic scales of systemic operations. Crucially, the conservation of Markov blankets (of Markov blankets) at every hierarchical scale enables the dynamics of the states at one scale to enslave the (states of) Markov blankets at the scale below, thereby ensuring that the organization as a whole is involved in the minimization of variational free energy." (p. 8)

In their paper, Kirchoff, et al. (2018) use an intuitive example, where a single blanket might say 'I model the world', an ensemble of blankets might say 'we model the world', and hierarchically nested blankets might say 'we model ourselves, modelling the world'. They also state that this hierarchical nesting of blankets also preserves Haken's

(1983/2004) slaving principle of fast macroscopic processes enslaving smaller microscopic ones:

> " ... this kind of self-assembling activity implies a separation of the dynamics involved into slow and fast time scales—a signature feature of the slaving principle in synergetics ... As a result it becomes possible to understand that slow ensemble dynamics arise from microscale dynamics unfolding over fast time scales." (p. 8)

While this HRO potentially applies to all living systems, regardless of their level complexity, substantial attention has been paid to the regulatory role of the nervous system, and in particular, to the levels of information processing and organization of the human brain.

Hierarchies of Organization in the Brain

Friston (2008, 2010) described the brain as consisting of hierarchical levels of organization, where each level in the hierarchy has Markov characteristics. He describes a hierarchy of message passing between levels, where lower levels pass prediction errors to the next highest level in the hierarchy, while higher levels pass down predictions. While some levels are supplied by genetic inheritance, new levels do emerge through developmental process over time. It is evident that the development of the brain preserves the principles of HRO (and the FEP), where each new emergent level is founded upon (and constrained by) sub-ordinate levels, yet comes to organize the degrees of freedom of those lower levels as well. Populations of neurons also support nested Markov blankets allowing encoding of slower and more complex neuronal activities, which involve progressively greater areas of the brain. In this perspective, consciousness is cast as some of the highest-level predictions the system can produce, though this is still speculative (Hobson, Hong & Friston, 2014).

This approach to hierarchical levels of function whose relationships are regulated by the FEP has already produced novel approaches in neuroscience. A paper by Diaconescu, et al. (2017) entitled 'A computational hierarchy in human cortex' has presented evidence for a correspondence between the sequence of evoked neuronal activity, and the predicted order of Bayesian inference computations. Specifically, a theory of mind task was divided into three hierarchical levels of integration. A model of Bayesian inference was developed which predicted a three-level computational hierarchy, with the simplest step being completed first, and the output of that first calculation entering a new computation at the second level, and so on to the third. Electrophysiological and neuro-imaging showed a sequence of activations occurring in the order predicted by the computation model. The authors contend that this approach may offer a new tool for investigating

164   *Patrick Connolly*

deficits in hierarchical processing in autism and schizophrenia, such as for the hierarchical theory of mind task in their study.

As indicated previously, while the FEP is a fundamental organizing principle of biological self-organization and living systems, there are further, higher-order principles founded upon it. A good example is that of evolution.

How Evolution Entrains the FEP

The principle of natural selection (NS henceforth) must be considered a regulatory principle of living systems that is super-ordinate to the FEP. Evolution by NS as we understand it is dependent on the existence of living systems, however it must operate invariantly upon all living systems. Just as the FEP imposes constraints on HRO in the sense that all new levels of organization are characterized by Markov blankets, so too NS imposes new constraints on the emergence of new levels of organization, which is a tendency towards increased survivability and adaptivity. This also implies a tendency towards greater complexity and diversity, reflecting the complexity of the environment and the potential diversity of ecological niches. Significantly, Haken's (1983/2004) slaving principle is preserved here too, in the sense that evolution is a much slower process, operating from one generation to the next over very long periods of time. Further, natural selection does not operate at the individual level, but rather at the level of populations (Connolly & Van Deventer, 2017; Hopkins, personal communication, 8th September 2017). As suggested by Ramstead, Badcock and Friston (2017), there is a Markov blanket around the entire population, and that regulation by NS operates at this level through limiting the degrees of freedom of the component blankets, such as individuals.

We might observe examples that demonstrates how these three principles (HRO, the FEP, and NS) are preserved in evolution. This could be seen in work by Eldar, et al. (2009) who attempt to explain the apparent 'stepwise' nature of evolution in the observation that changes in phenotypic expression are often 'complete' in the sense that a species may develop a new set of arms without appearing to move through a series of approximations or intervening stages on the way to developing a new morphological form. They address this though suggesting that genetic mutations in species often have unpredictable results that affect members of the population differently, a phenomenon called partial penetrance. In this situation, a particular mutation might make a 'complete' change (such as a new pair of arms, as described above) in only one or two individuals within a population while having a diverse range of effects on the others possessing the mutation, including no effect at all. Progressive changes in genetic replication and septations of such mutations may continue to produce this noise (in the sense of uncertain outcomes), until they gradually synergize and obtain stability. They demonstrate this effect in a study of how mutations in the bacilis subtilis bacteria (which typically produce single spores in the wild type) may, through perturbations in signaling and replication of the mutated gene, gradually achieve stabilization of a twin sporulation variety in the population, through the intervening steps of random variations through successive cycles of reproduction.

This may be understood as an expression of recursive organization, in which the stability reflects the new attractor state. More importantly, the regulation through NS is critical here, as the mutation only gains its stability through successive reproduction cycles operating at the population level. Only surviving mutations can attain stability. We clearly see the entrainment of these levels of organization, operating simultaneously.

Variational Neuroethology

Ramstead, Badcock and Friston (2017) have recently announced the field of variational neuroethology, which adopts precisely such an approach to making sense of how the FEP and NS have worked in concert to define the specific forms that organisms have, with a focus on understanding the evolution of the human brain. They outline the concept of the Hierarchically Mechanistic Mind (or HMM) which not only assumes the hierarchical organization of the brain in terms of nested Markov blankets and regulated by the FEP, but also the dependence of that structure on evolutionary processes working at various time scales.

The concern about different timescales is at the heart of the project of variational neuroethology that they outline in their paper (Ramstead, et al., 2017). This is not only because the FEP operates at different levels of hierarchical structure of the brain (from small-scale and fast processes operating at subcellular and cellular levels, to slower processes operating at the level of the organism, and beyond to cultural processes), but also because evolution through NS also seems to work through different time scales as well, which are described in the following paragraph.

In their formulation, Haken's (1983/2004) slaving principle is preserved, in that these various timescales of neural activity and are understood to limit the degrees of freedom of processes occurring at smaller spatial scales, and faster timescales. Specifically, the authors adopt Tinbergen's (1963) four levels of enquiry for explaining the behavior of living systems at the levels of mechanism, ontogeny, phylogeny and function (or adaptive value). In their treatment, Ramstead, et al. (2017) treat these four levels of enquiry as occupying ascending timescales (and spatial scales as well). At the lowest (smallest and fastest) level, mechanism refers to 'causation', the specific causes of behaviors referring to activities in the structure of the individual, including cellular and neural processes. At the second level, ontogeny refers to the development over the lifespan of the individual. Phylogeny refers to epigenetic mechanisms that work across generations, such as through kin groups. Finally, at the highest (slowest and largest) level, function refers to the adaptation of the species types to ecological niche. Critically, each of these changes minimizes free energy as well, whether actions are driven in short time by neuronal processes, or adaptation at evolutionary timescale - which minimizes the free energy of specific phenotypes (Ramstead, et al., 2017). Their description is reproduced below in Figure 3.

Process (temporal scale)	Level of enquiry	Psychological paradigm
Mechanism (real time)	*Neurocognition* (processes occurring within and around the individual)	Psychological subdisciplines
Ontogeny (development time)	*Neurodevelopment* (the individual)	Developmental Psychology
Phylogeny (intergenerational time)	*Neurophylogeny* (groups, e.g., kin)	Evolutionary developmental biology and psychology
Adaptation (evolutionary time)	*Neural evolution* (homo sapiens)	Evolutionary Psychology

Figure 3. The minimization of free energy at different timescales organized around Tinbergen's (1963) four levels of enquiry, after Ramstead, et al., 2017.

How Social Interaction and Culture Come to Regulate Living Systems

In the above example of variational neuroethology as well as earlier in the paper, it has been suggested that the organization at levels of recursion above that of individuals, such as that of social groups or cultures, are constrained by the FEP. It has been suggested that social phenomena may be regulated by their own principles of organization that are nonetheless founded on principles that regulate individuals. The scale-free nature of the FEP means that it should constrain all emerging higher-level regulatory organization, including beyond the individual mind, and to groupings of individuals as well (Friston, personal communication, 13 July 2015).

In other words, we could suggest that a given culture has a Markov blanket: *"cultural ensembles minimise free energy by enculturing their members so that they share common sets of precision-weighting priors" (Ramstead, et al., 2017)*

What this means is that socio-cultural interaction comes to constrain the degrees of freedom of individual humans' brains and behavior, and that social regulation emerges as a superordinate regulatory organization that entrains both evolution through NS as well as the FEP (Connolly & van Deventer, 2017).

In over four decades of research work, John Gottman and colleagues have shown that the emotions and arousal experienced by married partners in their interactions comes to be organized by set patterns of interaction. Based on an evaluation of positive and negative emotions experienced during a 15-minute interaction involving conflict, their model can predict relationship outcome with around 90% accuracy (Gottman, Murray, Swanson, Tyson & Swanson, 2002). This body of research work represents fairly powerful evidence that stable patterns of social interaction comes to organize the lower-order physiological, behavioral and affective states of human beings.

One could use an example to show how the levels of explanation being discussed here, HRO, the FEP, NS and organization by social interaction, are not in competition with one another as explanatory systems, but rather hierarchical. If I am telling my brother that my friend betrayed me, my behavior could be explained at different levels:

1. (Social) Because the system of language categorizes the experience of betrayal as shared meaning
2. (NS) Because evolution has equipped me with social behavior that mobilizes support against social attack
3. (FEP) Because this action has the lowest expected free energy
4. (HRO) Because my structure consists of layers of organization and all influence my behavior.

All of these explanations are true and all operate, there is no competition. However, if you were to select which of these best explains the specific behavior of standing in front of my brother, and moving through an incredibly complex series of movements of vocal chords, lungs, etc. it would be 1) linguistic organization that emerges from social interaction in the development of the individual. In this way the organization by social, linguistic or cultural influence (and these may be different forms of organization) is superordinate to NS and the FEP.

Regarding the influence of culture, Richerson and Boyd (2006) offer an interesting account of how culture has transformed human evolution. It has been suggested that human beings have crossed the 'cultural Rubicon', meaning that human survival and reproduction has overwhelmingly become dependent on our ability to succeed socially, and to behave in culturally adaptive ways.

While it may well be the case that social organization represents a new emergent regulatory tendency for living systems, there is not yet a 'principle' that has been developed to describe this social organization in the same way as the FEP describes biological organization, or even that NS has described evolutionary organization. Certainly, it is likely that this will be a tendency from members of a culture to behave the same as one another over time.

Interpersonal Synchrony

An interesting contemporary direction in research on social interaction refers to the concept of interpersonal synchrony. This is the idea that the neural activities of two interacting agents can come to synchronize with one another, which not only forms the basis for developing interpersonal awareness and empathy and developing relationships, but also minimizes the free energy of both participants in the interaction. Friston and Frith (2015) demonstrate how simulations of birdsong where two 'birds' take turns sustaining a birdsong become possible through a model suggesting synchrony based on mutual minimization of free energy. While this is just a simulation, and proof of principle at best, there is nonetheless a growing body of research evidence linking synchrony (in behavior, neural activity and physiological measures with higher ratings of interactions and interaction partners, increased cooperative task efficiency, and better outcomes in psychotherapy (Koole & Tschacher, 2016; Rennung & Göritz, 2016). Good parent-infant synchrony has been suggested as a critical component of healthy social and emotional development in infants (Feldman & Eidelman, 2004) and interactional synchrony predicts prosocial behavior in infants (Cirelli, Einarson & Trainor, 2014).

It is clear that social interaction and the role of culture are an important contemporary and future frontier in extending our understanding of regulatory principles that govern human living systems, and it is likely that new approaches will use computational methods utilizing mathematically defined regulatory principles.

CONCLUSION

From all of the above examples of neuroscience, evolution, variational neuroethology, social interaction and cultural influence, the vast potential for future scientific work which utilizes the free energy principle, should hopefully be demonstrated to the reader. It is likely that the amount of scientific work utilizing the FEP within a systems-based approach is likely to increase dramatically in the following decade(s). With regard to the central focus of this chapter which is HRO, the intention has been to describe a particular picture of reality as complex hierarchies of self-organization extending from the most granular level of subatomic organization, up to the highest principles organizing living systems and human life. Hierarchical computational models making use of in silico simulation are likely to play an ever increasing role in research, and are increasingly likely to support a systems-theory description of reality.

REFERENCES

Bateson, G. (1972). *Steps to an ecology of mind: collected essays in anthropology, psychiatry, evolution and epistemology.* Chicago: University of Chicago Press.

Cirelli, L. K., Einarson, K. M. & Trainor, L. J. (2014). Interpersonal synchrony increases prosocial behavior in infants. *Developmental Science, 17*(6), 1003-1011.

Connolly, P. & van Deventer, V. (2017). Hierarchical Recursive Organization and the Free Energy Principle: From Biological Self-Organization to the Psychoanalytic Mind. *Frontiers in Psychology, 8,* 1695, DOI: 10.3389/fpsyg.2017.01695.

Diaconescu, A. O., Litvak, V., Mathys, C., Kasper, L., Friston, K. J. & Stephan, K. E. (2017). *A computational hierarchy in human cortex.* Manuscript submitted for publication.

Eldar, A., Chary, V., Xenopoulos, P., Fontes, M. E., Loson, O. C., Dworkin, J., Piggot, P. J. & Elowitz, M. B. (2009). Partial penetrance facilitates developmental evolution in bacteria. *Nature, 460*(7254), 510–514. http://doi.org/10.1038/nature08150.

Feldman, R. & Eidelman, A. I. (2004). Parent-Infant Synchrony and the Social-Emotional Development of Triplets. *Developmental Psychology, 40*(6), 1133-1147.

Friston, K. J. (2010). A free energy principle for the brain. *Nature Reviews Neuroscience, 11,* 127-138. http://dx.doi.org/10.1038/nrn2787.

Friston, K. J. (2013). Life as we know it. *Journal of the Royal Society Interface, 10,* http://dx.doi.org/10.1098/rsif.2013.0475.

Friston, K. J. & Frith, C. (2015). A duet for one. *Consciousness and Cognition, 36,* 390-405. http://dx.doi.org/10.1016/ j.concog.2014.12.003.

Friston, K. J., Kilner, J. & Harrison, L. (2006). A free energy principle of the brain. *Journal of Physiology, 100,* 70-87.

Friston, K. J. & Stephan, K. E. (2007). Free-energy and the brain. *Synthese, 159*(3), 417-458.

Gottman J. M., Murray J. D., Swanson C. C., Tyson R. & Swanson K.R. (2002). *The mathematics of marriage: dynamic nonlinear models.* Cambridge: MIT Press.

Grobbelaar, P. W. (1989). *Freud and systems theory: An exploratory statement* (Unpublished doctoral dissertation). Rand Afrikaans University, Johannesburg.

Haken, H. (2004). *Synergetics: Introduction and advanced topics.* Berlin: Springer-Verlag (Original work published in 1983).

Hobson, J. A., Hong, C. C. & Friston, K. J. (2014). Virtual reality and consciousness inference in dreaming. *Frontiers in Psychology: Cognitive Science, 5,* 1133 doi: 10.3389/fpsyg.2014.01133.

Kirchhoff, M., Parr, T., Palacios, E., Friston, K. & Kiverstein, J. (2018). The Markov blankets of life: autonomy, active inference and the free energy principle. *Journal of the Royal Society Interface, 15,* 20170792. http://dx.doi.org/10.1098/rsif.2017.0792.

Koole, S. L. & Tschacher, W. (2016). Synchrony in psychotherapy: A review and an integrative framework for the therapeutic alliance. *Frontiers in Psychology.*, *7*, 862. doi: 10.3389/fpsyg.2016.00862.

Maturana, H. R. (2002). Autopoiesis, structural coupling and cognition: A history of these and other notions in the biology of cognition. *Cybernetics and Human Knowing*, *9*(3-4), 5-34.

Maturana, H. R. & Varela, F. J. (1980). *Autopoiesis and Cognition*. London: D Reidel.

Palacios, E. R., Razi, A., Parr, T., Kirchoff, M. & Friston, K. J. (2017). *Biological self-organization and Markov blankets*. Manuscript submitted for publication.

Prigogine, I. & Stengers, I. (1984). *Order out of chaos*. New York: Bantam.

Ramstead, M. J. D., Badcock, P. B. & Friston, K. J. (2010). Answering Schrödinger's question: A free-energy formulation. *Physics of Life Reviews*, (2017), http://dx.doi.org/10.1016/j.plrev.2018.01.003.

Rennung, M. & Göritz, A. S. (2016). Prosocial consequences of interpersonal synchrony: A meta-analysis. *Zeitschrift für Psychologie*, *224*, 168-189.

Richerson, P. J. & Boyd, R. (2006). *Not by Genes Alone: How Culture Transformed Human Evolution*. Chicago: University of Chicago Press.

Rovelli, C. (2016). *Reality is not what it seems: the journey to quantum gravity*. London: Allen Lane.

Von Bertalanffy, L. (2009). General systems theory: Foundations, development, applications. New York: George Braziller (Original work published in 1969).

Wiener, N. (1965). *Cybernetics: Or control and communication in the animal and the machine* (2nd ed.). Cambridge: MIT Press.

Wiener, N. & Schadé, J. P. (Eds.). (1965). *Progress in biocybernetics*, (Vol. 2). Philedelphia: Elsevier Publishing Company.

In: Focus on Systems Theory Research
Editors: Manuel F. Casanova and Ioan Opris

ISBN: 978-1-53614-561-8
© 2019 Nova Science Publishers, Inc.

Chapter 8

NEW DIRECTIONS IN OCCUPATIONAL ROADWAY SAFETY GROUNDED IN COMPLEX SYSTEMS THEORY AND SIMULATION MODELING

Michael Kenneth Lemke, PhD[1,2,] and Yorghos Apostolopoulos, PhD[2,3]*

[1]Department of Social Sciences, The University of Houston-Downtown,
Houston, TX, US
[2]Complexity & Computational Population Health Group
Texas A&M University, College Station, TX, US
[3]Department of Health & Kinesiology, Texas A&M University,
College Station, TX, US

ABSTRACT

Occupational characteristics, such as work organization, work content, and the workplace itself, can directly influence worker health and safety. This is especially evident among long-haul truck drivers, whose occupation places them at heightened risk for roadway accidents. Extant efforts to reduce occupational roadway accidents are primarily grounded in a reductionist paradigm, which limits the potential of resrach and action. In contrast, a complex systems paradigm – grounded in complex systems theory and computational modeling and simluation – can allow stakeholders in occupational roadway safety to embrace new theoretical perspectives and methodological approaches and identify better strategies to reduce accidents.

---

[*] Corresponding Author Email: LemkeM@uhd.edu.

Keywords: occupational safety, long-haul truck drivers, reductionism, complex systems theory, computational modeling and simulation

> *"We are accidents waiting to happen"*
>
> *-There, There (Radiohead)*

INTRODUCTION

Work organization, work content, and the workplace as a whole can directly influence the physical and psychological health of humans [1]. The role of occupation in health, disease, and safety outcomes is continually evolving. For example, while workplace safety has vastly improved, work-related energy expenditure has decreased [2, 3]. Further, vast disparities exist both across and within occupations with regard to risk exposures and acute and chronic health and safety outcomes [4-6]. Increased recognition of the importance of occupation in worker well-being has spurred occupational health and safety (OHS) efforts, which have the potential to benefit a wide array of stakeholders, from workers themselves to their families, communities, employers, and society as a whole [7, 8]. For many employers, OHS efforts have become essential to their overall strategic mission as they strive to increase worker productivity and reduce healthcare costs [9-11]. Increased emphasis on OHS efforts is reflected in federal policy, such as in the U.S. Affordable Care Act and the U.S. National Institute of Occupational Safety and Health's *Total Worker Health* program [12, 13].

Ongoing OHS efforts are marked by notable shortcomings. Extant programs are rarely comprehensive, employee-driven, fully customized for the unique milieu of each workplace, or integrated into the organizational culture – all of which are shown to maximize the effectiveness of OHS efforts [12, 14-16]. Further, and even more consequential, OHS efforts rarely address the root causes of occupation-induced health and safety outcomes, and as a result these programs have generally failed to yield long-term significant population-level impacts [17, 18]. Workplace wellness practitioners and others have been critical of these underwhelming efforts and have called for a transition away from "get well quick" schemes toward more holistic and sustainable efforts [17, 18]. However, to wholly accomplish such a shift, the guiding paradigm that shapes OHS theory, methodology, and analysis will likely need to change.

These limitations are indicative of an underlying worldview, or paradigm, which underlies most extant OHS research and action. Broadly, OHS efforts are grounded in a *reductionist paradigm*, which is based on the assumption that "the whole is the sum of the parts"; thus, in this view, we can wholly understand a problem by investigating its component parts separately [19]. While effective for relatively simpler problems, OHS problems are characterized by attributes of *dynamic complexity* – such as interdependence and interconnectedness among causal factors – which create a whole that is not the sum of its parts [20-22]. Thus, a *complex systems paradigm* has the potential to revolutionize OHS efforts and fulfill their potential to deliver broad and sustainable improvements to worker health and safety.

Occupational health and safety constitutes a broad field, so for the sake of clarity and brevity the focus for this chapter will be on occupational roadway safety, and, in particular, on U.S. long-haul truck driver (LHTD) roadway safety. There are nearly two million LHTD in the United States and they experience excessive disparities in nonfatal and fatal injuries compared to other occupations, many of which are due to roadway accidents [23-25]. Although roadway accident rates among LHTD reached a historic nadir in 2009, they have leveled off and even shown signs of increasing in recent years [26]. Of particular concern is the wider impact of LHTD roadway accidents on public health and safety: Among large truck crashes, the ratio of other vehicle, pedestrian, and bicyclist fatalities to large truck occupant fatalities was nearly six-to-one [26]. Efforts to mitigate roadway accidents among LHTD bear the hallmarks of OHS efforts more broadly [27], and the same attributes which limit the effectiveness of OHS in other contexts are present in this problem as well [28]. Thus, LHTD roadway safety can potentially serve as "proof-of-concept" for the proliferation of a complex systems paradigm across broader OHS efforts.

Complex systems approaches have become relatively more common on workplace safety and can substantively contribute to safety initiatives; further, these approaches have been successfully applied in other safety-critical domains, including among other transport operators [28-30]. These approaches have the potential to similarly improve LHTD roadway safety outcomes if thoroughly applied [28-31]. Here, we delve into the reductionist paradigm which shapes extant LHTD roadway safety efforts and its limitations. We then explicate the theoretical and conceptual contributions that a complex systems paradigm can bring to LHTD roadway safety research and action. Finally, we describe the methodological and analytical tools – in particular, *computational modeling and simulation* - that can be brought to bear by integrating a complex systems paradigm into LHTD roadway safety. Cumulatively, these implications are likely representative of more broadly integrating a complex systems paradigm into OHS efforts as a whole.

CONVENTIONAL THEORY AND METHODOLOGY IN OCCUPATIONAL ROADWAY SAFETY

Occupational safety efforts, including those pertaining to roadway safety, have primarily been grounded in a reductionist paradigm. As the name implies, reductionism is characterized by its theoretical assumptions regarding the value of reducing complicated and complex phenomena into component parts. In contrast to holism, which focuses on viewing phenomena holistically, reductionism is underpinned by theoretical assumptions that phenomena can be understood by investigating component parts in isolation, which can then be aggregated to provide a comprehensive understanding of the whole [32, 33]. As a paradigm, the reductionist perspective guides theory and methodology and has concurrent implications for both occupational roadway safety research and action.

Conventional Theory in Occupational Roadway Safety

Reductionism has been the dominant theoretical perspective in occupational roadway safety research [28], as the bulk of these efforts have been component-focused and have sought to explicate individual cause-and-effect relationships [28, 30]. For example, organizations typically implement an OHS management system to reduce roadway accidents, which has risk assessment as its foundation [34]. Risk assessment is focused on identifying, analyzing, and evaluating potential safety threats in the workplace, and then to take action to mitigate these risks [34]. Risk management is underpinned by reductionist prinicples in its focus on components – here, individual safety threats – in isolation [35]. Other approaches, such as the concept of "safety culture", superficially address occupational roadway safety from an ecological perspective [29]; yet, these approaches similarly view safety climate from a reductionist perspective [34]. Occupational roadway safety interventions grounded in reductionism are similarly component-focused, and often seek to modify a small number of individual components (especially driver-level factors) to improve safety outcomes [28, 30]. Further, occupational roadway safety policies issued by industry and government are shaped by reductionist perspectives, and occupational roadway safety data collection and monitoring systems are limited to relevant influences as assumed by these perspectives (e.g., driver- and vehicle-related factors), ignoring how structural and other factors and their interactions may influence LHTD and other occupational roadway accidents [28 30 31].

Conventional Methodology in Occupational Roadway Safety

Research methodologies and analyical approaches in occupational roadway safety are based on the underlying assumptions of the reductionism paradigm [28]. These approaches most commonly combine experimental or quasi-experimental research designs with inferential statistics [36] to derive understanding of the causal role of individual component parts. Methodologically, the principal goal is to evaluate focal cause-and-effect relationships by achieving variable isolation. Thus, experimental study designs which provide a high degree of internal validity and experimenter control – such as randomized clinical trials (RCTs) – are preferred [37-39]. Internal validity is the primary concern even in non-RCT designs (e.g., quasi-experimental), which are more common in occupational roadway safety and other OHS research [38].

Analytically, conventional approaches in occupational roadway safety rely heavily on inferential statistics, which assume linearity and independence among causal factors [40]. The general linear model broadly underlies statistical modeling and is grounded by a number of assumptions, including fixed entities with variable attributes and monotonic causal flow [41]. Statistical modeling approaches, especially regression modeling, assess the relationships between "independent" and "outcome" variables [42] and are designed to impose linearity onto often-nonlinear phenomena through the use of statistical adjustments (e.g., interaction terms) [43]. In other words, they deliberately simplify phenomena under question [39], such as LHTD roadway accidents, in a way that imposes linearity and independence amongst the variables under investigation.

Limitations of Conventional Approaches in Occupational Roadway Safety

Occupational roadway safety efforts grounded in reductionism ignore entrenched knowledge regarding the influence of broader influences, as well as the reciprocity and interactions between factors across levels of influence [28, 31, 44]. As a result, reductionism creates a "blame culture" which neglects underlying meso- and macro-level causal factors (e.g., corporate and federal policies) and focuses primarily on micro-level factors (e.g., LHTD behavior) [28, 44]. This perspective has been indicated as a key barrier in creating powerful change in LHTD roadway accident rates, as drivers act as "red herrings" while broader factors are overlooked [30, 31]. For example, among LHTD the importance of driver-level factors such as sleep quality, sleep duration, sleep disorders, and health status in roadway accidents have been established [45-48]; however, much less is known about the role of broader economic, social, financial, technological, political, and organizational forces, such as federal and corporate policies, work organization characteristics, and new in-vehicle technology (e.g., electronic logging devices) [29, 30], and their interactions. As a result, the body of knowledge in these domains is incomplete, and the understanding of professional driver behaviors only accounts for a relatively small amount of the overall variance in LHTD roadway safety outcomes [35, 49]. In practice, occupational roadway accident investigations are shaped by the "blame culture" induced by the narrow reductionist worldview, typically concluding that human error – usually that of the driver – is the culpit, and rarely look beyond micro-level factors [50].

From a methodological and analytical perspective, characteristics that shape causality in occupational roadway safety, such as interactions, interdependence, and nonlinearity, are deliberately ignored for the sake of internal validity [29]. Similarly, statistical modeling is unable to capture characteristics, such as individual and spatial heterogeneity, interactions, interdependence, feedback, nonlinearity, and emergence [33, 42, 51] which collectively induce occupational roadway accidents. Even more advanced statistical modeling techniques, such as multilevel modeling, are fundamentally limited by the same assumptions as regression modeling and are also incapable of capturing these influences [38, 42, 51]. Especially problematic are the ways in which methodological and analytical techniques in reductionism reciprocally shape how researchers think, theorize, and study safety phenomena [39, 41].

Pragmatically, the dominance of the reductionist paradigm in occupational roadway safety research has constrained action to mitigate roadway accidents. Actions to improve occupational roadway safety that are based solely in reductionism are weakened by an inaccurate and/or incomplete understanding of the underlying forces which induce roadway accidents, which typically leads to ineffective mitigation efforts [28]. Interventions are primarily restricted to addressing individual components, especially those related to drivers or vehicles [28]. These interventions have had often-underwhelming results; for instance, the aforementioned OHS management systems have had debatable effetivness, including those which emphasize newer concepts such as safety culture [34].

The term "policy resistance" describes a phenomenon seen in many intervention contexts where attempts to make a change for the better are ineffective, have unanticipated side-effects, or even exacerbate the very problems they attempt to solve [52]. While well-meaning, these attempts at change typically arise from a reductionist perspective [52], which is unable to account for the dynamic complexity which defines occupational roadway safety systems [49]. This has been seen among OHS managers, who typically adopt a "silo mentality" and attempt to improve the individual components which are believe contribute to occupational roadway accidents (e.g., LHTD training); as a result, they are often ineffective or even unintentionally compound the roadway safety problems they intend to solve [34]. Because of these limitations, it is likely that a paradigm shift away from reductionism, and towards complex systems approaches, is necessary to profoundly advance occupational roadway safety efforts [31].

A SHIFT TOWARDS COMPLEX SYSTEMS THEORY IN OCCUPATIONAL ROADWAY SAFETY

Over the past few decades, occupational roadway safety research has gradually shifted its paradigmatic orientation away from the component-focused reductionist perspectives and toward holistic approaches [53]. As researchers and practitioners have come to appreciate the role of underlying causes and the complexity of the numerous factors which contribute to occupational roadway accidents, complex systems approaches have become increasingly integrated into prevention research and action [53, 54] Although largely untapped [29], it appears that these approaches hold vast potential in explicating and reducing roadway accidents by changing the way occupational roadway safety is thought about, analyzed, and acted upon [29, 49].

Complex systems approaches in occupational roadway safety are somewhat heterogenous in their theoretical, methodological, and analytical characteristics; however, they share an emphasis on factors beyond those stressed in reductionism, especially those structural, systemic factors which induce occupational roadway accident risk [29, 30, 55]. These approaches can provide superior guidance in understanding causes of past accidents, identifying current accident risks, and intervening to reduce accident risks in the future [30, 44, 55]. Complex systems approaches also shift fault away from the "blame culture" targeted at LHTD and other professional drivers and towards finding root causes nested at structural levels [54]. Here, we describe complex systems theory and concepts in occupational roadway safety.

Complex Systems Theory in Occupational Roadway Safety

Although relatively new to occupational roadway safety research, complex systems-based theories have been called for in these domains since the 1980s [54]. While their popularity dramatically increased in the late 1990s, as the shortcomings of reductionist approaches became increasingly evident, their status as a mainstay in occupational roadway safety research is not evident, although certain system concepts are influential [28-30]. Further, the terms "system" or "systems thinking" are often used in occupational roadway safety research without a corresponding utilization of complex systems-based approaches [29, 30].

Complex systems theory has been delineated in multiple ways. In general, complex systems theory describes several key attributes of systems: Components, interrelationships and interdependencies between components, and the purpose of the system [29]. Alternately, complex systems theory may describe systems in terms of their structure (a hierarchy of subsystems and their functions), relationships (interactions between system components and subsystems), and behavior (system outputs, which are goal-driven) [54, 56]. Occupational roadway safety systems are typically conceptualized as consisting of systems-of-systems (SoS), which are arrays of interconnected individual systems (sometimes referred to as subsystems) [57].

Complex systems theory in occupational roadway safety views LHTD accidents as resulting from detrimental relationships, and especially unanticipated interactions, between diverse component parts within the system [30, 31, 53]. These relationships, defined by their interactions and interdependencies across multiple levels of influence and varying temporal scales, generate roadway accidents which are viewed as *emergent behaviors* [30, 54]. In this way, the blame for occupational roadway accidents is shifted away from professional drivers and towards the array of actors which ultimately contribute to these outcomes [30]. Exploring these theoretical perspectives requires research methodologies and analyses which generate holistic understanding of the system which generates occupational roadway accidents, which is necessary to capture and interpret key relationships within the complex system [58]. The knowledge generated from these approaches can transform occupational roadway safety interventions by targeting relationships between components across levels of influence within the system, instead of the components themselves [28, 30].

As suggested by its name, a key concept in complex systems theory is complexity, which refers to the aforementioned interactions and interdependencies between system elements, including subsystems [49]. In complex systems theory, these relationships are coupled in such a way as to obscure causal forces in the system and cause *nonlinear* effects [57, 59]. Because occupational roadway safety has been characterized as being inherently complex, complex systems thinking may be especially relevant in these contexts [31, 44, 59]. The role of time is also prevalent in complex systems theory, which focuses on *dynamic* system functioning. Here, various causal forces operate across different time scales, and cause and effect may be very distant in time (as well as space) and exhibit delays [56, 57, 59]. Together, complex systems theory highlights the *dynamic complexity* of systems, which often shrouds the specific roles of underlying causal forces [59].

In complex systems theory, system elements, including subsystems, continually evolve and adapt over time [44, 57]. These elements are autonomous, have their own goals, and often are in competition with one another in their pursuit of goals; further, as elements change over time, surrounding elements adapt and reciprocate, leading to these elements evolving over time in response to the system around them (i.e., *co-evolution*) [49, 57]. In occupational roadway safety, system elements often are in competition, which can be seen in organizations as trade-offs between roadway accident risk aversion and other competing forces, such as profitability [49]. These responses among system elements constitute *feedbacks* within the system and generate *circular causality* [60-62]. Combined with dynamic forces, and especially time-delayed effects, small evolutionary and adaptative steps can lead to minute changes over time which are not detected, but lead occupational roadway safety systems to "drift into failure" and generate roadway accidents later in time [57]. These instances of drift reflect *critical transitions* (or *tipping points*) and are indicative of the nonlinearity in outcomes that result from dynamic complexity [63].

Finally, as is the case with systems theory, *emergence* is a focal concept in complex systems theory in occupational roadway safety [21, 57]. Here, roadway accidents *emerge* from the dynamic complexity inherent to underlying occupational roadway safety systems [28, 49, 57]. In other words, the accident risk of LHTD is generated by – or *emerges* from – the dynamic complexity within the occupational roadway safety system [49]. Emergence generates outcomes which are often surprising, unpredictable, or uncertain, especially when these phenomena are explored from the reductionist perspective [44]. This is because, theoretically, emergence negates reductionism, as it cannot be predicted based on investigating individual components – or even subsystems – in isolation [57].

Complex systems theory remains chronically underutilized and unexplored in occupational roadway safety research [28, 30]. This may be partly attributed to the relative difficulty, compared to reductionist approaches, of investigating dynamic complexity, which is exacerbated by the sheer number of potentially relevant interacting components [29, 58]. However, to more effectively manage occupational roadway safety, it is necessary to understand the roles of dynamic complexity; nonlinearity; co-evolution, adaptation, feedbacks, and circular causality; emergence; and other complex systems properties – forces which ultimately shape roadway safety and induce roadway accidents [49, 55, 58]. For example, understanding time-delayed effects can lead to efforts to minimize delays (e.g., more rapid feedback for policies or behaviors which increase safety risk) or identify optimal interventions which are more effective in the long run [30 50]. Interventions which support safety-enhancing adaptive behavior among system elements also hold tremendous promise [30].

A SHIFT TOWARDS COMPLEX SYSTEMS METHODOLOGY IN OCCUPATIONAL ROADWAY SAFETY

The methodological and analytical approaches within the reductionist paradigm are inherently incapable of capturing the relevant theoretical and conceptual constructs in complex systems theory. Instead, these theoretical perspectives feature their own tools – grounded in diverse modeling approaches – which enable scientific exporation. In this section, we highlight just a handful of the rapidly-growing repertoire of techniques that can be utilized by researchers, including a special set of these techniques, called computational modeling and simulation, which are especially adept for investigating challenges and failures of complex systems.

Modeling of Occupational Roadway Safety Systems

While not exclusive to complex systems approaches, methodology and analysis in these domains often emphasize modeling. There are many types of modeling approaches, many of which continue to evolve and improve over time [29, 64]. Typically the considerations that go into deciding on a specific modeling approach are the purpose of the model, the availability of data to construct and test the model, and the "end users" who will ultimately use the model (e.g., company safety personnel) [64]. Models are constructed for a number of purposes, which include prediction, experimentation, group learning, decision-making, and conflict resolution [64]. Critically, models are constructed for specific purposes, which means that a model built for one context may not be valuable in other contexts [29].

Model development is typically an iterative process, as models are inherently inaccurate and can nearly always be continually improved [29, 63]. This is a crucial point, as models are deliberate simplifications of reality which can be used to overcome the limitations of stakeholders' "mental models" and meaningfully explore systems [29, 52]. In this sense, they can be extremely valuable, but their limitations need to be explicitly stated and understood by stakeholders to ensure that they are used appropriately [56]. Uncertainty is an inherent concern for any model, especially those that are designed toward more preceise prediction [64]. Adjusting models for uncertainty and establishing their validity can be accomplished in numerous ways, depending on the purpose of the model; for example, this may include establishing model plausibility or replicating time-series data of the phenomenon that is being modeled (i.e., the *reference mode*) [64, 65].

In general, systems modeling approaches in occupational roadway safety have often focused on accident analysis, with some of the more commonly-used techinques being Accimap, Systems-Theoretic Accident Modeling and Processes (STAMP), and Drift into Failure (DIF) [28, 44, 63]. These techniques can shed light on interacting factors across levels of influence – from drivers to federal policies – which contribute to roadway accidents [28]. Overall, many types of systems modeling approaches have, or can be, applied to occupational roadway safety [29, 30]. Modeling approaches that have been applied in these domains include component models, mathematical models, sequence models, and intervention models [29]. These models are usually developed to evaluate roadway accident risks, although they are commonly poorly defined [29]. Regardless, systems modeling approaches hold great potential for understanding and acting upon the underlying systems which induce occupational roadway accidents. Systems-based models tend to be more comprehensive than other approaches to understanding these outcomes, especially with regard to relationships between system elements [29]. However, the superior understanding gleaned from systems modeling can then translate to better decision-making to enhance occupational roadway safety [29, 50].

Modeling of Complex Systems: Computational Modeling and Simulation in Occupational Roadway Safety

Computational modeling and simulation represent a unique category of complex systems modeling approaches. These approaches share characteristics with the aforementioned modeling approaches, including the ability to capture elements of dynamic complexity such as interactions, interdependencies, and multi-level influences. However, these types of approaches offer the distnict advantage of simulation, which are computer-based (*in silico*) platforms which allow for various scenarios to be tested virtually [66]. These provide opportunties for testing countless counterfactuals in a thorough manner not available through conventional experimentation [33, 40, 67]. For example, numerous intervention configurations – many of which may not be testable in reality due to ethical or pragmatic concerns – can be tested across long time horizons within the same simulation model in a matter of seconds [68-70].

As is the case with other modeling approaches, computational modeling and simulation approaches are built for a specific purpose and typically are developed and improved in an iterative manner [29, 63]. Because they are more time- and labor-intensive to construct, these models especially aim for four suitability criteria: Usefulness, adequacy, plausibility, and understandability [29]. One particular challenge is striking an optimal level of detail: Models which are too complex can become difficult to test and understand, while models which are too simple may neglect important parameters which are vital to understanding system behaviors [29, 64]. To ensure trustworthiness in model structure and simulation results, models typically undergo rigorous calibration and testing to ensure their validity [50, 58, 64].

Two of the most common and powerful types of computational modeling and simulation techniques are system dynamics modeling (SDM) and agent-based modeling (ABM). System dynamics models are expressed as ordinary differential equations and use stocks, flows, auxiliary variables, delays, and balancing and reinforcing feedback loops as "building blocks" in model construction [70]. System dynamics models have been used in a wide variety of settings, including multiple contexts in occupational roadway safety [32, 34, 50, 56, 58, 59, 63, 71]. However, they remain untapped in the domain of LHTD roadway safety. Agent-based modeling is relatively newer than SDM [38]. The building blocks in ABM construction are autonomous agents, environments, rules, and networks [64, 72]. In contrast to SDM, ABM function as object-oriented programs, where the objects (i.e., agents) have "memory" that is recorded during the course of a simulation run [38, 72]. As with SDM, ABM has been used in multiple settings, including many contexts in occupational roadway safety; however, ABM has not been utilized in LHTD roadway safety [73-78].

Both SDM and ABM have unique strengths which can be utilized in the context of occupational roadway safety, including among LHTD [79]. SDM is most appropriately used for exploring problems from the aggregate, "top-down" level, as it facilitates the thorough investigation of nonlinear interrelationships among numerous causal factors, particularly through its emphasis on feedback loops [58, 59]. In contrast, ABM is most appropriate for exploring problems from the "bottom-up", as it allows for the incorporation of heterogeneity among agents and environment, as well as adaptation among these elements; additionally, it is especially adept at studying emergence [39, 65, 68]. Both approaches share many strengths as well; for example, both can be used to explore nonlinear phenomena, including critical transitions, and both can be successfully incorporated into participatory research approaches [68, 80, 81]. Finally, SDM and ABM can be combined together, or with other modeling approaches (e.g., discrete event simulation), in the form of hybrid models [67]. Hybrid models can combine the advantages of these approaches, which suggests their great – and, yet, largely untapped – potential in the study of complex systems such as occupational roadway safety [67].

CONCLUSION

Complex systems theory and methodologies constitute promising, yet vastly underappreciated and underutilized, approaches to understanding and significantly reducing persistent LHTD roadway accident rates. However, before these approaches can become commonplace in occupational roadway safety, a paradigm shift must take place towards wholly embracing and incorporating complex systems theoretical and methodological perspectives [28]. A complex systems paradigm – with its theoretical and conceptual grounding and methodological and analytical toolbox of computational modeling and simulation – appears to hold significant potential in transforming occupational roadway safety research and action. While the infusion of a complex systems paradigm into occupational roadway safety is not a panacea for alleviating roadway accidents altogether, it can provide OHS researchers, managers, policy-makers, and other stakeholders with a better understanding of the true nature of the systems which underlie roadway accident risks, which can lead to better decision-making to mitigate these adverse outcomes [28, 50, 51].

Moving Forward: Adopting a Complex Systems Paradigm in Occupational Roadway Safety

Although there has been increased emphasis on complex systems approaches in occupational roadway safety, there are several barriers that likely must be surmounted before such a paradigm shift can take place [30]. For one, occupational safety researchers and professionals need to be willing and open to embrace complex systems approaches and apply them in their own work [28]. This will require support, guidance, and revised data collection systems to gather systems-level data [28, 30, 31, 35]. At the organizational and policy levels, the temptation for addressing single components to improve occupational roadway safety must be resisted in favor of understanding and fixing the interactions and emergent consequeneces among multilevel components across different spatial and temporal scales [35]. To accomplish this, complex systems approaches must achieve buy-in from occupational safety stakeholders, and the unique strengths of these approaches (e.g., simulation modeling) need to be clearly laid out [31]. This is especially important, given the reluctance of stakeholders to reject well-established and understood approaches, such as those grounded in reductionism, in favor of complex systems approaches which are unfamiliar and resource-demanding [28, 54, 56].

While occupational roadway safety, especially among LHTD, was the "proof-of-concept" used here, the value of shifting toward a complex systems paradigm can be found in numerous other domains, both within and outside of OHS. Elements of dynamic complexity can be found across the social, health, and safety sciences, and these approaches have similar potential to transform research and action in other domains just as has been demonstrated here in the context of occupational roadway safety [36, 82]. Unfortunately, the pattern of underappreciation and underutilization of complex systems approaches is true in these other domains as well [36, 82]. Initiating a paradigm shift toward complex systems approaches across these broad fields will require overcoming numerous barriers, but the potential impacts of the innovative and impactful research and action that may follow is profound.

REFERENCES

[1]   Leka, S; Jain, A. *Health impact of psychosocial hazards at work: An overview.* Nottingham, UK: University of Nottingham Institute of Work, Health & Organisations, World Health Organization, 2010.

[2]   Schnall, PL; Dobson, M; Rosskam, E. *Unhealthy work: Causes, consequences, cures.* Amityville, NY: Baywood Publishing Company Inc. 2009.

[3]   Church, TS; Thomas, DM; Tudor-Locke, C; et al. Trends over 5 decades in US occupation-related physical activity and their associations with obesity. *PLoS One,* 2011, 6(5), 1-7.

[4]   Sorensen, G; Landsbergis, P; Hammer, L; et al. Preventing chronic disease in the workplace: A workshop report and recommendations. *Am J Public Health,* 2011, 101(S1), S196-S207.

[5] Luckhaupt, SE; Cohen, MA; Li, J; et al. Prevalence of obesity among US workers and associations with occupational factors. *Am J Prev Med*, 2014, 46(3), 237-48.

[6] Bureau of Labor Statistics. Occupational Injuries/Illnesses and Fatal Injuries Profiles Washington, DC: U.S. Department of Labor; 2016 [Available from: https://data.bls.gov/gqt/ProfileData accessed May 7 2017.

[7] Baicker, K; Cutler, D; Song, Z. Workplace wellness programs can generate savings. *Health Aff (Millwood)*, 2010, 29(2), 304-11. doi: 10.1377/hlthaff.2009.0626.

[8] Leka, S; Kortum, E. A European framework to address psychosocial hazards. *Journal of Occupational Health*, 2008, 50(3), 294-96.

[9] Chapman, LS. *Planning wellness*: Chapman Institute, 2007.

[10] Di Milia, L; Mummery, K. The associaton between job related factors, short sleep and obesity. *Ind Health*, 2009, 47(4), 363-68.

[11] Lemke, M; Apostolopoulos, Y. Health and wellness programs for commercial motor-vehicle drivers: Organizational assessment and new research directions. *Workplace Health Saf*, 2015, 63(2), 71-80. doi: 10.1177/2165079915569740.

[12] *Total Worker Health: Centers for Disease Control and Prevention; 2012* [Available from: http://www.cdc.gov/niosh/TWH/totalhealth.html accessed December 5 2012.

[13] Anderko, L; Roffenbender, JS; Goetzel, RZ; et al. Promoting prevention through the Affordable Care Act: Workplace wellness. *Prev Chronic Dis*, 2012, 9.

[14] Tu. HT; Mayrell, RC. *Employer wellness initiatives grow rapidly, but effectiveness varies widely*. Washington, D.C.: National Institute for Health Care Reform; 2010 [Available from: http://www.nihcr.org/Employer-Wellness-Initiatives.html accessed December 1 2014.

[15] Linnan, L; Bowling, M; Childress, J; et al. Results of the 2004 National Worksite Health Promotion Survey. *Am J Public Health*, 2008, 98(8), 1503-09.

[16] Burton, J. *WHO Healthy Workplace Framework and Model*. World Health Organisation, Geneva, 2010, 12.

[17] Lewis, A; Khanna, V. Is it time to re-examine workplace wellness "get well quick" schemes? *Health Affairs Blog*, 2013.

[18] Silberman, R. Workplace wellness programs: Proven strategy or false positive? *Michigan Journal of Public Affairs*, 2007, 4, 1-8.

[19] Best, A; Moor, G; Holmes, B; et al. Health promotion dissemination and systems thinking: towards an integrative model. *Am J Health Behav*, 2003, 27(Supplement 3), S206-S16.

[20] Chan, S. Complex adaptive systems Cambridge, MA: Massachusetts Institute of Technology; 2001 [Available from: http://web.mit.edu/esd.83/www/notebook/Complex%20Adaptive%20Systems.pdf accessed December 6 2015.

[21] Madey, G; Kaisler, SH. *Computational modeling of social and organizational systems 2008* [Available from: http://www3.nd.edu/~gmadey/Activities/CMSOS-Tutorial.pdf accessed October 25 2015.

[22] Leischow, SJ; Best, A; Trochim, WM; et al. Systems thinking to improve the public's health. *Am J Prev Med*, 2008, 35(2), S196-S203.

[23] Bureau of Labor Statistics. *Occupational outlook handbook: Heavy and tractor-trailer truck drivers*. Washington, DC: US Department of Labor; 2015 [Available from: http://www.bls.gov/ooh/transportation-and-material-moving/heavy-and-tractor-trailer-truck-drivers.htm accessed April 20 2016.

[24] Bureau of Labor Statistics. *Nonfatal occupational injuries and illnesses requiring days away from work, 2015*. Washington, DC: US Department of Labor, 2015.

[25] Smith, SM. Workplace hazards of truck drivers. *Mon Labor Rev*, 2015, 138.

[26] Federal Motor Carrier Safety Administration. *Pocket Guide to Large Truck and Bus Statistics Washington, DC: US Department of Transportation; 2014* [Available from: https://www.fmcsa.dot.gov/sites/fmcsa.dot.gov/files/docs/FMCSA%20Pocket%20Guide%20to%20Large%20Truck%20and%20Bus%20Statistics%20--%20October%202014%20Update%20%282%29.pdf accessed August 25 2016.

[27] Apostolopoulos, Y. *Work organization and the epidemiology of commercial driving: From monocausal to multilevel approaches*. Winston Salem, North Carolina, USA, 2012.

[28] Salmon, PM; McClure, R; Stanton, NA. Road transport in drift? Applying contemporary systems thinking to road safety. *Safety Science*, 2012, 50(9), 1829-38.

[29] Hughes, BP; Newstead, S; Anund, A; et al. A review of models relevant to road safety. *Accid Anal Prev* 2015, 74(Supplement C), 250-70. doi: https://doi.org/10.1016/j.aap.2014.06.003.

[30] Salmon, PM; Lenné, MG. Miles away or just around the corner? Systems thinking in road safety research and practice. *Accid Anal Prev*, 2015, 74, 243-49.

[31] Newnam, S; Goode, N; Salmon, P; et al. Reforming the road freight transportation system using systems thinking: An investigation of Coronial inquests in Australia. *Accid Anal Prev*, 2017, 101, 28-36.

[32] Egilmez, G; Tatari, O. A dynamic modeling approach to highway sustainability: Strategies to reduce overall impact. *Transportation Research Part A: Policy and Practice*, 2012, 46(7), 1086-96.

[33] El-Sayed, AM; Scarborough, P; Seemann, L; et al. Social network analysis and agent-based modeling in social epidemiology. *Epidemiologic Perspectives & Innovations*, 2012, 9(1), 1-10.

[34] Goh, YM; Love, PED; Stagbouer, G; et al. Dynamics of safety performance and culture: A group model building approach. *Accid Anal Prev*, 2012, 48, 118-25.

[35] Goode, N; Salmon, PM; Lenne, MG; et al. Systems thinking applied to safety during manual handling tasks in the transport and storage industry. *Accid Anal Prev*, 2014, 68, 181-91.

[36] Castellani B. Focus: *Complexity and the Failure of Quantitative Social Science: Discover Society; 2014* [Available from: http://discoversociety.org/2014/11/04/focus-complexity-and-the-failure-of-quantitative-social-science/ accessed April 1 2016.

[37] Glass, TA; McAtee, MJ. Behavioral science at the crossroads in public health: Extending horizons, envisioning the future. *Soc Sci Med*, 2006, 62(7), 1650-71.

[38] Luke, DA; Stamatakis, KA. Systems science methods in public health: Dynamics, networks, and agents. *Annu Rev Public Health* 2012;33:357-76.

[39] Auchincloss, AH; Diez Roux, AVD. A new tool for epidemiology: The usefulness of dynamic-agent models in understanding place effects on health. *Am J Epidemiol* 2008;168(1):1-8.

[40] Marshall, BDL; Galea, S. Formalizing the role of agent-based modeling in causal inference and epidemiology. *Am J Epidemiol*, 2015, 181(2), 92-99.

[41] Abbott, A. Transcending general linear reality. *Sociological Theory*, 1988, 6, 169-86.

[42] Galea, S; Hall, C; Kaplan, GA. Social epidemiology and complex system dynamic modelling as applied to health behaviour and drug use research. *International Journal of Drug Policy*, 2009, 20(3), 209-16.

[43] Philippe, P; Mansi, O. Nonlinearity in the epidemiology of complex health and disease processes. *Theor Med Bioeth*, 1998, 19(6), 591-607.

[44] Newnam, S; Goode, N. Do not blame the driver: A systems analysis of the causes of road freight crashes. *Accid Anal Prev*, 2015, 76, 141-51.

[45] Lemke, MK; Apostolopoulos, Y; Hege, A; et al. Understanding the role of sleep quality and sleep duration in commercial driving safety. *Accid Anal Prev*, 2016, 97, 79-86.

[46] Vennelle, M; Engleman, HM; Douglas, NJ. Sleepiness and sleep-related accidents in commercial bus drivers. *Sleep and Breathing*, 2010, 14(1), 39-42.

[47] Smolensky, MH; Di Milia, L; Ohayon, MM; et al. Sleep disorders, medical conditions, and road accident risk. *Accid Anal Prev*, 2011, 43(2), 533-48.

[48] Anderson, JE; Govada, M; Steffen, TK; et al. Obesity is associated with the future risk of heavy truck crashes among newly recruited commercial drivers. *Accid Anal Prev*, 2012, 49(0), 378-84. doi: 10.1016/j.aap.2012.02.018.

[49] Hettinger, LJ; Kirlik, A; Goh, YM; et al. Modelling and simulation of complex sociotechnical systems: Envisioning and analysing work environments. *Ergonomics*, 2015, 58(4), 600-14.

[50] Minami, N; Madnick, S. Using system analysis to improve traffic safety. Cambridge, MA: Massachusetts Institute of Technology, 2010.

[51] Galea, S; Riddle, M; Kaplan, GA. Causal thinking and complex system approaches in epidemiology. *Int J Epidemiol*, 2010, 39(1), 97-106.

[52] Sterman, JD. Sustaining sustainability: Creating a systems science in a fragmented academy and polarized world. In: Weinstein MP, Turner RE, eds. *Sustainability science: The emerging paradigm and the urban environment*. New York, NY: Springer 2012, 21-58.

[53] Branford, K. Seeing the big picture of mishaps: Applying the AcciMap approach to analyze system accidents. *Aviation Psychology and Applied Human Factors*, 2011, 1(1), 31-37.

[54] Underwood, P; Waterson, P. A critical review of the STAMP, FRAM and Accimap systemic accident analysis models. In: Stanton N, ed. *Advances in human aspects of road and rail transportation*. Boca Raton, FL: CRC Press 2012, 385-94.

[55] Marais, K; Saleh, JH; Leveson, NG. Archetypes for organizational safety. *Safety Science*, 2006, 44(7), 565-82.

[56] Goh, YM; Love, PED; Brown, H; et al. Organizational accidents: A systemic model of production versus protection. *Journal of Management Studies*, 2012, 49(1), 52-76.

[57] Harvey, C; Stanton, NA. Safety in System-of-Systems: Ten key challenges. *Safety Science*, 2014, 70, 358-66.

[58] Alirezaei, M; Onat, NC; Tatari, O; et al. The climate change-road safety-economy nexus: A system dynamics approach to understanding complex interdependencies. *Systems*, 2017, 5(6), 1-24.

[59] Goh, YM; Love, PED. Methodological application of system dynamics for evaluating traffic safety policy. *Safety Science*, 2012, 50(7), 1594-605. doi: https://doi.org/10.1016/j.ssci.2012.03.002.

[60] Miller, JH; Page, SE. *Complex adaptive systems: An introduction to computational models of social life*. Princeton, NJ: Princeton University Press 2009.

[61] Milstein, B; Homer, J. *System dynamics simulation in support of obesity prevention decision-making*. Institute of Medicine Committee on an Evidence Framework for Obesity Prevention Decision-Making. Irvine, CA: U.S. Centers for Disease Control and Prevention, 2009.

[62] Grimm, V; Railsback, SF. *Individual-based modeling and ecology*. Princeton: Princeton University Press 2005.

[63] Dulac, N; Owens, B; Leveson, N; et al. *Demonstration of a new dynamic approach to risk analysis for NASA's Constellation program: MIT CSRL final report to the NASA ESMD associate administrator*. Cambridge, MA: Complex Systems Research Laboratory, Massachusetts Institute of Technology, 2007.

[64] Kelly, RA; Jakeman, AJ; Barreteau, O; et al. Selecting among five common modelling approaches for integrated environmental assessment and management. *Environmental Modelling & Software*, 2013, 47(Supplement C), 159-81. doi: https://doi.org/10.1016/j.envsoft.2013.05.005.

[65] Marshall, DA; Burgos-Liz, L; Ijzerman, MJ; et al. Selecting a dynamic simulation modeling method for health care delivery research—Part 2: Report of the ISPOR Dynamic Simulation Modeling Emerging Good Practices Task Force. *Value Health*, 2015, 18(2), 147-60.

[66] Mabry, P. *Systems science: Past, present, and future.* Complex Systems, Health Disparities and Population Health: Building Bridges. Bethesda, MD, 2014.

[67] Osgood, N. *What tools does complex systems modeling provide for understanding population health and health disparities?* Conference on Complex Systems, Health Disparities and Population Health: Building Bridges. Washington, D.C., 2014.

[68] Hammond, RA. Complex systems modeling for obesity research. *Prev Chronic Dis*, 2009, 6(3), 1-10.

[69] Homer, J; Wile, K; Yarnoff, B; et al. Using simulation to compare established and emerging interventions to reduce cardiovascular disease risk in the United States. *Prev Chronic Dis*, 2014, 11(E195), 1-14.

[70] Sterman, JD. *Business dynamics: Systems thinking and modeling for a complex world.* Boston, MA: Irwin/McGraw-Hill 2000.

[71] Kumar, SN; Umadevi, G. *Application of system dynamic simulation modeling in road safety.* 3rd International Conference on Road Safety and Simulation. Indianapolis, IN, 2011.

[72] Wilensky, U; Rand, W. *An introduction to agent-based modeling: Modeling natural, social, and engineered complex systems with NetLogo.* Cambridge, MA: MIT Press 2015.

[73] Bosse, T; Mogles, NM. An agent-based approach for accident analysis in safety critical domains: A case study on a runway incursion incident. *Transactions on Computational Collective Intelligence XVII.* Berlin: Springer 2014, 66-88.

[74] SAFEPED: Agent-based environment for estimating accident risks at the road Black Spots. *Proceedings of the 11th International Conference on Autonomous Agents and Multiagent Systems*-Volume 3; 2012. International Foundation for Autonomous Agents and Multiagent Systems.

[75] Khalesian, M; Delavar, MR; Shiran, GR. A spatio-temporal GIS-based multi agent traffic micro-simulation for identifying the most important accident locations. In: Krek A, Rumor M, Zlatanova S, et al., eds. *Urban and Regional Data Management: UDMS 2009 Annual.* London: Taylor & Francis 2009, 427-38.

[76] Personal efficiency in highway driving: An agent-based model of driving behaviour from a system design viewpoint. *2014 IEEE 27th Canadian Conference on Electrical and Computer Engineering (CCECE)*, 2014, Toronto, ON.

[77] Road safety assessment using bayesian belief networks and agent-based simulation. *IEEE International Conference on Systems, Man and Cybernetics*, 2007, Halifax, NS.

[78] Song, TJ. Agent-based speed management strategy for freeway traffic safety (methodology and evaluation). *Journal of Korean Society of Transportation*, 2011, 29(4), 17-28.

[79] Lemke, MK; Apostolopoulos, Y. Policy, work organization and sleep health and safety of commercial drivers: Introducing a complex systems paradigm. *Journal of Ergonomics*, 2016, 6(1), 152-56. doi: 10.4172/2165-7556.1000151.

[80] Hovmand, PS. *Community based system dynamics*. New York, NY: Springer 2014.

[81] Hassmiller Lich, K; Minyard, K; Niles, R; et al. System dynamics and community health. *Methods for Community Public Health Research: Integrated and Engaged Approaches*, 2014, 129-70.

[82] Andersson, C; Törnberg, A; Törnberg, P. Societal systems: Complex or worse? *Futures*, 2014, 63, 145-57.

In: Focus on Systems Theory Research
Editors: Manuel F. Casanova and Ioan Opris

ISBN: 978-1-53614-561-8
© 2019 Nova Science Publishers, Inc.

Chapter 9

THE PART-SYSTEMS CONTINUUM IN MEDICINE

Patrick Finzer, MD, PhD[*]
Düsseldorf, Germany

ABSTRACT

Reductionism is a powerful concept in science and in the philosophy of science. It claims that nature is hierarchically structured, whereby the lower level can explain the higher one, e.g., molecules can be explained by their constituent atoms. But also in medicine, a reductionist research program has been initiated to reveal the molecular mechanisms of diseases.

Obviously, biological systems are generally open to reductionist explanations, whereby the systems parts explain the whole, resulting in an explanatory hierarchy: from the organism to organs, to tissues, to cells, and finally, to molecules, such as proteins or nucleic acids.

Although diseases can be explained by alterations of their constituents, the explanatory power of this respective level collapses when environmental factors become important in clinical situations, such as infections. Then, new interactions on less fundamental levels generate emergent properties, e.g., interactions of microorganisms with the immune system.

If we consider the development of diseases as the development of emergent system properties, the environment and the systems' self-organization come into account. Emergence claims that the micro-structure cannot explain the properties of the system and has been formulated as an anti-reductionist thesis. We will argue that in medicine and in different clinical situations both positions are the extreme endpoints of a continuum. Reductionism is able to describe diseases in which the parts can explain them, whereas emergentism is relevant when the self-organization of the system, due to new interactions with the environment,-accounts for the development of diseases. Emergent principles induce or maintain those new properties on a clinical level.

---

[*] Corresponding Author Email: finzerp@aol.com.

1. INTRODUCTION

Clinical medicine in most cases asks the question, why a patient becomes ill. Is it due to an infection or an accident? Is it a tumor causing the respective symptoms? It is obvious, that the answer to the 'why' question has serious consequences with respect to the prognosis and therapy.

There are certain forms of disease which can be explained by a chain of consecutive external events that ultimately cause an injury to the body. A paradigmatic example is a traffic accident where a car or a part of the car harms the skin or causes the fracture of bones. Such an event follows physical laws of forces of the collision energy and counterforces of the tissues and the organs.

The biological environment can cause illness as well by infection with microorganisms of different kinds, such as viruses, bacteria or parasites. But if we look more closely at infection patterns in populations epidemiologically, it can be seen that obviously, not everybody who is infected by a pathogenic microorganism becomes ill. On the contrary, in some clinical situations, harmless commensals can become pathogenic and may cause severe infections, e.g., in patients with leukemia or other forms of malignant diseases. This points to a whole and complex system regulating the biological reaction toward microorganisms: the immune system.

The immune system eliminating a microorganism generates a highly complex process, involving specialized cells, mediators, antibodies, etc. In contrast to an accident with a car, infection seems to depend much more on the immune system's concrete state and its specific organization. Whereas there is a clear correlation between the forces of the object hitting the body and the effects observed, e.g., a fracture, the immune system may react individually and dependent also on external factors, such as nutrition, climate or seasons. Therefore, the relation between microorganism exposure and specific reactions may not be in a linear relation. It would be complex, non-linear and even chaotic (Coffey, 1998).

However, in many cases, a reason for the appearance of a disease cannot be given, neither physically nor biologically. For example, why a cancer arises in one patient and not in another cannot be answered in most cases. This may be the case in so-called complex diseases in general, to which, besides cancer, heart diseases, diabetes, asthma or Parkinson belong. For the most part they seem to be caused by a combination of genetic, environmental and lifestyle factors. In some cases risk-factors have been identified, but causal models are still missing.

At least in complex diseases, the 'why' question cannot be answered in a causal manner. Therefore, it is worth addressing a different question: how do we become ill? This question can be addressed also in complex diseases and may give deeper insights relevant in research and clinical practice (Finzer, 2017).

2. REDUCTIONISM VERSUS EMERGENTISM

Reductionism is a powerful concept in science and in the philosophy of science. It claims that nature is hierarchically structured, whereby the lower level can explain the higher one, e.g., molecules can be explained by their constituting atoms. This approach is based on the assumption that the world consists of parts, and explanation therefore ends at the sub-atomic level of elementary particles (Oppenheim and Putnam, 1958). Although a reduction of a complex biological system to atoms or even elementary particles has not been successful up to now - which is finally a solution to the Schrödinger equation. However, micro-reductions in particular disciplines have been shown to be possible. The most common example is the reduction of classical thermodynamics to statistical mechanics - in this case, for example, the temperature of an ideal gas can be explained by the mean kinetic energy of its molecules (Carrier and Finzer, 2006). The aim of these reductions was to unify the sciences by deducing them from the laws and theory of physics together with contingent boundary conditions, and suitable correspondence principles translating concepts from higher-level into physics (Schurz, 2014).

Obviously, biological systems are generally open to reductionist explanations, whereby the system's parts explain the whole, together with anatomical and physiological knowledge. This results in an explanatory hierarchy: from the organism to organs, to tissues, to cells and finally to molecules, such as proteins or nucleic acids. Against this background medicine has implemented an enormous reductionist research program to reveal the molecular mechanisms of diseases. Nowadays, biomedical research tries to identify a part of the body, which can be causally linked to a biochemical mechanism of the disease under investigation (Finzer, 2017). This search starts on the level of macroscopic alterations of organs and goes to the microscopic tissues and cells. It ideally ends at the molecular level, which consists of macromolecular proteins, metabolic intermediates or genes. It groups phenomena into different hierarchical levels, such as organs, tissues, cells, etc., and tries to explain the so-called higher level by the next lower one (micro-reduction). In consequence, drug development, for example, searches for new therapeutic molecules by establishing binding assays in which the candidate substance interferes with a particular molecule or molecular mechanism. Along these lines, medical laboratories perform chemical analyses to enable or confirm diagnoses or to follow-up therapeutic interventions; in the meantime, most of the diagnoses in modern medicine are confirmed by lab analyses, which make this research program also practically a success story.

Despite these paradigmatic examples, reductionism faces serious problems: the extreme complexity in biology limits the reductionist approach significantly. Complexity increases enormously, even from atoms to molecules, which enables reductions only by assuming radical simplifications (Schurz, 2014). To handle complexity in sciences, empirical system laws are frequently established. In particular, the deduction of laws from fundamental sciences is strongly challenged by the fact that the different disciplines - such as biology, psychology, etc. - have discovered their own laws (Schurz, 2014). In medicine and biological sciences, concepts of reduction are therefore currently limited to biochemistry, cell biology or genetics: It addresses the question as to whether an organism or a disease can be explained by specific parts of the body, e.g., molecules, tissues or organs, and their alterations. Whether a reduction is successful can only be assessed practically; for example, if a treatment based on specific molecular interaction can improve the clinical situation of a patient.

Usually, emergence has been established as an antithesis to reductions. The classic concept has been provided by C. D. Broad, who stated that the properties of a whole cannot be deduced from the knowledge of their constituent parts in isolation or in less complex or simpler wholes (Broad, 1925). This notion will limit the power of reductions, since in biomedical research genes under investigation can be expressed in simpler systems, e.g., a human gene can be transferred into mice, yeast or other cells to be studied.

A distinction between different notions of emergence has to be mentioned. In its strong version, emergence describes a gap between scientific explanations, which cannot be bridged. The most relevant examples are the perception of sensory stimuli, such as colors or other qualities, and the physico-biological state of the brain: the mental representation of these qualities cannot be reduced to the brain or the function of the brain.

From examples like these, a vitalistic force has been postulated to govern biological processes. Rejection of vitalism has often undermined emergentism as being only a lack of current scientific understanding of reducible problems. However, Broad's notion of emergentism can be reformulated as a strong version such that properties of the system cannot be deduced from the behavior of parts, together with a most complete knowledge of the arrangement of the system's parts and the properties they have in isolation or in other less complex systems (Boogerd et al., 2005)

The weak version of emergentism accepts physicalism and the notion that the parts are determining the microstructure of the system; however, this does not entail the notion that the system's properties can be fully reduced to it (by micro-reduction - Schurz, p. 48). In contrast, complex systems such as biological organisms are able to reorganize their constituent parts, e.g., due to changes in environmental conditions: The system rearranges the parts to new properties (organizational properties). A dynamic process can be induced and maintained, which is in principle independent of the corresponding microstructure and therefore cannot be understood fully by micro-reduction.

The questions of reductionism and emergentism can be discussed fruitfully in the context of medical practice and research. Can diseases be understood as system properties or can they be reduced fully to their underlying microstructure. Or, in other words, is the development of diseases reducible to the behavior and function of their parts or do diseases appear as emergent properties of the system and as a reorganization of the constituent parts of the organism?

From this distinction complete different clinical foci arise - either on the parts of the body or on the system and its behavior: diseases and their development can either be explained, diagnosed and treated with regard to the parts of the body or, in contrast, by understanding the system and its organizational properties.

3. REDUCTIONIST RESEARCH PROGRAM IN MEDICINE

The subjects of medicine are the diagnosis and therapy of diseases (Scully, 2004). Cystic fibrosis (CF), for example, is a disease whose molecular basis was successfully revealed in recent years. It is worth considering first the symptoms and the clinical picture of disease, like a physician.

CF normally emerges during early childhood. In the initial course of the disease, intestinal symptoms appear, such as ileus, fatty stool and poor growth, together with difficulty breathing and coughing up sputum. In the further progress, bronchitis and lung infections are frequent symptoms, together with sinus infection.

According to the symptoms, alterations of organs and tissues can be found. Often, the pancreas is irreversibly damaged, often with painful inflammation (pancreatitis), as is the architecture of the lung with bronchiectasis (Davies, 2007).

Patho-physiologically, mucus of the pancreas is thickened and causes occlusion of ducts, delivering digesting enzymes to the gut, which causes poor growth and weight gain in infants. In the airways, thickened mucus reduces mucociliar clearance of the bronchi, which causes coughing and dyspnoe (Tang et al., 2014).

A molecular basis of CF has now been identified for most cases. Mutations in a gene encoding for the cystic fibrosis transmembrane conductance regulator (CFTR) can be found in more than 70% of cases - the corresponding protein is involved in the function of an ion channel regulating liquid volume through chloride secretion and inhibition of sodium absorption (Davis et al., 2007). Therefore, production of mucus, or airway-surface liquid, in cystic fibrosis is altered, leading to flaws in mucociliary transport and other lung-protection mechanisms (Stoltz et al., 2015).

As shown for the above levels, clinical findings can be explained by alterations of particular organs, both on a macroscopic and a microscopic level. The cough, for example, can be explained by thickened mucus and alterations of the airway architecture. Finally, on a protein gene level, a dysfunction of the mucus secretion has been described, which again explains microscopic, macroscopic and clinical findings, together with the anatomical and physiological conditions. Therefore, a successful reduction can be reconstructed from clinical to molecular level.

In this context, we will not argue that the gene is a reducing level, since genetic reductionism fails for general reasons (Carrier and Finzer, 2006). Therefore, we consider the gene as a structure, which corresponds to a protein, not at a more fundamental level. In addition, the correspondence between gene and protein allows the screening of unborn or newborn infants for genetic mutations using highly sensitive gene-based methodological assays, which is more sensitive than screening for proteins.

Subsequent Explanations on Reductive Level Fail

The reduction can be confirmed practically, since newborn babies can be diagnosed with CF by performing a DNA test. If a mutation of the CFTR-gene is detected in this procedure, the baby will develop CF, although the newborn baby may be clinically and phenotypically healthy. This reductive level - the DNA-protein-level - provides a prognosis as to whether the disease will become apparent or not.

Interestingly, external factors such as second-hand smoke exposure, air pollution or ambient temperature have been shown to have an impact on lung function in CF patients (Collaco et al., 2014). The situation of patients is profoundly impaired when infections of the airways and the lung occur: Difficulties breathing and dyspnoe increase, and infection with fever appears, which may lead to a highly critical clinical situation for the patient. Initially, more common bacteria are associated with infections. At a later stage, bacteria which are known to grow in water become dangerous, such as *P. aeruginosa* or *B. cepacia*. Those microorganisms colonize und infect the lung and may cause chronic recurrent infections (Tang et al., 2014).

It is important to note that an unequivocal reduction of this highly dangerous clinical situation to the micro-structure of the system cannot be performed, since microorganisms are not constituents of the human organism. They are clearly external, having their own genome, metabolism and reproduction. In addition, they are not stably linked with the organism. They can be a purely transient colonization or even absent during a patient's lifetime. Therefore, the microbiome and the effects it induces are clearly emergent to the human system: the attempt to reduce this clinical situation to the parts of the human body fails. As a consequence, the reduction to the molecular DNA-protein-level loses explanatory and practical power, when the disease develops clinical problems such as severe and recurrent infections.

CFTR-Mutations Favor Growth of Microorganisms

In recent years, progress has been made to work out the molecular bases of inflammation in CF airways, aiming to bridge the gap between the molecular level of CFTR-mutation and infection with particular microorganisms.

In the lung of CF patients, typically high levels of infiltrating immune cells such as neutrophils, but also inflammatory mediators such as cytokines, can be found (Tang et al., 2014). Interestingly, it has been reported that pulmonary inflammation in CF patients was observed early after birth, although common pathogens such as *P. aeruginosa* were not detectable (Khan et al., 1995). This points to a direct role of CFTR in pulmonary inflammation. And indeed, neutrophils have been shown to express the CFTR-protein, and that knock-down of this expression impairs the antimicrobial activities of those immune cells (Rieber et al., 2014). In addition, CFTR is thought to play a role in inflammatory cytokine production via activation of the nuclear transcription factor NF-kB (Tang et al., 2014). Therefore, the molecular basis of CF can explain why microorganisms find favorable growth conditions in the airways of the lung.

Alterations of the Microbial Pathogens

But besides the growth conditions of microorganisms, a second effect plays a role, which takes place on the level of the microbial pathogens themselves. Airways of infants with CF appear normal early after birth, but soon become infected. One of the first pathogens is *S. aureus*. During chronic infection, a phenotypic conversion of these bacteria can be observed, especially the formation of so-called small colony variants (Tang et al., 2014). *P. aeruginosa* appears later in CF patients and also undergoes phenotypic conversion. During this stage, they gain resistance to host antimicrobial peptides and evasion of host recognition and phagocytosis (Tang et al., 2014). These pathogens cause sustained inflammatory responses resulting in impaired pulmonary function.

Although CFTR is involved in many processes leading to immune dysfunction, it cannot explain the role of the pathogens in morbidity and death in CF patients. The molecular level of the disease - mutation of the CFTR-gene - can no longer explain the inflammation triggered by microorganisms colonizing the airways. Therefore, the explanatory power of the molecular level of the host collapses and fails to explain the appearance of recurrent and severe lung infection in CF patients.

Biofilms and Inflammation

One additional problem occurs during lung infections in CF patients. That is the clinical failure or impaired effects of antibiotic agents. Interestingly, this may happen although pathogenic bacteria have been tested sensitive or intermediate sensitive in the diagnostic laboratory.

The reason for this is, that the microorganisms not only interfere with the mucus and the epithelial level of the airways as well as the cells of the immune system, but in addition, they themselves build a complex system of interference. This phenomenon can be considered a complex system - the so-called biofilms.

Bacteria were isolated in pure culture on artificial media in the routine settings of laboratory testing. However, it became obvious that sessile cells differ significantly from their floating (planktonic) counterparts (Donlan and Costerton, 2002). It turned out that bacteria under particular conditions tend to grow in matrix-enclosed biofilms, themselves structurally and dynamically complex biological systems: These are surface-associated microbial communities, surrounded by an extracellular polymeric substance matrix produced on their own (Hall-Stoodley et al., 2004; Hall-Stoodley and Stoodley, 2009). This agglomeration shows intrinsic resistance to antibiotics and mechanisms of host defense (Donlan and Costerton, 2002). *P. aeruginosa* found in sputum grows in biofilms within the bronchi and lungs of CF patients (Hall-Stoodley et al., 2004).

In the context of our discussion, the formation of biofilms on the mucus of patients with CF is obviously an emergent phenomenon, extremely important for the clinical situation of severe and recurrent infections. The response to antibiotics cannot, in this case, be deduced from testing planktonic growing bacteria in the microbiological laboratory. Especially since the concrete composition of bacterial species within the biofilm is often unknown.

Broadening the Reduction Basis

The fact that the molecular level of the body cannot explain the clinical situation of recurrent infections in CF does not mean, that no reduction is possible at all. On the contrary, one could argue that the bacteria colonizing the body and building biofilms may be conceived as parts of the "patho-system" and therefore as parts of the underlying patho-mechanism of the disease: The microorganisms contribute significantly to many physiological functions of the body, e.g., digestion of food in the gut. Then, reduction would be intact again and the clinical situation would be explainable by the micro-level and the (micro)organisms involved.

From a mechanistic point of view, the clinical situation can be reduced to the specific parts involved. But with respect to the initial reduced level - mutated transporter molecule in the airways – the severe complications in patients suffering from CF - such as pneumonia - point clearly to additional factors, such as air pollution or environmental microorganisms. As a conclusion, although CF is a disease which can be defined on a molecular level, the emergent clinical situations are strongly dependent on external factors.

External Factors in Complex Diseases

The situation in other complex diseases can be analog (Finzer, 2017). Plenty of different cancer types have been described, and it is believed that they are based on genetic alterations. Today, hereditary cancers are known which show higher frequency in particular families and which can, in some cases, be defined on a molecular level, e.g., familial adenomatous polyposis (FAP). FAP is a genetic condition, passed from generation to generation. Patients develop intestinal polyps, which can transform into colon cancer. The APC(adenomatous polyposis coli)-gene is linked to this disease.

However, the vast majority of colon cancers appears sporadic. Only a transformation model involving many different genes has been established (Fearon and Vogelstein, 1990), although in most other cancers no clear gene basis has been found at all.

In addition, the current literature points to the importance of external risk factors in the development of cancer: little physical exercise, low fruit and vegetable intake, high body mass index, alcohol use and smoking (Murray and Lopez, 2013). This stresses the importance of environmental factors that strongly impact the organism.

But a significant burden of cancer comes from infection, mainly by viruses such as hepatitis or herpes viruses, but also from bacteria (e.g., *H. pylor*) or parasites such as Schistosoma (Kuper et al., 2000). Similar to the CF situation, an external microorganism can be casually linked to these forms of infection-related cancer and therefore these diseases cannot be explained by the parts of the body alone. Per definition, the development of cancer in these cases is an emergent property of the organism. But from a mechanistic point of view, as in the case of CF, the parts relevant to the cancer can be identified, which restores a reduction and keeps it intact on a mechanistic level. Nevertheless, it additionally points to the impact of environmental factors.

Furthermore, it becomes evident that cancer development goes along with the morphological reorganization of particular tissues of the body: new blood vessels can be built and the histologically distinguishable formation of cancer can be found - a new and emergent microscopic and macroscopic part of the body. Inflammation is a major step in the development of many cancers, which causes migration of immune cells, secretion of mediators of inflammation and, in the long run, chronic changes in the architecture of the corresponding tissue (Philip et al., 2004). In addition, interaction of cells transforming into tumor cells and of components of the immune system is considered to be an important step toward the development of cancer (Hanahan and Weinberg, 2000; Finzer et al., 2000). These steps of inflammation and change in tissue architecture can be seen as new properties of the organism.

4. GENERAL APPEARANCE OF EMERGENCE

Having discussed the above biomedical research examples, the value of a reductionist explanation cannot be denied: the initial clinical situation of CF can be deduced from disturbance at the molecular level - namely the dysfunction of the CFTR-molecule. Together with knowledge of the physiological - the role of mucus and its function in airway clearance - and the anatomic situation of the bronchi and the pancreatic ductus, the initial clinical symptoms of patients suffering from CF can be explained. Although from a formalistic point of view, the relevant microorganisms are not part of the body, they can explain the pathological basis of the disease. Even though the complexity of diseases such as cancer is also extremely high, they are generally accessible to reductionist research and explanation (Finzer, 2003; Finzer, 2014).

However, with respect to the development of diseases or the instability of clinical situations, emergence plays a crucial role. The organism generates a new property - namely a symptom or a disease – by interfering with external factors, such as microorganisms. In the first example, the system generates chronic infections and inflammation by reacting to bacteria and biofilms in altered airway mucus; in the second example, infection with an oncogenic microorganism finally leads to the development of cancer. In both cases, the molecular parts of the body, the immune system and tissues and organs involved cannot fully explain the development of the discussed diseases: the microorganisms, together with external factors, such as dietary factors, etc., contribute as well.

Systems theory provides a framework to understand the generation of new properties (Mazzocchi, 2008). Biological systems are characterized by a flow-through of material and energy from their environment. With this flow, they are able to rearrange themselves and change the organization of their parts. This may finally result in new properties of the system, independent of the properties of the isolated parts (Misteli, 2001). The development of these new properties corresponds to what we call emergence.

The appearance of biofilms is an example of emergence within the environmental factors, which also show change in organization of the parts: microorganisms organize themselves in a self-produced matrix, which again consists of different chemical and biological compounds. They gain new properties such as resistance to antibiotic agents. In this case, cultivation and analysis of bacteria on and in classic agar cannot explain the appearance of antibiotic resistance of this kind. Emergence can therefore be characterized as "horizontal" since the systems' property cannot be deduced from the property of their constituents in isolation or in more simple systems (Boogerd et al., 2005).

In analogy, a "vertical" emergence indicates that systemic properties cannot be deduced from the properties of the systems' parts: the micro-structural base - together with the relevant laws - are not able to explain the higher-level properties (Boogerd et al., 2005). This can be assumed in cancer development induced by chronic inflammation: Infective agents together with external factors, such as food rich in calories, favor the appearance of inflammation in the organism. Mutations within this milieu can inactivate growth control, which finally allow particular cells to proliferate and become the nucleus of a tumor (Hanahan and Weinberg, 2000).

Emergent Principles

As shown in the case of CF, some diseases can be explained by alterations of their constituents. However, the explanatory power of this respective level collapses when environmental factors become important in clinical situations, such as infections. Then, new interactions on less fundamental levels generate emergent properties, e.g., interaction of microorganisms with the immune systems.

If we consider the clinical development of diseases as the development of an emergent system property, the environment and the systems' self-organization come into account. There are obviously shifts from one level to another and the establishment of new interactions (Finzer, 2017): In the cases mentioned, microorganisms interact with the immune system, which correlates clinically with the appearance of systematic signs of inflammation. For example, the shift from dysregulated production of saliva favoring the growth conditions for microorganisms to new interaction of microorganisms with the immune system. In addition, the shift of microorganisms evolving to more resistant variants within the airways of CF patients can be observed. Shifts appear also when the disease or particular symptoms perpetuate: For example, when inflammation turns from an acute into a chronic or recurrent form. Such a shift is not only relevant in CF, but also in the development of cancer: in this case, chronic inflammation seems to be a permissive environment for the emergence of malignant tumor cells (Mueller and Fusenig, 2004).

These shifts could be caused by accidental processes finally creating new and emergent system properties. However, since they can be observed in most CF patients, it is also conceivable that those shifts are governed actively, either by intrinsic mechanisms or by external factors influencing the organism or relevant sub-systems. Hence an active shift from one property of the system to another by generating new interactive relationships or new level-interactions can be called emergent principles (Finzer, 2017). They can be presented as clinical symptoms when the system properties become phenotypically apparent in the context of a disease.

5. System and Its Parts – Implications in Medicine

Interestingly, the development of diseases or clinical situations can be explained in two ways: On the one hand, some diseases are open to reductionist explanations, e.g., cystic fibrosis by the molecular setting - together with anatomical and physiological knowledge. Accordingly, some diseases can also be explained by the parts of the body, for example, a hereditary mutation in FAP patients, which causes intestinal symptoms over time. On the other hand, the development of other diseases and many dynamic clinical situations may be defined as new and emergent system properties. The environment - pollution, nutrition, noxii, microorganisms, etc. - allows or even forces the systems to reorganize. Therefore, we can call a clinical situation reducible to the parts of the body mereologic. If the development of a disease can be explained as a reorganization of the system, it can be considered emergent.

Organisms are in general open to reductionist explanations. But complexity, in contrast, is a strong practical limitation since the body consists of countless parts and interactions. Empirical system laws therefore help to bridge confusion generated by complexity. The assessment of clinical situations often relies on those laws; for example, if in case of doubt a particular diagnosis is favored due to knowledge of the distribution and frequency of particular diseases within the population.

At least the following conclusions can be drawn from these considerations. First, some diseases or clinical situations are mainly determined by the parts of the system, e.g., a monogenic hereditary syndrome; others are more open to be modulated by the environment, for example, complex diseases such as cancer. Second, in some clinical situations, the biological systems seem resistant to external factors, e.g., exposure to *P. aeruginosa* in healthy people or even patients at an early stage of CF. Normal dosages of exposure to these bacteria causes no health-compromising effects, whereas at a later stage of CF, the airways can be highly colonized or even infected by these microorganisms, which induces chronic infections. Third, biological systems are able to create new and unpredictable states by reorganizing their constituents.

Therefore, both positions are the extreme end-points of a continuum in medicine: Reductionism is able to describe diseases in which the parts can explain them, whereas emergentism is relevant when the self-organization of the system, due to new interactions with the environment, accounts for the development of diseases and clinical situations. Mechanisms which induce or maintain a shift to new properties on a clinical level can consequently be called emergent principles.

To understand the system's ability of self-organization and the environmental influences would allow to improve the management of diseases. Keys to this understanding could be the system biology and environmental medicine. The identification and analysis of emergent principles would be extremely worthwhile, to better understand the possible clinical outcomes of particular clinical situations. These principles may help to reduce complexity in the understanding of situations, and to interfere with them may advance therapy.

Life has been defined as an organizational phenomenon: amino acids, nucleic acids and other molecules become "alive" when organized in a specific way. This may explain why emergence is so often relevant in medicine. For example, in oncology, most tumors emerge spontaneously; in addition, the burden of complex or even functional diseases is high compared to monogenic syndromes. Therefore, it is very likely that emergence is of utmost importance, with a great impact on medicine, namely the dynamics of clinical situations or the field of preventive medicine. In any case, our considerations suggest that monocausal explanations for diseases are extremely rare. For the majority of diseases, medicine needs to respect the complexity, for their diagnostic process as well as for their therapy and prognosis.

REFERENCES

Boogerd, F. C., Bruggemann, F. J., Richardson, R. C. Stephan, A., and Westerhoff, H. V. Emergence and its Place in Nature: A Case Study of Biochemical Networks. *Synthese,* 145, 131 – 164. 2005.

Broad, C. D. *The Minde and Its Place in Nature.* Trubner & Co, London. 1925.

Collaco, J. M., Blackman, S. M., Raraigh, K. S., Morrow, C. B., Cutting, G. R. and Paranjape, S. M. Self-reported exercise and longitudinal outcomes in cystic fibrosis: a retrospective cohort study. *BMC Pulmonary Medicine.* 14, 159. 2014.

Carrier, M and Finzer, P. Explanatory Loops and the Limits of Genetic Reductionism. *International Studies in the Philosophy of Science.* 20 (3), 267 – 283. 2006.

Coffey, D. S. Self-organization, complexity and chaos: The new biology for medicine. *Nat. Med.,* 4 (8), 882 – 885. 1998.

Davies, J. C., Alton, W. W. F. W. and Bush, A. Cystic fibrosis. *BMI,* 335, 1255 – 1259. 2007.

Donlan, R. M. and Costerton J. W. Biofilms: Survival Mechanisms of Clinically Relevant Microorganisms. *Clinical Microbiology Reviews,* 15 (2), 167 – 193. 2002.

Fearon, E. R. and Vogelstein, B. A genetic model for colorectal tumorgenesis. *Cell,* 61, 759 – 767. 1990.

Finzer, P. *Zum Verständnis biologischer Systeme. Reduktionen in Biologie und Biomedizin.* [Understanding of biological systems. Reductionism in biology and biomedicine.] Centaurus Verlag Herbolzheim. 2003.

Finzer, P. *Systemorganisation und Emergenz in der Medizin. Wie wir krank werden.* [Systems organization and emergence in medicine. How we become ill.] Springer Spektrum. 2014.

Finzer, P. How we become ill. *EMBO reports,* 18 (4), 515 – 518. 2017.

Finzer, P., Soto, U., Delius, H., Patzelt, A., Coy, J. F., Poustka, A., zur Hausen, H. and Rösl, F. Differential transcriptional regulation of the monocyte-chemoattractant protein-1 (MCP-1) gene in tumorigenic and non-tumorigenic HPV 18 positive cells: The role of the chromatin structure and AP-1 composition. *Oncogene,* 19, 3235 – 3244. 2000.

Hall-Stoodley L., Costerton J. W. and Stoodley, P. Bacterial Biofilms: From the Natural Environment to Infectious Diseases. *Nature Reviews Microbiology,* 2, 95 – 107, 2004.

Hall-Stoodley, L. and Stoodley, P. Evolving concepts in biofilm infections. *Cellular Microbiology,* 11(*l*), 1034 – 1043. 2009.

Hanahan, D. and Weinberg, R. A. The hallmarks of cancer. *Cell,* 100, 57 – 70. 2000.

Khan, T. Z., Wagener, J. S., Bost, T., Martinez, J., Accurso, F. J., Riches, D. W. Early pulmonary inflammation in infants with cystic fibrosis. *Am J. Respir. Crit. Care Med,* 151, 1075 – 1082. 1995.

Kuper, H., Adami, H.-O. and Trichopoulos, D. Infections as a major preventable cause of human cancer. *J. Int. Med.,* 248, 171 – 183. 2000.

Mazzocchi, F. Complexity in biology. *EMBO reports,* 9 (1), 10 – 14. 2008.

Mueller, M. M. and Fusenig, N. E. Friends or foes – bipolar effect of the tumour stroma in cancer. *Nat. Reviews Cancer,* 4, 839 – 849. 2004.

Murray, C. J. L. and Lopez, A. D. Measuring the Global Burden of Disease. *N Engl J Med,* 369 (5), 448 – 457. 2013.

Misteli, T. The concept of self-organization in cellular architecture. *The Journal of Cell Biology,* 155 (2), 181 – 185. 2001.

Oppenheim, P. and Putnam, H. Unity of science as a working hypothesis. In: H. Feigl, M. Scriven and G. Maxwell (Hrsg.), *Minnesota Studies in the Philosophy of Science. Vol. II. Concepts, Theories, and the Mind-Body Problem* (S. 3 – 36). Minneapolis: University of Minnesota Press. 1958.

Philip, M., Rowley, D. A. and Schreiber, H. Inflammation as a tumor promoter in cancer induction. *Seminars in Cancer Biology,* 14, 433 – 439. 2004.

Rieber, N., Hector, A., Carevic, M. and Hartl, D. Current concepts of immune dysregulation in cystic fibrosis. *The international journal of biochemistry & cell biology,* 52, 108 – 112. 2014.

Schurz, G. Philosophy of Science. A unified approach. Routledge, New York and London. 2014.

Scully, J. L. *What is a disease? EMBO reports,* 5, 7, 650 – 653. 2004.

Stoltz, D. A., Meyerholz, D. K. and Welsh, M. J. Origins of Cystic Fibrosis Lung Disease. *N. Engl. J. Med.,* 372, 351 – 362. 2015.

Tang, N. C., Turvey, S. E., Alves, M. P., Regamey, N., Tümmler, B. and Hartl, D. Current concepts: host-pathogen interactions in cystic fibrosis airways disease. *Eur. Respir. Rev.,* 23, 320 – 332. 2014.

In: Focus on Systems Theory Research
Editors: Manuel F. Casanova and Ioan Opris

ISBN: 978-1-53614-561-8
© 2019 Nova Science Publishers, Inc.

Chapter 10

SYSTEMS THEORY AND THE CEREBRAL CORTEX

Manuel F. Casanova, MD[1,2,], Ioan Opris, PhD[3], Estate M. Sokhadze, PhD[1] and Emily L. Casanova, PhD[1]*

[1]Department of Biomedical Sciences,
University of South Carolina School of Medicine, Greenville, SC, US
[2]Department of Pediatrics, Greenville Health System, SC, US
[3]University of Miami Miller School of Medicine, FL, US

ABSTRACT

The brain is a complex system whose functionality reflects the hierarchical arrangement of its components. Evolution has tinkered with the arrangement of its parts so as to lay newer constructs on top of atavistic anatomical elements. The largest region of the mammalian brain is the cerebral cortex. Its development is based on self-organization accrued to the migration of periventricular stem cells along a gliophilic pathway leading to the cerebral plate. The end result is a vertical or radial structure called the minicolumn. Researchers acknowledge the minicolumn as a unit of information processing and a source of emergent cognitive operations. The basic symmetry of the minicolumns provides for the preservation of several morphometric quantitites (e.g., changes in cell size *vs.* minicolumnar width, translation of cells along the central axis of the minicolumns) which constrain how the brain develops, ages and evolves.

---

[*] Corresponding Author: Manuel F. Casanova, MD, Department of Pediatrics, Section of Developmental Behavioral Pediatrics, 200 Patewood Drive, Building A, Suite A200, Greenville, SC 29615.

INTRODUCTION

Systems theory refers to the body of work that attempts to understand and explain how things come together in order to form parts of a whole. In terms of living organisms, it defines how different organs are physiologically and anatomically related together so as to form the musculoskeletal, circulatory, digestive, endocrine, integumentary, urinary, lymphatic, immune, respiratory, nervous and reproductive systems. The focus of systems theory on biology, specially living organisms, stems from Karl Ludwig von Bertalanffy (1902-1972), one of the most important theoretical biologists of 20th century. Von Bertalanffy was one of the originators of general system theory which posits the interdependence of all phenomena whether they are physical, biological, or belong to the social sciences.

Von Bertalanffy proposed that human beings were not merely robots acting to satisfy their biological needs, but rather, active personality systems creating their own universe. This point of view was borne as a reaction against the reductionistic ways of thinking that permeate science and occasionally are taken to an extreme. Indeed, in The Astonishing Hypothesis, a book by Nobelist Francis Crick, there is an attempt to establish the basis of consciousness by asserting that, "Y*ou, your joys and your sorrows, your memories and your ambitions, your sense of personal identity and free will, are in fact no more than the behaviour of a vast assembly of nerve cells and their associated molecules"* (Crick, 1994). It has been argued that the words used in Crick's hypothesis, "no more than", deny the actual existence of consciousness which he was trying to investigate (http://www.consciousentities.com/crick.htm). Crick was a major proponent of the reductionist approach which proved widely successful in the early days of molecular biology but has otherwise underestimated the complexity of biological systems (Van Regenmortel, 2004).

Reductionism stands opposite to systems theory in its attempts to understand the whole of reality by breaking it apart and focusing on its components. For systems where its elements have the holistic properties of the whole, this approach may provide for significant breakthroughs. In studying the liver, for example, you can gain a lot of knowledge by studying its main parenchymal cell, the hepatocyte. These cells, make 70-85% of the liver's mass, and mirror the liver's function in regards to protein synthesis and storage, transformation of carbohydrates, synthesis of cholesterol and detoxification and excretion of substances, and initiating the formation of bile. Surgeons have found that you can remove a large portion of the liver, up to 70% of its volume, when performing a lobectomy for a tumor. The large regenerative capacity of the liver along with the monolithic functions of its representative cell, the hepatocyte, allows for recovery in many of these cases. The same can't be said for studying the brain where neurons differ among each other in regards to shape, location, and transmission so as to be considered different cells (*vide infra* minicolumns). Contrary to the liver, a surgical resection of the brain won't provide for regeneration and resulting symptoms may differ according to the location of the intervention.

Methodological reductionism has provided important scientific insights by simplifying the object of its study. However, by taking for granted that parts of the system are independent of each other they fail to explain emergent phenomena. The dangers are illustrated in the Indian parable of the blind men and an elephant. In examining an elephant, a blind man touching its tail, believed it was a rope. Another blind man touching one of its leg thought it was a pillar, while another one examining its tusks believed they were pipes. The moral of the story is that conclusions based on limited perception and life experiences may provide for overreaching misinterpretations. Sometimes when you break down an organism it is difficult to put it back together. Humpty Dumpty, the character of the nursery rhyme, is portrayed as an egg that is irreparably damaged as it falls from a wall. Not all of the king's men could put Humpty Dumpty back together again after it broke in to pieces.

Humpty Dumpty sat on a wall,
Humpty Dumpty had a great fall.
All the king's horses and all the king's men
Couldn't put Humpty together again.

Reductionism and system theory stand in close analogy to bottom-up and top-down processing. Bottom-up processing starts at the level of the sensory input and is data driven. Individual elements are first identified and then linked together. How this binding is achieved in the brain has given rise to endless speculations. Neuroscientists believe that the cognitive experience of the whole is derived from binding together the activities of different parts of the brain through high frequency synchronized oscillations in the gamma bandwidth (Llinas, 2002).

James Gibson (1904-1980), a strong advocate of the bottom-up (data-driven) approach, articulated the theory of direct perception, also known as the ecological approach. The theory argues that perception is the direct result of gathering information from the environment. No learning is required with the presupposition that there is enough information in the environment to make sense of the world. The bottom-up approach suggests that throughout evolution perception has been necessary for survival (https://www.simplypsychology.org/perception-theories.html).

Contrary to Gibson's views that perception relied primarily on the information present on the stimulus, Richard Gregory (1923-2010) supported a top-down (constructivist) approach to perception. Gregory espoused the importance of prior knowledge and experience in making inferences regarding perception. This was a throwback to Hermann von Helmholtz who regarded perception as a Bayesian (probabilistic) inference. According to Helmholtz we "attain knowledge of the lawful order in the realm of the real, but only in so far as it is represented in the tokens within the system of sensory impressions" (Westheimer, 2008, p. 642). The classical example is that you best understand a difficult handwriting by trying to make sense out of the individual sentences rather than the isolated words. The reason being that the neighboring words add context and an aid to understanding.

Top-down *vs.* bottom-up processing introduces us to the spectrum of cognitive styles observed in neurodevelopmental disorders. In one of these conditions, dyslexia, affected individuals have difficulties in learning words, letters, and symbols despite normal general intelligence. Dyslexic individuals find it difficult to extract meaning out of individual words as they exhibit both fixation instability at the end of saccades and poor smooth pursuit eye movements (Eden et al., 1994). Researchers believe that the dyslexic phenotype reflects a difference in the way they process information. For many affected individuals, this alternate strategy manifests itself as a unique cognitive style rather than a deficit (Aaron et al., 1993). Dyslexics learn from looking first at the big picture and then go for specific details; they are top-down processors of information. They also exhibit strengths in higher level thinking processes and tend to be above average conceptualizers (http://www.dyslexiafoundation.org.nz/info.html).

At the opposite end of the dyslexic cognitive spectrum, autistic individuals, bombarded by sensory cues, tend to isolate details and analyze them individually before grasping a given concept. In an article for The New Idealist (http://magazine. thenewidealist.com/2015/07/09/issue-6-online-extra-with-temple-grandin-on-autism-innovation-the-secrets-of-silicon-valley/) Dr. Temple Grandin stated:

> *"I am good at trawling through the internet through vast amounts of journal artciles and then pick out what are the really important things. I then synthesize all of this resource down into one short paragraph...That's something that I'm good at doing...I'm a bottom-up thinker- I take the details and put them together."*

Researchers have proposed that the cognitive styles observed in autism and dyslexia is defined by differences in minicolumnar morphometry (Williams and Casanova, 2010). In autism, smaller minicolumns and a narrowed gyral window favors local hyperconnectivity (e.g., more arcuate or mu fibers) and long-range hypoconnectivity (e.g., a diminution of commissural projections). The inverse arrangement is seen in dyslexia. The reported anatomical findings argue for changes within the cerebral cortex and its connectivity with little or no alterations at other levels of organization within the nervous system.

THE TRIUNE BRAIN

Contrary to the paradigmatic shifts that have brought about great advances in science over the past few decades, evolution has tinkered with the organization of the brain at a glacial pace. According to Richard Emes, lecturer in Bioinformatics at Keele University, "It is amazing how a process of Darwinian evolution by tinkering and improvement, has generated from a collection of sensory proteins in yeast, the complex synapse of mammals associated with learning and cognition" (https://crev.info/2008/06/evolution146s_tinkerer_creates_the_brain_that_creates_evolutionary_theory/). Indeed, evolution has not replaced brain structures but rather rearranged and added on to ancestral structures thus creating layers of increasing complexity to its organization.

A basic understanding of how the nervous system evolved to its present complexity was provided by the American physician and neuroscientist Paul MacLean (MacLean, 1990). According to MacLean three different structures stratigraphically arranged themselves to form the brain. The innermost and oldest layer is the reptilian complex primarily comprised by the basal ganglia. These structures account for instinctual behaviors involved in dominance, exploration, and territoriality. On top of the reptilian layer, evolution provided the paleomammalian strata consisting of the limbic system (i.e., septum, amygdalae, hippocampus, hypothalamus, and cingulate cortex). These structures account for the way our motivations and emotions shape our behaviors. Finally, and most recently, the neomammalam complex (cerebral cortex) is the most superficial strata that conferred upon us the abilities for language, planning and sensory perception. The cerebral cortex, or more specifically the neocortex, provides the largest relative expansion for cetaceans (whales and porpoises) and hominids (orangutans, gorillas, chimpanzees, bonobo and Homo). The fact that the neocortex has been the newest portion of the cerebral cortex to evolve gives rise to its name (prefix *neo* meaning new).

The Triune brain model is of importance to Systems Theory as it describes a putative hierarchical arrangement to the brain with three interdependent modules. This organization has been studied in laboratory animals by decortication (i.e., the removal of the neocortex). Rats that have undergone this surgical procedure can walk, drink, mate and have a normal sleep-wake cycle. Their behavior seems normal to the casual observer thus proving that lower strata of organization are sufficient for self-maintenance. Human patients who suffer severe and widespread brain injury damaging their neocortex may awaken from a coma and show reflex movements without response to commands. This condition was called persistent vegetative or apallic (meaning without pallium or cortex) state. The pejorative connotation of calling somebody a vegetable has led to renaming the condition unresponsive wakeful syndrome. In this condition, the preservation of attentional-conscious functions in the absence of the cortex detracts from suggesting a role for the thalamocortical complex in consciousness and relegates the same to the conserved areas of the brain, i.e., the upper brainstem (Merker, 2007).

Behavioral psychologists who adopted the Triune model of brain evolution have used the same to explain why humans are emotional actors on the world's stage. Jonathan Haidt (https://getlighthouse.com/blog/the-elephant-and-the-rider-motivate-your-team/) used to illustrate this point with a story of a man riding an elephant. In this metaphor, the man represents the rational side or the cerebral cortex while the elephant is the emotional side or limbic system. The man believes he is in-charge of the direction taken by the elephant along a predetermined route. He holds the reins and steers the animal and, in effect, he seems to be in control. However, the elephant with its poor eyesight is startled by a mouse (the situational side or environmental influence) darting across its path. The spooked elephant frantically abandons its path and hurriedly walks to the surrounding jungle bush. The man realizes that he is at a precarious disadvantage to the more powerful elephant. The metaphor illustrates how intuition and reasoning are dyads of brain function which are codependent on environmental factors.

MacLean's model is presently regarded as instructive but overly simplistic. The Triune brain emphasizes the relatively long periods of evolutionary stability that were followed by explosions of emergent skills caused by accreted strata. However, behaviors, whether primal, emotional or rational, are not neatly broken down into the three different levels of organization espoused by the Triune brain.

CEREBRAL CORTEX

The cerebral cortex is the largest areal extension within the mammalian brain. It is associated with higher brain functions such as the ability to hold multiple tracks of information at the same time, to "think in the future", verbal communication, attention, and judgement. Its ontogeny is complex and dependent on a highly-choreographed interplay between genes and the environment. The cerebral cortex develops from the embryonic ectoderm at the anteriormost portion of the neural tube. Many of the cells in the cerebral cortex originate from a ventricular zone teeming with precursor cells. Although the ventricular zone is often called the germinal matrix, this is a misnomer. The cells per se do not give rise to gametes and should not be considered germinal in origin. They are stem cells that in dividing replenish the stem cell pool and provide the precursors for either neurons or glia. The matrix that supports the stem cells is a highly-vascularized region that lacks parenchymal support and gives it the appearance of granulation tissue. Under magnification in a hematoxylin and eosin stained slide the periventricular germinal zone resembles a blue cell tumor, without the attached pleomorphism. The lack of parenchymal support and overabundance of thin vessels makes the ventricular zone susceptible to injury. Small vascular ruptures, e.g., birth trauma, may lead to large intraventricular bleeds especially in premature infants.

Gradients of expression for two homeobox genes define the cytoarchitecture of different brain regions (Muzio and Mallamaci, 2003). A high concentration of Pax6 and a low concentration of Emx2 promote the organization of motor regions characterized by large neurons having long projections. Brain regions of the motor archetype predominate in the frontal aspect of the brain. Their long projection enable coherence in function among disparate brain regions and with anatomical elements outside of the brain. Due to their long-range connectivity, some motor regions (e.g., dorsolateral prefrontal cortex) act as hubs of information processing that help integrate and modulate different cognitive functions of the brain. Other motor regions whose projections go outside of the cerebral hemispheres help control muscle movement. The opposite gradient, one where Emx2 predominates over Pax6, provides for an overall architecture where granule (small) cells predominate. These cells are proficient at short intraregional connections. A granular cell archetype is characteristic of the caudal regions of the brain with the visual cortex being the best example. Sensory areas, like the visual cortex, function by adding complementary information together from closely adjacent cortices through arcuate fibers. The midportion of the brain, going from front to back, is occupied by brain regions having cellular characteristics of both motor and sensory regions.

The cerebral cortex can be parcellated into different areas by using techniques that allow for distinguishing cellular, vascular, chemical, pigmentary, and/or pathological characteristics. Contrary to the cookie cutter borders of brain regions reported in cytoarchitectural maps, there are no sharp borders between different brain regions and researchers may argue their correctness even when viewing the same brain (Casanova and Kleinman, 1990). Similarly, although accepted in most textbooks that the neocortex has a six-layer, the many variations to this theme among different brain regions is seldom discussed or acknowledged. Two thirds of the cerebral cortex lays buried within sulci. The scarcity of studies detailing this brain region makes it *terra incognita*. It is therefore noteworthy that despite all of the variations and confusing observations, connections to the different layers follow a similar pattern throughout the cerebral cortex: layers II and III serving in capacity similar to that of an associational cortex, layer IV as sensory cortex (the "inbox" for information), and layers V and VI as the "outbox" or motor cortex (Calvin, 1997). The repetitiveness of this pattern along with other observations may have led Douglas and Martin to conclude that, "...each technical advance over the past century has reaffirmed that repeated patterns of structure and function are seen at every level, from molecule to cell to circuit, and that many of these patterns are common across cortical areas and species. In this context, the concept of a canonical circuit, like the concept of hierarchies of processing, offers a powerful unifying principle that links structural and functional levels of analysis across species and different areas of the cortex" (Douglas and Martin, 2010, p. 20).

MINICOLUMNS

The human brain contains some 100 billion neurons each one making from 1,000 to 10,000 connections to other neurons. These cells differ from each other in terms of shape, location, connectivity, and transmission. Modern studies have added to this variety by defining subtypes according to single-cell RNA-seq (Fuzik, et al., 2016). Still, representative illustrations in textbooks describe neurons as having a canonical structure consisting of a dendrite, cell body, and an axon with currents propagating according to Cajal's Law of Dynamic Polarization (from dendrites to axon). Arguably there are too many exceptions for this to be an accepted model. It is now known that axons can conduct in both directions and electrical synapses formed by gap junctions are much more common than previously thought. Furthermore, the release of more than one neurotransmitter from a synaptic ending adds to the complexity and singularity of neurons. Researchers now advocate that variances between neurons indicate differences in kind rather than degree. In this regard, the neuron does not stand as the representative element of the brain; rather, the anatomical structure which best illustrates the holistic properties of the brain is the minicolumn. This idea was first introduced by Cajal's disciple Rafael Lorente De No (1902-1990) when talking about an elementary cortical unit of operation comprised of small cylinders of tissue containing vertically arraigned chains of neurons (Lorente de No, 1938). "All the elements of the cortex are represented in it, and therefore it may be called an elementary unit, in which, theoretically, the whole process of transmission of impulses from the afferent to the efferent axon may be accomplished" (Lorente de no, 1938). This anatomical concept provided the first inkling of a modular organization to the cerebral cortex.

A module is a unit used to construct a whole. It is meant to represent a semi-independent element that can be exchanged with other similar modules without altering the operability of the systems to which it belongs. Because modules exhibit a tendency to be autonomous, the connectivity within the module far outpaces the connectivity between modules. Some people describe this fact by saying that the interdependence or linkage between modules is weak or loosely coupled. An advantage of a loosely coupled system is the alternative implementation of modules in order to provide a given service or function.

Otto Creutzfeldt thought that minicolumns throughout the cerebral cortex processed information in a similar manner with the resultant output dependent on both the source of the information (where it is coming from) and modulatory influences peculiar to each brain region (Creutzfeldt, 1977). The analogy is to an electrical outlet where the same circuitry coming to a house from a generator factory is able to power devices that differ among themselves markedly in terms of their own internal circuitry and function, e.g., a television set, radio, coffee maker, laptop, microwave oven. In the brain, this capacity to process information in a similar way regardless of brain region denotes plasticity.

Similar to an electrical outlet, minicolumns perform the same basic operations regardless of their location within the cerebral cortex. A person who is born blind no longer has a need for a visual cortex. In this case, the place usually allotted to the visual cortex is coopted to receive and process other sensory information whether auditory or tactile. Under these circumstances neuroimaging studies have found that the visual cortex activates when the blind person reads Braille (Sadato et al., 1996). Similarly, a person born deaf does not have a need for an auditory cortex, and the region of the brain finds alternate use in processing visual information. Bola, et al., 2016). The expanded area for visual processing in this case, confers the recipient with superior peripheral vision and motion detection. This cross modal plasticity denotes the capacity of the brain to adaptively reorganize itself and even to strengthen a sensory modality in order to compensate for the loss of another sensory modality. Minicolumns, in this regard, are akin to universal logic gates (e.g., NAND, NOR) which can be connected among themselves to construct any other logic gate and implement any required programming. According to Bach-y-Rita, this meant that, "...any part of the cortex should be able to process whatever electrical signals were sent to it, and that our brain modules were not so specialized after all" (Doidge, 2007, p. 18).

Using electrode recording from within the cerebral cortex Mountcastle was the first person to investigate the functionality of columnar processes within the somatosensory cortices of cats and monkeys. This organization was later confirmed in some of his experiments using slanted penetrations (at an angle of 45° to the surface of the brain) whose results showed changes in modality as the microelectrode transversed neighboring tissue (Mountcastle, 1957). This basic organization of vertically arranged cellular structures was later described in different parts of the cerebral cortex. The findings indicate a certain homogenenity of the cerebral cortex in its anatomical and physiological architecture.

The vertical organization of cellular elements described by Mountcastle are arranged as modules whose basic function is information processing. This has found a clinical application in a surgical procedure called multiple subpial transection. Sometimes when an epileptic focus is refractory to all forms of medical interventions a surgical resection may be considered. A decision on surgical intervention is usually dependent on the type and frequency of seizures, degree of disability and psychological makeup of the patient. Multiple subpial transection is a surgical technique used to control seizures when the affected area of the brain can't be removed safely or without causing major disability. This is of particular importance when the epileptogenic focus affects the language region of the brain (i.e., epileptic aphasia or Landau-Kleffner syndrome). In this procedure, the surgeon transects (cuts across) the cerebral cortex in a grid-like pattern. The cuts interfere with connection among neighboring modules of the brain in a way that interferes with the propagation of seizures; otherwise, processing of information within the columnar cellular structure is preserved. In a report of 14 children with Landau-Kleffner syndrome multiple subpial transection eleven children demonstrated postoperative improvement on measures of receptive or expressive vocabulary (Grote et al., 1999).

By using a biomorphic multi-electrode array and recording from the premotor cortical area 6 in nonhuman primates Opris and colleagues were capable of simultaneously sampling cells from supra- and infra-granular layers from adjacent minicolumns, (Opris et al., 2011, 2012ab, 2013, 2015b; Opris and Casanova, 2014) (Figure 1). It was shown that inter-laminar correlated firing between prefrontal cortical cells plays a role in the integration of perceptual and action information (Opris et al., 2011, 2012ab, 2013, 2017). The cortical minicolumn appears to be endowed with the ability to enhance cognitive performance (Opris, 2013, Opris et al., 2017) or, to decrease such performance when either the number of distractor images decreased (Opris et al., 2012b) or when under cocaine use (Opris et al., 2012a, 2015a) (Figure 2). These results, corroborated by studies of Sokhadze et al. (2014, 2017), pave the way towards uncovering the circuitry linking minicolumnar inputs and outputs initially sought by Mountcastle (1997).

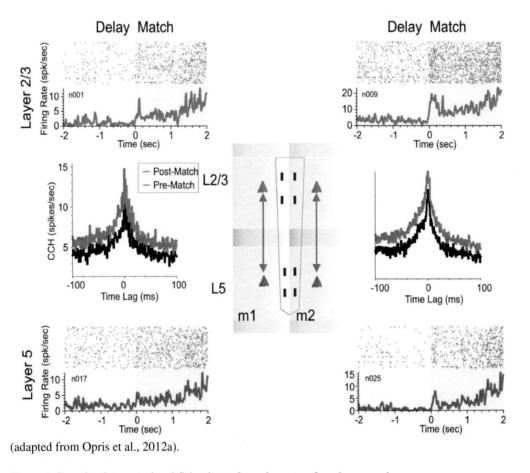

(adapted from Opris et al., 2012a).

Figure 1. Inter-laminar correlated firing in prefrontal cortex of nonhuman primates.

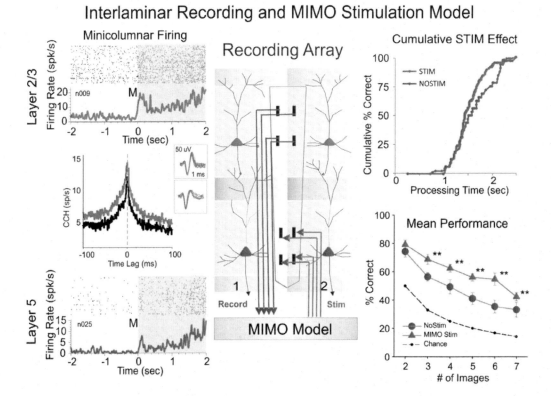

Figure 2. Augmented cognitive performance following stimulation in layer 5 with MIMO (multi-input multi-output) model extracted signals from layer 2/3 (Taken from Opris, 2013).

LAWS OF CONSERVATION

"It is increasingly clear that the symmetry group of nature is the deepest thing that we understand about nature today" Feyman and Weinberg, 1999 p. 73.

The term "Laws of Conservation" makes reference to a particular characteristic of a closed or isolated (i.e., not subject to external forces) system that does not change over time. Some common examples are the laws of conservation of energy, linear momentum, and electric charge. Amalia Emmy Noether (1882-1935), a German mathematician who did seminal work in abstract algebra, discovered the relationship between symmetry and conservations laws. Symmetries (also called the principles of simplicity) limit the possible forms taken by conservation laws independent of initial conditions.

Symmetry operations summarize the regularities of how the brain transforms itself during growth and aging. Indeed, it would be impossible to consider the astronomical permutations dictating the possible interactions among different neurons without the existence of certain symmetries (Casanova 2010; Casanova et al., 2011; in press). The ability to reproduce results of studies among different places and times attest to the invariance of these laws under space-time translations. In this section, we examine how laws of physics defined by symmetry operations help explain aspects of the cerebral cortex organization.

Laws of conservation make reference to particular measurable properties that do not change when looking at them from different referential perspectives. The ingrained symmetry and transformational inertia imply a basic geometrical organization to the system. In the brain, subcortical structures tend to have a nucleoid organization; that is, one lacking laminar or columnar structures. Those subcortical structures that have a laminar organization (e.g., lateral geniculate nucleus) acquire the same through reciprocal connections to the cortex. In this regard, the mammalian neocortex is remarkable for its periodic arrangement of cellular elements that allow its parcellation into different cortical regions. This arrangement has long been recognized by neuroanatomists. Von Economo and Koskinas (1925) devoted one section of their book on the cytoarchitectonics of the human cortex to the vertical arrangements of cells and other anatomical elements. They called these arrangements *Radii*, because of their radial disposition transversing the cortex, from top (pial surface) to bottom (junction of gray white matter junction). Peters et al. (1991a, b) showed that apical dendrites from pyramidal cells bundled together on their way to the molecular layer. The periodicity of these bundles was similar to those of pyramidal cells. Piecing together all of these elements along with other vertical constructs (e.g., axonal bundles, double bouquet cells) gives us the minicolumn (Casanova and Tillquist, 2008; Peters and Sethares, 1996, 1997). It is within the minicolumns that we see he emergence of functions that its individual elements did not possess. According to Mountcastle (1998) the minicolumns is a system that provides operational transforms to its input stimuli. Some candidate functions to these transforms include (Casanova, 2005):

- Thresholding: a nonlinear relation between the level of presynaptic input and cortical neuronal discharge.
- Amplification of inputs: as in the example of when a single impulse in a single myelinated fiber of a peripheral nerve in an attending human suffices to evoke a conscious perception.
- Derivative function: cortical operations tend to accentuate and amplify transient inputs, adapt to constant ones.
- Feature convergence: the creation of a neural representation of a complex feature or set of features by combining signals of two or more simpler ones.
- The distribution function: some areas receive the neural signals of certain simpler features of sensory stimuli and distributed then separately to other cortical areas. Areas 3b and V1 in addition to having other functions, serve as distribution centers.
- Coincidence detection: by convergence of excitation, linking together two events that occur closely in time.

- Synchronization and coherence of activity in the different nodes of distributed system.
- Pattern generation: creation of spatial and temporal patterns in output signals that are not present in inputs (e.g., induced rhythms).

The symmetry of the minicolumns is evident from its isotropy in space. Different morphometric measurements remain the same regardless of the plane of section used to probe them (i.e., sagittal, coronal, transverse) (Casanova et al., 2011). This is possible because the neuropil of the minicolumn acts in a permissive manner to preserve its geometry (Casanova et al., 2007). A linear contact distribution mapping distances from random points within the neuropil to nearby stained cellular elements provides similar values regardless of the cortical area examined or age of patients. (Casanova et al., 2011) The end result of this malleability is that we can perform transformative functions to space coordinates of the minicolumn and the final product will be independent of the amount of the transformation. As an example, translation of pyramidal cells around the central axis of the minicolumns is constrained so that the vectorial addition of their distances is zero regardless of brain parcellation or age of the patient (Casanova et al., 2011). Another conserve quantity is that of the relative size of pyramidal cells as related to their minicolumnar width. Dilation or resizing of cell size follow concurrent changes to the width of the minicolumns. This correlation is evident in the granular cortex (i.e., smallest neurons and minicolumnar widths) as well as in the motor cortex (i.e., largest pyramidal cells and widest minicolumns) reported for the human brain.

In conclusion, the cerebral cortex is an evolutionary hodgepodge whose emergent properties arise from its capacity for self-organization. Gliophilic migration define the core of the cell minicolumns, establish its symmetry, and emergent functions. Transformative actions that preserve the isolation of the system (e.g., aging) are constrained by laws of conservation. This constraint is not feasible when the system is no longer isolated (e.g., trauma).

REFERENCES

Aaron, PG; Wleklinski, M; Wills, C. Developmental dyslexia as a cognitive style. R Malatesha Joshi, CK Leong (eds). *Reading disabilities: diagnosis and component processes.* Springer: New York, ch. 42, pp. 3017-317, 1993.

Bola, L; Zimmermann, M; Mostowski, P; Jednorog, K; Marchewka, A; Rutkowski, P; Szwed, M. Task-specific reorganization of the auditory cortex in deaf humans. *PNAS*, 114(4), E600-E609, 2016.

Calvin, WH. *How Brains Think: Evolving Intelligence, Then and Now.* Basic Books, 15th ed, 1997.

Casanova, MF; Kleinman, JE. The neuropathology of schizophrenia: a critical assessment of research methodologies. *Biol Psychiatry*, 27(3), 353-62, 1990.

Casanova, MF. An apologia for a paradigm shift in the neuroscience. In MF Casanova (ed) *Neocortical Modularity and the Cell Minicolumn*. Nova Science Publishers, Inc. New York: New York, ch 3, pp. 33-55, 2005.

Casanova, MF; Trippe, J; Switala, A. A temporal continuity to the vertical organization of the human neocortex. *Cereb Cortex*, 17(1), 130-7, 2007.

Casanova, MF. Cortical organization: a description and interpretation of anatomical findings based on systems theory. *Translational Neuroscience*, 1(1), 62-71, 2010.

Casanova, MF; Tillquist, CR. Encephalization, emergent properties and psychiatry: a minicolumnar perspective. *Neuroscientists*, 14(1), 101-18, 2008.

Casanova, MF; El-Baz, A; Switala, A. Laws of conservation as related to brain growth, aging, and evolution: symmetry of the minicolumns. *Frontiers in Neuroanatomy*, 5(56), 1-9, 2011.

Casanova, MF; Opris, I; Sokhadze, E; Casanova, EL. Systems theory, emergent properties and the organization of the central nervous system. In Opris I and Casanova MF (eds). *The Physics of the Mind and Brain Disorders*. Springer Series in Cognitive and Neural Systems. Springer, New York, ch 3, pp. 55- 68, 2017.

Creutzfeldt, O. Generality of the functional structure of the neocortex. *Naturwissenschaften (Natural Sciences)*, 64, 507-517, 1977.

Doidge, N. *The Brain that Changes Itself*. Viking Penguin, New York, 2007.

Douglas, RJ; Martin, LAC. Canonical cortical circuits. In GM Shepherd and S Grillner (eds) *Handbook of Brain Microcircuits*, Oxford University Press, New York, p. 15-21, 2010.

Eden, GF; Stein, JF; Wood, HM; Wood, FB. Differences in eye movement and reading problems in dyslexic and normal children. *Vision Res*, 34(10), 1345-58, 1994.

Feynman, RP; Weinberg, S. *Elementary Particles and the Laws of Physics*, Cambridge University Press, Cambridge, 1999.

Fuzik, J; Zeisel, A; Mate, Z; Calvigioni, D; Yanagawa, Y; Szabo, G; Linnarsson, S; Harkany, T. Integration of electrophysiological recording with single-cell RNA-seq data identifies neuronal subtypes. *Nature Biotechnology*, 34, 175-183, 2016.

Grote, CL; Van Slyke, P; Hoeppner, JA. Language outcome following multiple subpial transection for Landau-Kleffner syndrome. *Brain*, 122(3), 561-566. 1999.

Llinas, R. *I of the Vortex: From Neurons to Self*. MIT Press, 2002.

Lorente de No. Architectonics and structure of th cerebral cortex. JF Fulton (ed.) in *Physiology of the Nervous System*. Oxford University Press, New York, pp. 291-330, 1938.

MacLean, P. *The Triune Brain in Evolution: Role in Paleocerebral Function*. Plenum Pres, New York, 1990.

Merker, B. Consciousness without a cerebral cortex: a challenge for neuroscience and medicine. *Behav Brain Sci*, 30(1), 63-81, 2007.

Mountcastle, VB. Modality and topographic properties of single neurons of cat's somatic sensory cortex. *J Neurophysiol*, 20, 408-434, 1957.

Mountcastle, VB. (1997). The columnar organization of the neocortex, *Brain*, 120 (4), 701-22.

Muzio; Mallamaci. Emx1, emx2 and pax6 in specification, regionalization and arealization of the cerebral cortex. *Cereb Cortex*, 13(6), 641-7, 2003.

Opris, I; Chang, S; Noga, BR. (2017). What is the evidence for inter-laminar integration in a prefrontal cortical minicolumn? *Frontiers in Neuroanatomy*, 11, 116.

Opris, I; Casanova, MF. (2014). Prefrontal cortical minicolumn: from executive control to disrupted cognitive processing. *Brain*, 137 (7), 1863-1875.

Opris, I. (2013). Inter-Laminar Microcircuits across the Neocortex: Repair and Augmentation. Research Topic: "Augmentation of brain function: facts, fiction and controversy", Lebedev MA, Opris I and Casanova MF (ed.), *Front. Syst. Neurosci.*, 7, 80. doi: 10.3389/fnsys.2013.00080.

Opris, I; Gerhardt, GA; Hampson, RE; Deadwyler, SA. (2015a). Disruption of columnar and laminar cognitive processing in primate prefrontal cortex following cocaine exposure. Research Topic: "Structural and functional organization of the prefrontal cortex" Tinsley CJ (ed.). *Front. Syst. Neurosci.*, 9, 79.

Opris, I; Fuqua, JL; Gerhardt, GA; Hampson, RE; Deadwyler, SA. (2015b). Prefrontal cortical recordings with biomorphic MEAs reveal complex columnar-laminar microcircuits for BCI/BMI implementation. *J Neurosci Methods.*, 244, 104-13. doi: 10.1016/j.jneumeth.2014.05.029.

Opris, I; Hampson, RE; Stanford, TR; Gerhardt, GA; Deadwyler, SA. (2011). Neural activity in frontal cortical cell layers: evidence for columnar sensorimotor processing. *J Cogn Neurosci.*, 23(6), 1507-21. doi: 10.1162/jocn.2010.21534.

Opris, I. (2013). Inter-laminar microcircuits across neocortex: repair and augmentation. *Front Syst Neurosci.*, 2013 Nov 19, 7, 80. doi: 10.3389/fnsys.2013.00080. eCollection 2013.

Opris, I; Santos, L; Gerhardt, GA; Song, D; Berger, TW; Hampson, RE; Deadwyler, SA. (2013). Prefrontal cortical microcircuits bind perception to executive control. *Sci Rep.*, 3, 2285. doi: 10.1038/srep02285.

Opris, I; Hampson, RE; Gerhardt, GA; Berger, TW; Deadwyler, SA. (2012a). Columnar processing in primate pFC: evidence for executive control microcircuits. *J Cogn Neurosci.*, 24(12), 2334-47. doi: 10.1162/jocn_a_00307.

Opris, I; Fuqua, JL; Huettl, PF; Gerhardt, GA; Berger, TW; Hampson, RE; Deadwyler, SA. (2012b) Closing the loop in primate prefrontal cortex: inter-laminar processing. *Front Neural Circuits.*, 6, 88, doi: 10.3389/fncir.2012.00088. eCollection 2012.

Peters, A; Palay, SL; Webster, HF. *The Fine Structure of the Nervous System: Neurons and Their Supporting Cells*, 3rd Edn. New York: Oxford University Press, 1991a.

Peters, A; Sethares, C. Organization of pyramidal neurons in area 17 of monkey visual cortex. *J. Comp. Neurol.*, 306, 1–23, 1991b.

Peters, A; Sethares, C. Myelinated axons and the pyramidal cell modules in monkey primary visual cortex. *J. Comp. Neurol.*, 365, 232–255, 11996.

Peters, A; Sethares, C. The organization of double bouquet cells in monkey striate cortex. *J. Neurocy-tol.*, 26, 779–797, 1997.

Sadato, N; Pascual-Leone, A; Grafman, J; Ibanez, V; Deiber, MP; Dold, G; Hallet, M. Activation of the primary visual cortex by Braille reading in blind subjects. *Nature*, 380, 526-528, 1996.

Sokhadze, EM; Lamina, EV; Casanova, EL; Kelly, DP; Opris, I; Khachidze, I; Casanova, MF. (2017) Atypical Processing of Novel Distracters in a Visual Oddball Task in Autism Spectrum Disorder. *Behav Sci (Basel)*. 2017 Nov 16, 7(4). pii: E79. doi: 10.3390/bs7040079.

Sokhadze, EM; El-Baz, AS; Sears, LL; Opris, I; Casanova, MF; (2014). rTMS neuromodulation improves electrocortical functional measures of information processing and behavioral responses in autism. *Front Syst Neurosci.*, 2014 Aug 6, 8, 134. doi: 10.3389/fnsys.2014.00134. eCollection 2014.

Van Regenmortel, MHV. *Reductionism and complexity in molecular biology*. EMBO Rep 5(11):1016-1020, 2004.

Von Economo, C; Koskinas, GN. *Die Cytoarchitektonik der Hirnrinde des erwachsenen Men- schen*. Wien: Springer.

Westheimer, G. Was Helmholtz a Bayesian? *Perception*, 37(5), 642-50, 2008.

Williams, EL; Casanova, MF. Autism and dyslexia: a spectrum of cognitive styles as defined by minicolumnar morphometry. *Med Hypothesis*, 74(1), 59-62, 2010.

In: Focus on Systems Theory Research
Editors: Manuel F. Casanova and Ioan Opris

ISBN: 978-1-53614-561-8
© 2019 Nova Science Publishers, Inc.

Chapter 11

FROM QUORUM SENSING TO DYNOME THROUGH MITOCHONDRIA

Jean Ciurea and Tatiana Ciurea
Clinical Emergency Hospital "Bagdasar Arseni"
Functional Neurosurgery Department, Bucharest, Romania

ABSTRACT

Beyond cell powerplant role, mitochondrion, considered a symbiont of bacterial origin, is a source of cells light emission which may be an epiphenomenon of chemical reactions or/and an information channel, as observed in bacterial colonies where limited nutrients level is inducing bioluminescent activity, possible a signal determining a slower colony growth. If this is the case, then this message is received, analyzed and the action of limitation is taken by the population "quorum sensing" smart ability. The complex multiple roles of mitochondria are analyzed from this point of view. If biophotons contain information, then pathways must exist, receivers may be genetic and epigenetic structures organized in a sophisticated dynamic holographic analysis and memory system. This is grounding an audacious approach from mitochondria to connectome till dynom.

HISTORY

The mitochondrion is the only organelle having genetic material outside cell nucleus. This organelle is surrounded by a double membrane and a circular chromosome of DNA as that typical of prokaryotes and bacteria. It was observed in the mid 19th century short after the discovery of the nucleus. Its name comes from *mitos* (thread in the Greek language) and *chondros* (granule in Greek language). Altmann in 1890, described mitochondria as "bioblasts" (i.e., a hypothetical unit of living matter) existing in a symbiotic relationship with the host cell (Altmann, 1890). The term mitochondria was introduced by Benda (Benda, 1898).

The idea that the mitochondria have a bacterial origin generated important scientific debates. The respiratory function of mitochondria was demonstrated only in 1925 when cytochromes were observed by Keilin. Later (1941), Lipmann grounded their role in metabolism by introducing the concept of phosphate macroergic bonds in adenosine triphosphate (ATP). A few years later (1948), oxidative phosphorylation was described by Lehninger. However, it was not until 1976 when mitochondrial DNA was completely mapped (Ernster et al. 1981).

ORIGINS, EVOLUTIONARY TIMELINE AND AGE CLOCK

Generally, it is accepted that a proto-eukaryotic cell without mitochondria (anaerobic archaebacteria) captured an a-proteobacterium by endocytosis around 1–2 billion years ago. This statement is based on genetic and structural data (Sagan L. 1967). As an endosymbionts, the mitochondria are unique among cellular organelles. Mitochondria evolved from a bacterial origin, as evidenced by the mitochondrial genomic sequences that have been retained throughout evolution (Anderson S et al. 1981). Within mitochondria, new genetic mutations accumulate in a clock-like manner thus provid away for dating genetic events (Bromham et al. 2003, Zuckerkandl et al. 1961, Kumaret al. 2005). Indeed, the aging clock involves the gradual accumulation of sequential changes in thousands of copies of the same gene or genes. Mitochondrial DNA mutates every 8000 years (Loogvali et al., 2009). It is important to note however, that mitochondrial DNA is less precise for genealogical dating than Y-chromosome DNA (Poznik et al., 2013).

A team of researchers using molecular clock methods found that mutation in human mitochondrial deoxyribonucleic acid (mtDNA) is 5–10 times faster than in nuclear DNA. This high rate may be due, in part, to an elevated rate of mutations in mitochondrial DNA and high cell energy needs. Because of the high rate of evolution, mitochondrial DNA is likely to be an extremely useful molecule to employ in the high-resolution analysis of evolutionary processes (Brown et al., 1979).

Phylogenetic and geographic studies of human mitochondrial DNA (mtDNA) have revealed fundamental information concerning the origins of our species and human population migration on our planet (Avise 2000; Torroni et al., 2006; Underhill et al., 2007). A human mtDNA study revealed only one population source for all mankind transpiring in Africa, approximately 140,000 to 200,000 years ago (Cann et al., 1987).

The mtDNA has a very high mutation dynamic. Heteroplasmy is a state where new mtDNA mutation arises in a cell resulting a mixed intracellular population of mtDNAs.

The mutant and normal genetic information are randomly distributed in daughter cells when a heteroplasmic cell divides, thus creating a homoplasmic mutant or wild type derivate. It has also been reported that there is a tendency of modified mtDNAs (with mutations) to be amplified within cells. The latter phenomena has been hypothetically explained as a need of the nucleus to compensate for an energy deficiency by making more mitochondria. Consequently, cells with modified mitochondria preferentially replicate. As the amount and influence of mutant mtDNAs increases, the mitochondrial efficiency declines, reactive oxygen species ROS production increases, and the propensity for apoptosis increases. In this way tissue function declines and diseases manifest themselves. This cycle of progression gives rise to the aging clock (Wallace et al., 2001; Wallace et al., 2002).

NUCLEAR DNA VS MT DNA

Mitochondria can control cell nuclear activity by unknown gene expression mechanisms. Ancient human nuclear DNA is common to all individuals within our species. On the other hand, the mitochondrial genetic system is present in thousands of copies in every living cell of the organism. The mitochondrial respiratory chain is the result of cooperation between the mitochondrial and nuclear genomes. There is great geographical variation due to individual energetic needs mainly interconnected to temperature variation and seasonal feeding habits. This diversity is why humans adapted so well to different global environments that had different climates and seasons.

There are about 900 mitochondrial proteins which are encoded by the nuclear genome and imported into the mitochondria. The circular (bacterial resemblance) mtDNA genome contains 37 genes. Thirteen of these genes encode protein subunits of respiratory complexes I, III, IV, and V; only complex II is composed of proteins encoded by nuclear genes. The high rate of mutation of mitochondrial genome is poorly understood, even when the genetic organization appears to be rather simple (Wallace, 2005).

Mitochondrial DNA mutations have the potential to provoke cell death. More than 200 documented mutations in the 37 mtDNA-encoded genes, and an equal number in almost 100 nDNA-encoded genes are capable of inducing apoptosis (Smits et al., 2010). The signaling cascades that coordinate the dialog between mitochondria and cell structure are identified as key regulators for normal function (Karbowski et al., 2007). Mitochondria may signal within their network in ways similar to that of a bacterial colony. It is accepted that the coordinated activity of the reticulum involves signaling cascades to the organelles, an example being the apoptotic waves of cytochrome c release and calcium flux during a triggering cell death (Pacher et al., 2001; Szabadkai et al., 2004).

Retrograde signals are sent from the mitochondria back to the nucleus in the yeast model organisms (Sik et al., 2004). Retrograde signaling informs the nucleus of changing metabolic demands initiated at the mitochondria, leading to an up regulation of mitochondrial metabolism (Civitarese et al., 2010; Neuspiel, 2008). The mitochondria then send "pods" to another intracellular organelle, the peroxisome, thus instituting a communicative system of membrane transport (Andrade-Navarro et al., 2009; Hyde et al., 2010; Zunino et al., 2004).

STRUCTURE AND FUNCTION

Anatomically the mitochondria is bound by an outer membrane enclosing an inner one. The inner membrane is folded by invaginations called cristae. Its size ranges between 0.75 and 3 µm in diameter (Wiemerslage et al., 2016). Different cells exhibit different cristae morphologies, e.g., tubular, lamellar, helical, or even triangular cristae. They are situated at a right angle to the longitudinal axis of the mitochondria (Fawcett, 1981). Vertebrate neurons show typically filamentous mitochondria associated with the microtubules (MTs) of the cytoskeleton, forming together a continuous network known as the mitochondrial reticulum (Skulachev, 2001). The outer mitochondrial membrane is 75 angstroms (Å) thick and has a protein-to-phospholipid structure similar to that of the eukaryotic cell membrane. The porins are channels that allow molecules of 5000 Daltons or less in molecular weight to freely diffuse from one side of the membrane to the other (Bruce et al., 1994). Larger proteins can enter the mitochondrion by an actively coupled mechanism controlled by translocase (Herrmann et al., 2000).

The mitochondrial outer membrane can become associated to the endoplasmic reticulum (ER) membrane, in a structure called MAM (mitochondria-associated ER-membrane). This is of importance in the ER-mitochondria calcium signaling system (Hayashi et al., 2009).

The intermembrane space is the space between the outer membrane and the inner membrane. Small molecules (less then 5000 Daltons) are found in similar concentrations to the cytoplasm due to free trans membranal circulation. Larger molecules circulate by the active mechanisms previously mentioned (Bruce et al., 1994). Cytochrome C is localized within this space (Chipuk et al., 2006).

The inner mitochondrial membrane performs a redox reaction of oxidative phosphorylation and ATP synthesis. It contains cardiolipin which makes it impermeable to all molecules. Molecular transport is performed by translocators. This membrane shows a high potential (200 microV) due to the electron transport chain (Bruce et al., 1994). The inner mitochondrial is folded into many cristae. These cristae offer a large surface for energy production reactions (Mannella, 2006). The inner mitochondrial membrane and cristae (IMMC) are one of the most active area of research in cellular biology (Cogliati et al., 2013; Cogliati et al., 2016).

The diaphragmatic muscle is an important muscle responsible for sleep respiration and maintaining proper blood oxygen levels. Resistance to fatigue put it in a special category with myocardium. The rat diaphragm muscle present a characteristic as in muscle tissue reticula actually extend across neighboring cells resulting in a supracellular mitochondrial network. They look like cable-like structures (Bakeeva et al., 1978).

THE POWERPLANT OF THE CELL

The mitochondria generate most of the cell's supply of adenosine triphosphate (ATP) by means of chemical reactio (Campbell et al., 2006). The human brain represents only 2% of the body's weight, but it accounts for 20% of its resting metabolism (Kety, 1957; Rolfe and Brown, 1997).

Known as the "power-house" of the cell, mitochondria use the oxidation of reduced substrates with molecular oxygen and a proton force across the inner membrane. This force is in turn utilized by membrane bound enzymes which phosphorylate adenosine diphosphate (ADP) to adenosine triphosphate (ATP), the latter being the universal energy-providing molecule for biochemical reactions. Otherwise, these organelles provide a highly efficient route for eukaryotic cells to generate ATP from energy-rich molecules. Electrons from oxidative substrates are transferred to oxygen via a series of redox reactions. Protons are pumped from the matrix across the mitochondrial inner membrane through respiratory complexes I, III, and IV. When protons return to the mitochondrial matrix down their electrochemical gradient, ATP is synthesized via complex V and ATP synthase (Mitchell, 1977).

The brain signaling-related energy use is 30 micromol ATP/g/min which equals that of the human leg muscle running in a Marathon race. Energy economy is essential for the neocortex. An increase in mean firing rate of 1 Hz increases consumption (in rodent) by 6.5 micromol ATP/g/min, so that a mean firing rate of 18 Hz for all neurons would increase consumption to the maximum of 120 micromol ATP/g/min (Hochachka, 1994). Unsurprisingly, anoxia or ischemia can easily damage the brain. Understanding these energy demands may help institute targeted therapy (Ames, 1995). Some therapies target brain energy consumption in an attempt to restore the ion movements generated by postsynaptic currents, action potentials, and neurotransmitter uptake (Siesjö, 1978; Ames, 2000).

A promising investigation tool is based on combining PET and Deuterium MR to measure mitochondrial function in health and disease. The principle is to simultaneously measure, via Dynamic Deuterium MR (DDMR), the glucose consumption and the formation of nascent metabolic water for ATP generation. FDG -PET yields information regarding the quantity of glucose that reaches different sites and its rate of consumption. After its formation in mitochondria, HDO (water containing Deuterium) enters the blood flow. Subsequently, labeling of various molecules in the metabolic process can beneficially be identified by DDMR. It was demonstrated by Mateescu et al. in 2017 that *in vivo* Dynamic Deuterium MR can simultaneously determine glucose consumption and the corresponding mitochondrial water formation. It is possible to combine DDMR with PET by building MRI scanners that would include low gamma nuclei. This will lead to a better multi-voxel characterization of mitochondrial function in health and disease. Moreover, corroboration with functional MRI results would greatly enhance the diagnostic power of these techniques (Pichler et al., 2008; Avril et al., 2016; Mateescu et al., 2011 and 2015; Lu M et al., 2017).

The brain's grey matter activity is mainly dominated by glutamatergic excitatory synapses (Braitenberg and Schüz, 1998). Mitochondria are observed close to synapses having major energetic needs (Wong-Riley, 1989; Wong-Riley et al., 1998). Glucose utilization is proportional to the rate at which glutamate is converted to glutamine in the brain as demonstrated by magnetic resonance studies. It seems that glutamatergic activity is responsible for the major energy consumption in the brain, and that energy use on glutamate uptake and conversion to glutamine controls glucose usage and cortical blood flow (Sibson et al., 1998).

IMMUNOLOGY

There are many reports of importance to the present topic on the mammalian protein called MAVS (mitochondrial anti-viral signaling protein). MAVS is an integral outer membrane protein that plays a central role in the signal transduction cascades that lead to the nuclear factor Nf-kB stress and type 1 interferon response. The Nf-kB and interferon(IFN) responses are critical for the cellular production of cytokines that alert the body as to a viral infection (Sethet al., 2005; Xu et al., 2005; Kawai et al., 2005; Meylan et al., 2005).

Mitochondria are involved in immunological and septic shock-related mechanisms. They are responsible for the identification of a key component required to signal viral infection and activate the immune response. MAVS (mitochondrial antiviral signaling protein) function as the "launchpad" for the Nf-kB and interferon type 1 IFN antiviral transcriptional response (Scott, 2010). Localization in the mitochondria of this essential component may be due to the proximity to the apoptotic machinery existing there. The goal of the infected cell is to alert the neighboring cells of the viral infection (Castanier et al., 2010). MAVS activity is to induce mitochondrial fusion, which is known to be protective against cell death (Yasukawa et al., 2009).

Due to the evolutionary origins of the mitochondrion as a primordial bacteria, it may be perceived by the organism as a potential pathogen when in direct contact with blood as in the case of massive traumatic lesions (Manfredi et al., 2010). Finally, it has been observed that various bone fractures or trauma injuries inducing a toxic shock response, utilize the same molecular pathways as those engaged in severe bacterial infections. Mitochondria released from the ruptured cells are responsible for this toxic shock response (Zhang et al., 2010). In summary, the mitochondrion is mainly known for its role in supplying cellular energy but it is also of importance in information generation and transmission, cellular growth, division, differentiation, fight against infection and death (McBride et al., 2006).

PLANT *VS.* ANIMAL WORLD MITOCHONDRION

Plant mitochondria function the same way as animal mitochondria by means of an electron transport chain that translocate protons and generate adenosine triphosphate ATP (Dudkina et al., 2006). This process also generates reactive oxygen species (ROS) with similar effects on plant cell as in animals. In excess, ROS can damage the cells, but they are also an important signal produced in response to varied stresses. Because mitochondria depend on proteins encoded by both mitochondrial and nuclear genomes, a sophisticated two-way communication between organelles exists to ensure correct mitochondrial biogenesis and function (Amirsadeghi et al., 2007; Laloi et al., 2004).

Pollen development is dependent on a balance of fusion and fission which controls the morphology and number of plant mitochondria. When affected, this balance may cause cytoplasmic male sterility (Hanson and Bentolila, 2004).

A complex interaction between chloroplasts, mitochondria and peroxisomes during photorespiration involves the oxygenase activity of the carbon dioxide fixing enzyme ribulose- 1,5- bisphosphate carboxylase/oxygenase (Maurino and Peterhansel 2010).

But, chloroplasts and mitochondria are different. Photosynthesis occurs in two steps, the light-dependent reaction and the Calvin cycle. The light dependent reaction captures solar photons to generate potential energy. The resulting products are then introduced into the Calvin cycle, which turns CO2 into the carbohydrate glyceraldehyde 3-phosphate. This carbohydrate is important to metabolism and generates complex sugars for structure and energy production. Cornelius van Niel suggested in 1931 that photosynthesis consists of general reactions wherein a photon is used to obtain a hydrogen donor and the hydrogen being used to reduce CO_2. The light-dependent reactions takes place on the thylakoid membranes. The inside of the thylakoid membrane is called the lumen, and the outside thylakoid membrane is the stroma. The light is trapped inside this complex by a reflection- refraction mechanisms, very efficient when wave length and intensity of light are adequate. There are membrane protein complexes that catalyze the light reactions. Water activated by a photon acts on pigment P680 and a poorly understood structure called the "water-splitting complex". This starts a reaction that splits water into electrons, protons and oxygen. The electrons are transferred to chlorophyll molecules that are pushed to a higher-energy state by photons. This is a very efficient process in photosynthesis. This efficiency is due to the fact that, in addition to direct excitation by light at 680 nm, the energy of light is harvested by proteins acting as antennas for other wavelengths which are transferred to these special chlorophyll molecules and captured for potential energy generation. This is the second core process in photosynthesis. The initial stages occur within picoseconds, with an efficiency of 100%. This, almost impossible efficiency, is due to a highly ordered spatial placement of molecules within the reaction core. In other words, particles are occupying fixed positions with respect to one another and unable to move freely. This is not a chemical reaction. It occurs within an essentially crystalline environment created by the macromolecular structure of Photosystem II (PSII). It is a solid-state process and the usual rules of chemistry do not apply in these environments. PS II is a transmembrane structure found in all chloroplasts. It splits water into electrons, protons and molecular oxygen as mentioned. The electrons are transferred to plastoquinone, which carries them to a proton pump. Consequently, molecular oxygen is released into the atmosphere as a by-product. This amazing complex structure is a macromolecule that converts the energy of sunlight into potentially energy with efficiencies that are impossible in ordinary conditions (Vass et al., 2009; "Photosynthesis". McGraw Hill Encyclopedia of Science and Technology, 2007).

Chloroplasts synthesize sugars by converting carbon dioxide (CO_2), water (H_2O) and solar energy into carbon sources, principally, glyceraldehyde 3-phosphate; whereas mitochondria convert carbon sources into cell energy (ATP), with CO_2 and H_2O as a by-product.

FISSION AND FUSION

Elegant studies in Drosophila and yeast initially revealed that the mitochondria are continually reshaped through ongoing fusion and fission events. Mitochondrial fusion and fission processes remain partly unknown. In neurons, where mitochondrial activity is intense due to high energetic necessities, the activation of signaling cascades are able to orchestrate the long-range motility along microtubules, followed by the arrest and anchoring of mitochondria to the actin cytoskeleton precisely where required (Chada and Hollenbeck 2003, Chada and Hollenbeck 2004).

Mitochondrial fragmentation was noticed during mitosis, where it is thought to facilitate the segregation of the reticulum into daughter cells, the mitochondria become highly fused during the growth phase of G1, and in response to multiple forms of stressors (Zunino et al., 2009; Frank et al., 2001; Tondera et al., 2009; Margineantu et al., 2002). Fragmentation also occurs during ischemia-reperfusion injury (Youle and Karbowski, 2005). Collective fragmentation of the mitochondria is the initial phase of programmed cell death, where the smaller fragments seem to accelerate the release of cytochrome c (Suen et al., 2008; Mitra et al., 2009).

It has also been shown that mitochondrial fission is a response to hyperglycemia (Yu et al., 2006; Makino et al., 2010; Gao 2010). Mitochondrial fusion is essential for the maintenance of mitochondrial DNA (Hermann et al., 1998; Rapaport et al., 1998). The local control of mitochondrial dynamics is considered functionally essential in signaling (reactive oxygen species fulfill this task before inducing oxidative damage), fission and fusion accomplished under complex protein guidance, removing the dysfunctional units by autophagy which is a mechanism of quality control and also a crucial role in embryogenesis but also counteracting aging process (Ishihara et al., 2009; Wakabayashi et al., 2009; Hoppins and Nunnari 2009).

The mitochondrial fusion biology and mtDNA stability were initially demonstrated in yeast model organisms (Hermann et al., 1998). It was hypothesized that fusing the mitochondria will dilute any mutant mtDNA and allow the wild type genomes to contribute functional electron transport chain components (Chen et al., 2010; de Brito and Scorrano, 2008). In the absence of fusion, accumulated mutations can induce dysfunction and autophagic clearance (Ehses et al., 2009).

Mitochondrial fission induces the depolarization of one of the "daughter" mitochondria and hyperpolarization of the other (Twig et al., 2009). This may be due to charged particles leakage during membrane scission, but this will recover as soon as the respiratory function is activated and later fuse back into the reticulum. If respiratory function is not reestablished, the protease Oma1 would become activated within the mitochondrial inner membrane and cleave the fusion GTPase Opa1, effectively exiling the depolarized organelle from the collective (Head et al., 2009; Vives-Bauza et al., 2010). Mathematical modeling of fission and fusion in the context of quality control would indicate that the process is likely stochastic in nature (Taguchi et al., 2007). Movement and docking of mitochondria, fission and fusion allows energy supply even in long pyramidal neurons.

CALCIUM (CA2+)

The influence of mitochondrial calcium sequestration on synaptic transmission has important implications for nervous functions. Neurotransmitter release is triggered by Ca2+ influx through voltage-gated channels (Katz, 1969). Factors regulating the spatiotemporal profile of the presynaptic cytoplasmic calcium transient influence release probability, vesicle recycling, and information processing in the brain. Mitochondria are capable of having an important effect on these processes because they can sequester large quantities of calcium (Duchen 1999, Nicholls and Budd 2000).

In cultured neurons, exposure to glutamate typically leads to three distinct phases of cytoplasmic Ca^2_+ elevation. First there is a spike, which may be followed by a recovery until an elevated plateau is attained. This recovery may reflect the partial desensitization of NMDA receptors (Legendre et al., 1993; Rafiki et al., 1997; Rosenmund et al., 1995), a component due to fast-desensitizing voltage-activated Ca2+ channels (Courtney et al., 1990), the delayed activation of Ca2+ extrusion pathways (Klishin et al., 1998), or mitochondrial sequestration (Vicario, 1991; Werth and Thayer, 1994). After the second, plateau, phase, an uncontrolled, essentially irreversible failure of cytoplasmic Ca2+ homeostasis, delayed Ca2+ deregulation (DCD) occurs (Tymianski et al., 1993).

Delayed Ca2+ deregulation precedes plasma membrane lysis (since the fluorescent probe is still retained in the cytoplasm) but reliably predicts subsequent cell lysis. The second and third phases of cytoplasmic Ca^2_+ elevation can proceed even after the removal of extracellular glutamate (Wang et al., 1996). Reduced calcium sequestration by mitochondria is associated with aging (Leslie et al., 1985) and neurodegenerative conditions such as amyotrophic lateral sclerosis, Huntington's disease, and Alzheimer's disease (Beal, 2000). In addition, symptoms similar to Parkinson's disease can result from inhibition of mitochondrial respiration by rotenone (Betarbet et al., 2000).

NITRIC OXIDE (NO)

There are reports suggesting that these mitochondria may act as signaling devices for the regulation of cytoprotective mechanisms and adaptive responses to hypoxia. Earlier observations indicating that nitric oxide (NO) at physiological concentrations modulates respiration through the reversible inhibition of the mitochondrial enzyme cytochrome C oxidase, in competition with O2, gave rise to the hypothesis that NO may have an important function in the regulation of such mechanisms (Cleeter et al., 1994; Brown and Cooper 1994; Schweizer and Richter, 1994; Moncada and Erusalimsky, 2002).

Experimental support for this hypothesis comes from a number of studies showing that the interaction of NO with cytochrome C oxidase in different types of cells is associated with the resistance to apoptosis induced by various kinds of stressors, including growth factor deprivation, O2 limitation, or intracellular calcium overload (Beltran et al., 2000; Almeida et al., 2001; Xu et al., 2004).

Excessive production of NO and mitochondrial dysfunction have been associated with pathophysiological mechanisms. However, the fact that NO inhibits mitochondrial respiration suggests that there may be instances in which NO production, mitochondrial dysfunction, and pathology could be intimately related (Brealey 2002).

The concept that NO is involved in cytoprotection is based on the hypothesis that it is controlled by the interaction between NO and cytochrome C oxidase. Considering that the majority of experimental work investigating the mechanisms of action of NO has been carried out with cells cultured at ambient [O2], the signaling consequences of the interaction between the enzyme and physiologically meaningful levels of NO have so far remained largely undetected and is important for future studies to be carried out in cells kept at 3% O2, a concentration which more closely reflects the situation *in vivo*.

ROS REACTIVE OXYGEN SPECIES

Radical production takes predominantly place in mitochondria, where redox-reactions of the mitochondrial respiration chain permanently produce reactive oxygen species (ROS) It was estimated that under normal conditions 1–2% of the cell's oxygen consumption is converted into ROS A normal amount of ROS is crucial for the physiological control of a variety of cell functions, whereas pathological increased levels of ROS cause oxidative damage to many cell

FROM HUNTER -GATHER FEEDING CONDITION TO "FAST FOOD" EATING HABITS

Cooperation between a small group of humans for food acquisition and the sharing the same with other members of the community is an important evolutionary drive meant to adapt to food season fluctuations. Fasting and physical efforts, liver glycogen stores are drained and ketones are produced from adipose tissue fatty acids. This metabolic switch in cellular fuel source is accompanied by adaptations of neural networks in the brain, enhancing their functionality and improving their resistance to aggression and disease. A rodent experimental model proved that a diet of reduced calories diet is associated with better life quality, longer life and less cancer (Sohal et al., 1994).

Food seasons fluctuations flexibility is based on a switch from the main glucose fuel to fatty acids and ketones. Fasting regularly may maintain an advantage during the lifespan of individuals. Mitochondria efficiently breaks down macromolecules, such as carbohydrates or lipids, into ATP. The inner mitochondrial membrane and cristae (IMMC) proteome perform essential biochemical reactions such as oxidative phosphorylation and mitochondrial biogenesis. The energy released by the flow of electrons is used to pump protons out of the mitochondrial inner membrane. This creates a capacitance across the mitochondrial inner membrane, the electrochemical gradient (Nicholls 1977; Nicholls and Bernson, 1977). The potential energy stored is coupled to

ATP synthesis. As protons flow back into the matrix through a proton channel, ADP and stored potential energy are bound, condensed, and released as ATP. Matrix ATP is then exchanged for cytosolic ADP by the adenine nucleotide translocator. The efficiency by which dietary calories are converted to ATP is determined by the coupling efficiency of oxidative phosphorilation. Pumping protons highly efficient out of the mitochondrial inner membrane is correlated with highly efficient ATP synthesis and mitochondria will generate the maximum ATP and the minimum heat per calorie consumed. These mitochondria are described as *tightly coupled*. If the efficiency of proton pumping is reduced, then each calorie burned will generate less ATP but more heat. Such mitochondria are identified as loosely coupled. The coupling efficiency is the proportion of calories utilized by the mitochondrion to perform work versus those to maintain body temperature in an endothermic being (Rolfe and Brand, 1997; Nicholls and Budd, 2000).

AGEING

Longevity and aging are different terms. Longevity refers to the average life span, whereas aging is defined by the appearance of a set of aging-induced phenotypes that may or may not affect life span, including reduced fertility, frailty, loss of hearing and eyesight, and changes in hair/fur color. The mitochondria are the only human genetic system that embodies the features necessary to explain the observed characteristics of the common age-related diseases. Ageing is also followed by changes in energy metabolism. Two key enzyme complexes are involved in the control of aging: rapamycin complex 1 (mTORC1) and the AMP-dependent protein kinase (AMPK). These two enzymes are reciprocally regulated, in that AMPK is activated during nutrient deprivation and low energy charge, whereas mTORC1 is activated by growth factors and in states of nutrient abundance (Inoki et al., 2012).

Studies demonstrated more longevity in several genetic systems including Saccharomyces cerevisiae, Drosophila Melanogaster, Caenorhabditis elegans, and mice (Lamming et al., 2013). Metabolism is related to age-induced pathophysiology. However, the aging process is difficult to understand. Evidence suggests that improved metabolic efficiency with reduced nutrient storage and enhanced fuel oxidation serves to combat age-related disease processes, resulting in enhanced healthy longevity.

APOPTOSIS

Apoptosis is also controlled by mitochondria. The essentials factor controlling the path to cell death has been proposed to be the extent to which cytoplasmic ATP levels is lowered by the bioenergetic consequences of glutamate exposure. Consequently, the energetic status of mitochondria "in vivo" may be an important factor in deciding the fate of the cell in terms of survival, apoptosis, or necrosis. Each of the mutually interacting energetic parameters may be involved, including substrate availability, respiratory chain activity, Ca2+ accumulation, generation of ROS, mitochondrial swelling, release of cytochrome c, and cellular ATP generation. The challenge is to sort out the individual functions and to identify the causal chain of events leading finally to cell death (Ankarcrona et al., 1995; Leist et al., 1997; Nicotera and Leist, 1997).

DISEASE

Neurological and neurodegenerative disorders are often associated with disruption of mitochondrial function. Patients with OxPhos dysfunction could present mutations in either mtDNA or nDNA. They present neurological clinical features such as seizures, myoclonus, ataxia, progressive muscle weakness, cognitive impairment, stroke-like episodes, etc. Psychiatric illness including mood disorders are frequent in modern humans. Lifelong illnesses affecting young individuals means a burden for family and society. These are chronic disorders with devastating consequences. Genetic vulnerability may be involved in different degrees. Meanwhile, mitochondrial DNA presents high genetic stability. Mitochondria has a direct maternal lineage transmission and some inherited diseases will be transmitted on this path. Despite the mutations present already from birth, they show, in some cases, delayed onset, being compensated by unknown factors. Although most patients with these disorders do not have typical mitochondrial disorders, there is a growing body of evidence to suggest that impaired mitochondrial function may underlie the deteriorating long-term course of these illnesses. Enhancing mitochondrial function could represent an important therapeutic direction.

The most frequent neurodegenerative disorders are Parkinson's disease, Huntington's disease and Alzheimer's disease. They have distinct pathological etiologies, but are also associated with mitochondrial dysfunction (Henchcliffe and Beal 2008; Turner and Schapira, 2010; Galindo et al., 2010). Indeed, mitochondrial dysfunction could form the basis of psychiatric changes that occur before neuronal loss. More than 25% of patients with neurodegenerative diseases receive some psychiatric diagnosis years before their neurodegenerative disorder is identified (Woolley et al., 2011).

Depression is a common manifestation of Parkinson's disease; a study showed that 19% of patients with Parkinson's disease presented with a major depressive disorder (Reijnders et al., 2008). Depression is an early symptom and is associated with an increased risk of Parkinson's disease. Autosomal recessive forms of Parkinson's disease are a consequence of mutations in the genes encoding the proteins PINK1 and Parkin known to be involved in mitophagy. Individuals who carry these mutations have a higher than expected incidence of mood disorders than others (Ishihara and Brayne 2006; Steinlechner et al., 2007).

Huntington's disease is associated with early mood disorders like psychological distress, irritability depression, obsessive compulsiveness, anxiety, interpersonal sensitivity, phobic anxiety and hostility (Berrios et al., 2002; Duff et al., 2007; Kirkwood et al., 2002). It is also associated with depression and a high risk of suicide (Paulsen et al., 2001; Fiedorowicz et al., 2011; Di Maio et al., 1993).

Alzheimer's disease patients manifest behavioral and psychological symptoms (Lyketsos et al., 2000). Many patients develop depression, apathy, anxiety, delusions and hallucinations (Lyketsos et al., 2001; Bassiony et al., 2002; Zubenko et al., 2003). Elevated glucocorticoid levels are associated with depression and also interfere with the ability of neurons to adapt to cellular insults, which could lead to neuronal damage and apoptosis finally inducing Alzheimer's disease (Aznar and Knudsen, 2011; Barnes and Yaffe, 2011; Goosens and Sapolsky, 2007).

Senile plaques and neurofibrillary tangles are associated with mitochondrial dysfunction (Swerdlow et al., 2010; Du et al., 2010; Li et al., 2004). Amyloid-β and tau also contribute to impaired axonal transport of mitochondria, which leads to synaptic degeneration (Calkins and Reddy, 2011; Sydow et al., 2011). Alzheimer's disease may present as synaptic damage due mitochondrial dysfunction as prove by cortex biopsy and fundamental experimental data (DeKosky and Scheff, 1990; Li et al., 2004).

Rare Mitochondrial Disorders

Impairment of one or more biochemical steps of mitochondrial metabolism based on genetic mutations is found in a group of diseases. These patients usually present with psychiatric symptoms such as depression, psychosis, bipolar disorder and personality change (Kato, 2001). One type is caused by a maternally inherited mutation in mitochondrial DNA inducing mitochondrial lactic acidosis, encephalomyopathy and stroke-like episodes. Another is caused by multiple deletions of mitochondrial DNA secondary to mutations in nuclear genes including chronic progressive ophthalmoplegia (Schapira, 2006). Mild mutations could give rise to a slowly progressive, late-onset neurodegenerative disease, such as Parkinson disease. Such mild mutations typically arise in one of two ways: either because the mutation does not cause a severe OxPhos impairment (e.g., mutations in complex I subunits cause Leber's hereditary optic neuropathy (Sadun et al., 2011), or because the proportion of mutated mtDNAs coexists with normal mtDNAs as heteroplasmy, within affected neurons and the deficit in ATP production is only partial, as is typically the case in oligosymptomatic mothers of affected children (DiMauro and Schon, 2003).

There are only few mutations associated with adult-onset neurodegenerative disease and only two well-documented mtDNA mutations are associated with adult-onset neurodegeneration: one with Parkinsonism (De Coo et al., 1999) and one with progressive encephalopathy and cytochrome c oxidase deficiency (Silvestri et al., 2000). A deficit of synthesis of mitochondrial iron-sulfur proteins that are components of respiratory complexes is responsible for Friedreich's ataxia (Schmucker and Puccio, *2010).* Thus psychiatric and neurodegenerative disorders are frequent in patients presenting mitochondrial disfunction. Their study could reveal pathological mechanisms involved in and understanding the cure of those disease.

Ischemic Glutamate Release

The ability of glutamate to act both as a universal metabolite and a specific neurotransmitter is dependent on the compartmentation of the amino acid within the cytoplasm and synaptic vesicles by specific active transport mechanisms. A primary bioenergetic restriction induced by anoxia, ischemia, hypoglycemia, and metabolic restriction disturbs this compartmentation. The release of glutamate from neurons during ischemia *in vivo* can be mimicked *in vitro* during chemical anoxia (respiratory chain inhibition), hypoglycemia (inhibition of glycolysis), or ischemia (combined respiratory chain and glycolytic inhibition). With cultured neurons (Perez-Pinzon, 1997) and brain slices (Calo et al., 1997) the Ca^{2+} - independent release of cytoplasmic glutamate predominates during chemical anoxia, ischemia, and hypoglycemia. In neuronal culture, an initial exocytotic component can be detected after chemical ischemia, consistent with a period of network firing before ATP decreases below the level required for exocytosis.

MITOCONDRIA AS INFORMATIONAL HUB BETWEEN MOLECULE TO CONTECTOM AND DYNOM

Bacterial colonies are able to communicate on trophic substrate availability, coordinating gene expressions in complex behaviors (Picard and, Burelle, 2012; Goo et al., 2015). There are nanotubes that extend up to 1 micrometer out of the surface of the cell walls. These tubules have a diameter of 30 to 13 nm (Dubey and Ben-Yehuda, 2011). Mediating information is exchanged between bacteria but also between mitochondria. Only immobilized mitochondria send nanotubes (Bowes and Gupta, 2008). This growth seems to be an incomplete fission of the mitochondrion (Zhang et al., 2016).

Retrotransposons are genetic elements that utilize an RNA intermediate to copy and paste themselves throughout the genome. There are two groups: long-terminal repeats

(LTRs) and those without (non-LTR). In the human genome, non-LTR retrotransposons consist of long interspersed elements (LINEs) and short interspersed elements (SINEs) (Cordaux and Batzer 2009).

Alu are primate specific genetic elements and are key factors in the formation of neurological networks, they may have contributed to the origin of human cognition. Billions of neurons that are organized into functional hubs, collectively forming the brain connectome (Van Den Heuvel and Sporns 2013). Alu elements could serve an important role in its formation and function of the brain connectome (Oliver and Greene 2011; Li and Church 2013; Smalheiser 2014; Linker et al. 2017; Bitar and Barry, 2017).

HEAT AND LIGHT PRODUCTION

Redox reactions are responsible for both heat and light production (Wise, 2006; Campbell & Reece 2008). An important consequence of the endosymbiotic theory of mitochondria is that all important action such as mitosis, meiosis, rough life conditions or welfare flexibility are consequences of nucleus mitochondria population dialog, where mitochondria has a final decision. In other words, mitochondria seem more independent then other organelles or even dominant in cell hierarchy. As bacteria are able to communicate within their colonies, the mitochondrial research community was equally surprised to learn that the mitochondria are not individual structures, but rather, they exist within an interconnected reticulum. An interesting example is bioluminescent bacteria growing in culture where luciferase synthesis occurs not in the early stage when nutrients are enough, but later. This is a consequence of activation at the level of deoxyribonucleic acid transcription which is attributed to an effect of a "conditioning" of the medium by the growing of cells. Since the phenomenon occurs without external intervention, it must be attributed to a conditioning of the medium affected by the growing cells (Kempner and Hanson, 1968).

One recent mathematical modeling study has suggested that the optical properties of the cristae in filamentous mitochondria may affect the generation and propagation of light within the tissue (Thar et al., 2004). The matrix is the space enclosed by the inner membrane. It is rich in proteins, enzymes and genetic material. It is responsible for the citric acid cycle, pyruvate and fatty acids oxidation (Bruce et al., 1994).

The ratio between the volume of the matrix and the one of the intramembrane space is dependent on the physiological state of the mitochondrion. When the mitochondrion is supplied with sufficient metabolic fuel and oxygen, two states can be distinguished. At low ADP concentrations the mitochondria are in a resting state with low oxygen consumption, whereas at high ADP concentrations the mitochondria respire oxygen at their full capacity. Both states are traditionally termed state 4 and state 3, respectively (Hackenbrock, 1972). During state 4, the matrix occupies about 90% of the mitochondrial volume, i.e., the cristae appear as thin infoldings. On the transition to state 3 the cristae swell until the matrix volume is finally almost halved, i.e., mitochondria in state 3 show an approximately equal distribution between the matrix and the intramembrane space volume. The contraction of the matrix volume during state 3 of respiring mitochondria increases the protein concentration further. This high protein concentration approaches the densest possible packaging for protein molecules with minimal water content. The protein content influences the optical properties of the compartments. The index of refraction is linearly dependent on the protein concentration (Halestrap, 1989; Srere, 1980).

REFRINGENCE

ER and mitochondria are an intracellular system known as mitochondrial reticulum, with a higher optical refraction coefficient than the surrounding cytoplasm. It can be hypothesized that they may serve as an electromagnetic wave guide. The distance between neighboring mitochondria is often much less than the wavelength of visible light and this would allow radiation propagating through a mitochondrion to cross the gap to a neighboring mitochondrion where it can propagate further (Lipson et al., 1995).

The closed contacts of filamentous mitochondria with the microtubules of the cytoskeleton (Ball, 1982; Heggeness et al., 1978) can be optically described as two parallel waveguides in close proximity. The theoretical decay length of the evanescent field of *circa* 30nm enables electromagnetic waves propagating within a mitochondrion to be coupled via the momentary field into the microtubule. Thus, even if filamentous mitochondria are not in close contact to each other, microtubules could provide light guiding along the cellular network of microtubules and filamentous mitochondria.

BIOPHOTONS

Information is transmitted in the nervous system in a way that is only partially revealed to our current knowledge. The basic nervous function can be explained by traditional theory, but complex brain function such as consciousness, mental activities, memory, emotions are not well understood. An alternative approach is communication by fast electrical synapses and biophotons, also called ultra-weak photon emissions also an electromagnetic field. This has been demonstrated in several plants, bacteria and certain animal cells. Recently, both experimental evidence and theoretical speculation have suggested that biophotons may play a potential role in neural signal transmission and processing, contributing to the understanding of the higher functions of nervous system

(Tang and Dai, 2014). Neurons also incessantly emit biophotons (Isojima et al., 1995; Kobayashi et al., 1999). A permanent weak light emission throughout the ultra-violet (UV), visible, and near-infrared (NIR) parts of the electromagnetic spectrum, can be detected by highly sensitive photo-multiplier-tubes. It was postulated that the emitted light, named as "biophotons", could be a part of signaling and information transfer between cell or even in the whole organism (Mei, 1994).

Briefly, the transmittance of light within mitochondria is in principle not confined to a single mitochondrion or cell. Structures such as the chemical and electrical synapsis or cardiac syncytium are good examples. Generally it is considered that this light emission is linked to the production of radicals accompanying the cell's metabolism (Cilento and Adam, 1995).Another possibility is that biophoton emission from neural tissue depends on the neuronal membrane depolarization and Ca^{2+} entry into the cells (Kataoka et al., 2001).Biophotons were directly measured from isolated mitochondria, where peroxidation of mitochondrial membrane lipids was the presumable light-producing mechanism in spinach leaf (Hideg et al., 1991). Specific substrates were shown to increase mitochondrial chemiluminescence significantly, as was demonstrated for the aerobic oxidation of aldehydes (Boh et al., 1982; Nantes et al., 1995). The role of ultra-weak chemiluminescence is generating a debate in the scientific community. Some consider it as a epiphenomenon of metabolic activity with no functional relevance; others speculated that biophotons are involved in triggering photochemical reactions within the cell (Cilento, 1982).

More audacious is the idea of information transfer as formulated by several researchers, including Mei in 1994. Filamentous mitochondria and microtubules can act as optical waveguides. Phase microscopy allows the measurement of the index of refraction for different intracellular components (Spencer, 1982). Measurements yielded values of $n_{cyto}=1.35$ (Johnsen and Widder, 1999) for the cytoplasm and $n_{mito}=1.4$ for whole mitochondria (Beuthan et al., 1996). The refractive index of microtubules was measured as $n_{mt}=1.51$ (Sato et al., 1975). Pure water index of refraction is 1.33. The shape of a typical filamentous mitochondrion can be regarded as an elongated cylinder with a diameter of 300nm, surrounded by a medium with a lower index of refraction. An analogy to optic fiber waveguides has been made which allow the transmission of light through bent paths total internal reflection is the basic principle on which the optic fiber cable functions. Paradoxically, a waveguide presenting a core diameter smaller than the wavelength of the light is still able to transmit light. Light is transmitted along optic fiber waveguides but it is not totally confined to the inner core, being partly also located as an "evanescent field" in the surrounding medium. The intensity of the transient field decreases exponentially with increasing distance to the center of the core. Furthermore, the spectrum of the transmittance and the reflectance can be analyzed by the transfer-matrix method. An ideal filamentous mitochondria will transmit light from 300 nm to 800nm if neither light amplification nor absorption is assumed. The main mechanisms for photon emission from an excited molecule are: spontaneous and induced emission. In the first case, the excited molecules emit the photons. Assuming that the excited molecules have a random spatial orientation, the emitted photons will not exhibit a preferred propagation direction, i.e., the emission is isotropic. The angle between the propagation direction and the long axis of an ideal mitochondrion determines whether the emitted photon is actually "captured" within the mitochondrion and guided by the optical properties of the mitochondrion. That is why only photons with a smaller than the critical angle of entrance in the guide will be transferred. Only a small fraction of biophotons will propagate towards both its ends of the ideal model chosen. In the second case, induced emission provides a possible mechanism for the proposed amplification of the internal light field. Induced emission takes place when an excited molecule is hit by a photon inducing the emission of a second photon with the same characteristics (vector and phase inducing temporal coherence) as the first considered generator photon. Tubulin dimer is a fluorescent molecule due to 8 tryptophan residues it contains (Nogales et al., 1998). The conformation of tubulin is responsible for the absorption (ca. 280 nm) and fluorescence (ca. 335 nm) wavelength. Probing absorption and fluorescence of tubulin is a standard method to determine the polymerization state. This can be considered one of the possible qualitative connections between the fluctuations of MT growth and its corresponding biophoton absorption and emission characteristics. Additionally, there exist other energy states (of both optical and vibrational nature which tubulin dimers and the whole MT can support (Pokorný et al., 1997; Jelínek and Pokorný, 2001; Deriu et al., 2010). Using as analogy the design of distributed feedback lasers and similar multi-layer system presenting different indices of refraction, high temporal coherence, high directivity, monochromatic light, mitochondria would act like lasers (Kneubuhl and Sigrist, 1999; Tannhauser, 1995). Induced light emission is a tempting working hypothesis for future research. However, it seems too speculative by critical evaluation. Meanwhile, considering that light is measured several centimeters outside mitochondrion as ultra-weak chemiluminescence, the real level of intensity inside might be much higher (Cadenas, 1988; Inaba, 1988; Thar and Kühl, 2004).

In general, the scientific consensus is that light propagation is mainly based on random absorption and scattering events (e.g., Yamada, 2000). In contrast, light guiding properties of the mitochondrial network could indicate that the light propagation can be essentially non-random. It is tempting to speculate that mitochondria function not only as power generator, but also as an important information hub interconnected by light with cell perikaryon, between cells, tissues, organs and organism itself. Last but not least, due to large numeric and spatial representation, speculation is extended to a complex holographic memory by the author. If quorum sensing was described in different system (microorganisms colonies, social hexapods, human group cultural behavior), why should it not be accepted it for the mitochondrial *"ego"*.

Mitochondrial oxidative metabolism generates heat and light as ultra-weak chemiluminescence. Due to its optical properties and multilayer structure, mitochondrial reticulum could be a wave guide working as lasting effect as seen tylakoide structure in chloroplast and in technical distributed feedback laser. There are data supporting that external illumination on the mitochondria could induce some kind of long-range interaction between individual units probably mediated by electromagnetic radiation itself (Thar and Kühl, 2004; http://www.sciencedirect.com/science/article/pii/ S0022519304002498).

Ultra-weak photon emissions known as biophotons (*vide supra*) could inform on living bodies biology in a non invasive way both in medicine and agriculture. Due to the complexity of the problem, large scale application is limited for now (Kobayashi, 2014). Efforts for whole human body biophotons scan are in progress (Van Wijk et al., 2014).

FROM CONNECTOM TO DYNOM

The human brain is an amazingly complex structure whose functionality, including higher-order cognitive functions, is determined by intricate connectivity patterns between tens of billions of neurons (Azevedo et al. 2009). The signaling between neurons uses binary-like electrical impulses, such that the multitude of brain functions, that are often performed concurrently, are the result of connectivity patterns across various spatial scales (Budd and Kisvarday 2012) that implement a mixed sequential, parallel or hierarchical architecture. Different functions are performed by well-defined areas of the brain (i.e., visual stimuli are processed solely by the primary visual cortex), some higher level functions (i.e., speech production, problem solving, music performance) can only be accomplished by various brain areas working together in a serial or, more likely, in a parallel or distributed design (Sigman and Dehaene 2008; Donos et al., 2017; Donos et al., 2016a; Donos et al., 2016b).

Connectome is a map of neural connections in the brain compared to a "wiring diagram" and it contains all neural connections within an organism's nervous system. This emerging field is focused on neurons and synapsis spanning microscale to large macroscale interactions but also targeting higher brain functions. Connectomics study the human brain as a network (Sporns, 2013). Networks contain nodes and edges. An edge connects two nodes and represents an anatomical connection between two brain active areas. In a functional network, an edge represents the statistical association between activities recorded from separate brain elements (Park and Friston, 2013).

The term "connectome" is used primarily in scientific efforts to capture, map, and understand the organization of neural interactions within the brain. The first mapped being was the round worm C. elegans (Varshney et al., 2011).

Extending the acquired knowledge from C. elegans, Bargman et al. (2013) found that neuronal dynamics, neuromodulation and parallel circuits, jump across systems, so the vertebrate retina wiring has common features with invertebrate nervous organization, suggesting that they expose common features to many living creature and data from small circuits may be useful to understand the large ones (Bargmann and Marder, 2013).

The living matter characteristics arise from complex interactions between its numerous constituents. That is the reason why it is crucial to understand the structure and the dynamics of the complex interactions that build up the structure and the derived functions of living organisms. None of these networks are independent, instead they form a 'network of networks' that is responsible for the behavior from the subcell level to organisms and society. It is accepted that similar laws may govern most complex phenomena in our known universe. A few principles are common and they must be deciphered. Evolution and natural selection reuse existing "winner solution" to further increase the organism's survival probability and its complexity. This fundamental observation will significantly support our understanding of biology (Hartwell et al., 1999; Kitano, 2002; Strogatz, 2001). The ultimate goal of connectomics is to map the human brain. This effort is pursued by the **Human Connectome Project**, sponsored by the National Institutes of Health (http://www.humanconnectomeproject.org/)

Dynome as defined by Kopell et al. (2014): "This expanded description of brain activity is what we call the "dynome." The dynome is the collection of experimental and modeling observations having to do with dynamical structure (and its physiological and pathophysiological implementation) in the brain and its relationship to cognition. It includes what is usually known as the functional connectome but expands the notion to go beyond statistical associations to the mechanisms involved in producing and processing signals within the brain. In the dynome context, understanding brain activity means uncovering the functions and dysfunctions provided by the brain's temporal dynamics. Like the connectome, the dynome proposes a framework for a broad research program. Yet the dynome does not have to be constructed *de novo*: there is already a body of work on which further efforts can be based. However, we note that, though much cognitively important dynamical structure has been uncovered, the field is still in its infancy."

Understanding signals, how are they produced, routed, combined in different patterns and hierarchical orders, generating complex electromagnetic fields could be compared to a symphony were neurons or organelles activity are the notes and the refined intellectual affective and subjective individual perception of the music is an astonishing accomplishment.

CONCLUSION

Mitochondria, far from being perfect machines, are fragile structures operating near their functional limits. Their pathology appears to underlie a host of degenerative disease states in the brain. Furthermore, it has been discovered that mitochondria have a role in the signaling pathways that culminate in apoptosis.

Mitochondrial function is complex. Several events can compromise mitochondrial function and integrity. The most important is the damage or mutation of mitochondrial DNA (mtDNA). An increase in reactive oxygen species (ROS) and abnormal elevation of cytosolic Ca^{2+} (caused by endoplasmic reticulum (ER) stress and dysfunction, and by Ca^{2+} over-influx through NMDA receptors (NMDARs) and calcium channels are responsible for other major disfunctions. Mitochondria have an important role in several processes that are essential to neuronal function based on ATP production which is essential for maintaining neuronal integrity and responsiveness, as well as neurotransmission, especially fast neurotransmission. These processes are also modulated by ROS, which can be produced by mitochondria. Furthermore, mitochondria can take up Ca^{2+} (released by the ER), and release Ca^{2+} and thereby play a part in maintaining intracellular Ca^{2+} homeostasis. Mitochondria are also crucial for neurite outgrowth and the regeneration of neuronal processes. Finally, leakage of mitochondrial intermembranous contents, such as cytochrome c, into the cytosol causes caspase activation, DNA damage and apoptosis. This process has been linked to neuron loss in ischaemia, traumatic brain injury and neurodegenerative diseases, but is critical in neurogenesis, in which the majority of newborn cells do not survive to become mature neurons.

The complex and frequently bewildering mutual interactions between mitochondrial and cellular bioenergetics presented here allows some general principles to be derived. First, the mitochondrial membrane potential is at the center of the cell's interactions, controlling ATP synthesis, mitochondrial Ca^{2+} accumulation, superoxide generation, and redox reactions. Second, mitochondria are intimately involved with both necrotic and apoptotic cell death. In the former mode, modeled by exposing cultured neurons to pathological glutamate, mitochondrial Ca^{2+} loading and consequent generation of ROS appear to play a central role. The generation of ROS and the maintenance of a reduced environment are both favored by a high mitochondrial membrane potential, and the damaging effects of the one, have to be balanced against the beneficial effects of the other. The mitochondria themselves appear to retain bioenergetic competence and the capacity to generate ATP until a late stage, characterized *in vitro* by delayed cytoplasmic Ca^{2+} deregulation. Mitochondrial release of proapoptotic factors, such as cytochrome c, is integral to apoptosis induced by a wide variety of cellular effectors of programmed cell death. Understanding the intact brain functions remain a goal for this generation and perhaps the next generations. Although there are considerable opportunities on the horizon for breakthroughs that may have a substantial impact on basic research an organized unitary and standardized approach is foreseen as necessary. Technological developments across many modalities, including progress in anatomical tracing and molecular-profiling techniques, innovations in optogenetic control, and advances in diverse activity readouts, are driving fundamental changes in the way that neuroscientists work. Organized thinking about communication in neural circuits may in itself help in organizing ties among researchers operating within these different modalities and from other biology and engineering disciplines.

REFERENCES

[1] Almeida A, Almeida J, Bolanos JP, Moncada S. Different responses of astrocytes and neurons to nitric oxide: the role of glycolytically generated ATP in astrocyte protection. *Proc Natl Acad Sci U S A*. 2001;98: 15294–15299.

[2] Altmann, R 1890. *Die Elementarorganismen und ihre Beziehungen zu den Zellen.* [*The elemental organisms and their relationships to the cells*]. Veit, Leipzig.

[3] Ames A 3rd (1992) Energy requirements of CNS cells as related to their function and to their vulnerability to ischemia: a commentary based on studies on retina. *Can J Physiol Pharmacol* 70:S158S164.

[4] Ames A 3rd (2000) CNS energy metabolism related to function. *Brain Res Rev* 34:42–68).

[5] Amirsadeghi S, Robson CA and Vanlerberghe GC (2007) The role of the mitochondrion in plant responses to biotic stress. *Physiologia Plantarum* 129: 253–266.

[6] Anderson S, Bankier AT, Barrell BG, de Bruijn MH, et al. 1981. Sequence and organization of the human mitochondrial genome. *Nature* 290: 457–65.

[7] Andrade-Navarro MA, Sanchez-Pulido L, McBride HM 2009. Mitochondrial vesicles: an ancient process providing new links to peroxisomes. *Curr Opin Cell Biol* 21: 560–7.

[8] Ankarcrona M, Dypbukt JM, Bonfoco E, Zhivotovsky B, Orrenius S, Lipton SA, Nicotera P. Glutamate-induced neuronal death: a succession of necrosis or apoptosis depending on mitochondrial function. *Neuron* 15: 961–973, 1995.

[9] Avise JC. (2000) *Phylogeography: The History and Formation of Species.* CambridgeMassachusetts: Harvard University Press.

[10] Avril S, Muzic RF Jr, Plecha D, Traughber BJ, Vinayak S, Avril N. 18F-FDG PET/CT for monitoring of treatment response in breast cancer. *J Nucl Med.* 2016 Feb; 57(Suppl 1): 34S–39S.,

[11] Azevedo FAC, Carvalho LRB, Grinberg LT, Farfel JM, Ferretti REL, Leite REP, Jacob Filho W, Lent R, Herculano-Houzel S (2009) Equal numbers of neuronal and nonneuronal cells make the human brain an isometrically scaled-up primate brain. *J Comp Neurol* 513:532–541.

[12] Aznar S and Knudsen GM. Depression and Alzheimer's disease: is stress the initiating factor in a common neuropathological cascade? *J. Alzheimers Dis.* 23, 177–193 (2011).

[13] Bakeeva LE, Chentsov Yu S, Skulachev VP. 1978. Mitochondrial framework (reticulum mitochondriale) in rat diaphragm muscle. *Biochim. Biophys. Acta* 501 (3), 349–369.

[14] Ball EH 1982. Mitochondria are associated with microtubules and not with intermediate filaments in cultured fibroblasts. *Proc. Natl Acad. Sci. USA* 79, 123–126.

[15] Bargmann, CI and Marder E (2013) From the connectome to brain function. *Nat. Methods* 10, 483–490.

[16] Barnes DE and Yaffe K. The projected effect of risk factor reduction on Alzheimer's disease prevalence. *Lancet Neurol.* 10, 819–828 (2011).

[17] Boh EE, Baricos WH, Bernofsky C, Steele RH 1982. Mitochondrial chemiluminescence elicited by acetaldehyde. *J. Bioenerg. Biomembr.* 14 (2), 1982.

[18] Bassiony MM et al. The relationship between delusions and depression in Alzheimer's disease. *Int. J. Geriatr. Psychiatry* 17, 549–556 (2002).

[19] Beal MF (2000) Energetics in the pathogenesis of neurodegenerative diseases. *Trends Neurosci* 23:298–304.

[20] Beltran B, Mathur A, Duchen MR, Erusalimsky JD, Moncada S. The effect of nitric oxide on cell respiration: A key to understanding its role in cell survival or death. *Proc Natl Acad Sci U S A.* 2000;97: 14602–14607.

[21] Benda C 1898. Ueber die Spermatogenese der Vertebraten und höherer Evertebraten. II. Theil: Die Histiogenese der Spermien. *Arch. Anal. Physiol.* 393-398.

[22] Berrios GE et al. Psychiatric symptoms in neurologically asymptomatic Huntington's disease gene carriers: a comparison with gene negative at risk subjects. *Acta Psychiatr. Scand.* 105, 224–230 (2002).

[23] Betarbet R, Sherer TB, MacKenzie G, Garcia-Osuna M, Panov AV, Greenamyre JT (2000) Chronic systemic pesticide exposure reproduces features of Parkinson's disease. *Nat Neurosci* 3:1301–1306.

[24] Beuthan J, Minet O, Helfmann J, Herrig M, Muller G 1996. The spatial variation of the refractive index in biological cells. *Phys. Med. Biol.* 41 (3), 369–382.

[25] Bitar M, Barry G (2017) Multiple innovations in genetic and epigenetic mechanisms cooperate to underpin human brain evolution. *Mol Biol Evol.* msx303.

[26]   Bowes T and Gupta RS (2008) Novel mitochondrial extensions provide evidence for a link between microtubule-directed movement and mitochondrial fission. *Biochem. Biophys. Res. Commun.* 376, 40–45.

[27]   Braitenberg V, Schüz A (1998*) Cortex: statistics and geometry of neuronal connectivity*, 2nd ed. Berlin: Springer.

[28]   Brealey D, Brand M, Hargreaves I, Heales S, Land J, Smolenski R, Davies NA, Cooper CE, Singer M. Association between mitochondrial dysfunction and severity and outcome of septic shock. *Lancet.* 2002; 360:219–223.

[29]   Bromham L, Penny D (2003) The modern molecular clock. *Nat Rev Genet* 4:216–224.

[30]   Brown WM, George M Jr, Wilson AC; George; Wilson (1979), "Rapid evolution of animal mitochondrial DNA", *Proc Natl Acad Sci U S A,* 76 (4): 1967–71,

[31]   Brown GC, Cooper CE. Nanomolar concentrations of nitric oxide reversibly inhibit synaptosomal respiration by competing with oxygen at cytochrome oxidase. *FEBS Lett.* 1994;356:295–298.

[32]   Bruce A, Johnson A, Lewis J, Raff M, Roberts K, Walter P (1994). *Molecular Biology of the Cell*. New York: Garland Publishing Inc.

[33]   Budd J, Kisvarday Z (2012) Communication and wiring in the cortical connectome. *Front Neuroanat* 6:42.

[34]   Cadenas E 1988. Biological chemiluminescence. *NATO ASI Ser, Ser. A* 146, 117–141.

[35]   Calkins, MJ and Reddy PH. Amyloid beta impairs mitochondrial anterograde transport and degenerates synapses in Alzheimer's disease neurons. *Biochim. Biophys. Acta* 1812, 507–513 (2011).

[36]   Calo G, Sbrenna S, Bianchi C and Beani L. Immediate and delayed effects of in vitro ischemia on glutamate efflux from guinea-pig cerebral cortex slices. *Brain Res.* 751: 300–306, 1997.

[37]   Campbell, Neil A, Williamson B, Heyden RJ (2006) *Biology: Exploring Life.* Boston, Massachusetts: *Pearson Prentice Hall.* ISBN 0-13-250882-6.

[38]   Campbell & Reece. Biology 8th edition. Benjamin Cummings. 2008. pp. 196–197.

[39]   Cann RL, Stoneking M, Wilson AC (1987), "Mitochondrial DNA and human evolution", Nature, 325 (6099): 31–36, *Nature.* 1987 Jan 1-7;325(6099):31-6.

[40]   Castanier C, Garcin D, Vazquez A, Arnoult D 2010. Mitochondrial dynamics regulate the RIG-I-like receptor antiviral pathway. *EMBO Rep* 11: 133–8.

[41]   Chada SR, Hollenbeck PJ 2004. Nerve growth factor signaling regulates motility and docking of axonal mitochondria. *Curr Biol* 14: 1272–6.

[42]   Chada SR, Hollenbeck PJ 2003. Mitochondrial movement and positioning in axons: the role of growth factor signaling. *J Exp Biol* 206: 1985–92.

[43] Chen H, Vermulst M, Wang YE, Chomyn A et al. 2010. Mitochondrial fusion is required for mtDNA stability in skeletal muscle and tolerance of mtDNA mutations. *Cell* 141: 280–9.

[44] Chipuk JE, Bouchier-Hayes L, Green DR (2006). "Mitochondrial outer membrane permeabilization during apoptosis: the innocent bystander scenario". *Cell Death and Differentiation*. 13 (8): 1396–1402.

[45] Cifra M, Pospíšil P. Ultra-weak photon emission from biological samples: Definition, mechanisms, properties, detection and applications, *Journal of Photochemistry and Photobiology B: Biology, Volume 139,* 5 October 2014, Pages 2-10.

[46] Civitarese AE, MacLean PS, Carling S, Kerr-Bayles L et al. 2010. Regulation of skeletal muscle oxidative capacity and insulin signaling by the mitochondrial rhomboid protease PARL. *Cell Metab* 11: 412–26.

[47] Cleeter MW, Cooper JM, rley-Usmar VM, Moncada S, Schapira AH. Reversible inhibition of cytochrome C oxidase, the terminal enzyme of the mitochondrial respiratory chain, by nitric oxide. Implications for neurodegenerative diseases. *FEBS Lett.;* 345:50–54.

[48] Cilento G, Adam W 1995. From free radicals to electronically excited species. *Free Radical Biol. Med.* 19 (1), 103–114.

[49] Cilento G 1982. Electronic excitation in dark biological processes. In: Adam W, Cilento G (Eds.), *Chemical and Biological Generation of Excited States.* Academic Press, New York.

[50] Cogliati S, Frezza C, Soriano M E, Varanita T, QuintanaCabrera R, Corrado M, Cipolat S, Costa V, Casarin A, Gomes L C, Perales-Clemente E, Salviati L, Fernandez-Silva P, Enriquez JA, Scorrano L. *Cell* 2013, 155, 160–171.

[51] Cogliati S, Enriquez J A, Scorrano L, *Trends Biochem. Sci.* 2016, 41, 261–273.

[52] Cordaux R, Batzer MA (2009) The impact of retrotransposons on human genome evolution. *Nat Rev Genet* 10:691–703.

[53] Courtney MJ, Lambert JJ, Nicholls DG. The interactions between plasma membrane depolarization and glutamate receptor activation in the regulation of cytoplasmic free calcium in cultured cerebellar granule cells. *J. Neurosci.* 10: 3873– 3879, 1990.

[54] David G Nicholls and Samantha L Budd. Mitochondria and Neuronal Survival: *Physiological Reviews* Vol. 80, pp 315- 360No. 1, January 2000.

[55] De Brito OM, Scorrano L 2008. Mitofusin 2 tethers endoplasmic reticulum to mitochondria. *Nature* 456: 605–10.

[56] De Coo, IF, Renier, WO, Ruitenbeek, W, Ter Laak, HJ, Bakker M, Schagger H, Van Oost BA and Smeets HJ (1999). A 4-base pair deletion in the mitochondrial cytochrome b gene associated with parkinsonism/MELAS overlap syndrome. *Ann. Neurol.* 45, 130–133.

[57] DeKosky ST and Scheff SW. Synapse loss in frontal cortex biopsies in Alzheimer's disease: correlation with cognitive severity. *Ann. Neurol.* 27, 457–464 (1990).

[58] Deriu MA, Soncini M, Orsi M, Patel M, Essex JW, Montevecchi FM, Redaelli A, Anisotropic Elastic Network Modeling of Entire Microtubules, *Biophys J* 99:2190 – 2199, 2010.

[59] Di Maio L et al. Suicide risk in Huntington's disease. *J. Med. Genet.* 30, 293–295 (1993).

[60] Donos C, Barborica A, Mindruta I, Maliia M, Popa I, Ciurea J (2017) Connectomics in Patients with Temporal Lobe Epilepsy. In: Opris I, Casanova M (eds) *The Physics of the Mind and Brain Disorders*. Springer Series in Cognitive and Neural Systems, vol 11. Springer, Cham.

[61] Donos C, Mălîia MD, Mîndruţă I, Popa I, Ene M, Bălănescu B, Ciurea A, Barborica A (2016a) A connectomics approach combining structural and effective connectivity assessed by intracranial electrical stimulation. *Neuro Image* 132:344–358

[62] Donos C, Mîndruţă I, Ciurea J, Mălîia MD, Barborica A (2016b) A comparative study of the effects of pulse parameters for intracranial direct electrical stimulation in epilepsy. *Clin Neurophysiol* 127:91–101.

[63] Dubey GP and Ben-Yehuda S (2011) Intercellular nanotubes mediate bacterial communication. *Cell* 144, 590–600.

[64] Duchen MR (1999) Contributions of mitochondria to animal physiology: from homeostatic sensor to calcium signalling and cell death. *J Physiol (Lond)* 516:1–17.

[65] Dudkina NV, Heinemayer J, Sunderhaus S, Boekema EJ and Braun H- P (2006) Respiratory chain complexes in the plant mitochondrial membrane. *Trends in Plant Science* 11: 232–240.

[66] Du, H et al. Early deficits in synaptic mitochondria in an Alzheimer's disease mouse model. *Proc. Natl Acad. Sci. USA* 107, 18670–18675 (2010).

[67] Duff, K, Paulsen JS, Beglinger, LJ, Langbehn, DR and Stout JC. Psychiatric symptoms in Huntington's disease before diagnosis: the predict-HD study. *Biol. Psychiatry* 62, 1341–1346 (2007).

[68] Ehses S, Raschke I, Mancuso G, Bernacchia A et al. 2009. Regulation of OPA1 processing and mitochondrial fusion by m-AAA protease isoenzymes and OMA1. *J Cell Biol* 187: 1023–36.

[69] Ernster Lars, Schatz Gottfried (December 1981) Mitochondria: a historical review. *The Journal of Cell Biology.* 91 (3 Pt 2): 227–255.

[70] Fawcett D 1981. *The Cell.* Saunders, Philadelphia.

[71] Fiedorowicz JG, Mills JA, Ruggle A, Langbehn D and Paulsen JS. Suicidal behavior in prodromal Huntington disease. *Neurodegener. Dis.* 8, 483–490 (2011).

[72] Frank S, Gaume B, Bergmann-Leitner ES, Leitner WW et al. 2001. The role of dynamin-related protein 1, a mediator of mitochondrial fission, in apoptosis. *Dev Cell* 1: 515–25.

[73] Galindo MF, Ikuta I Zhu, X, Casadesus G and Jordan J. Mitochondrial biology in Alzheimer's disease pathogenesis. *J. Neurochem.* 114, 933–945 (2010).

[74] Gao CL, Zhu C, Zhao YP, Chen XH et al. 2010. Mitochondrial dysfunction is induced by high levels of glucose and free fatty acids in 3T3-L1 adipocytes. *Mol Cell Endocrinol* 320: 25–33.

[75] Goo E et al. (2015) Control of bacterial metabolism by quorum sensing. *Trends Microbiol.* 23, 567–576.

[76] Goosens KA and Sapolsky RM. *Stress and Glucocorticoid Contributions to Normal and Pathological Aging in Brain Aging: Models, Methods, and Mechanisms* (ed. Riddle DR.) Ch.13 (CRC Press, Boca Raton, 2007).

[77] Hackenbrock CR 1972. States of activity and structure in mitochondrial membranes. *Ann. NY Acad. Sci.* 195, 492–505.

[78] Halestrap AP 1989. The regulation of the matrix volume of mammalian mitochondria in vivo and in vitro and its role in the control of mitochondrial metabolism. *Biochim. Biophys. Acta* 973 (3), 355–382.

[79] Hanson MR and Bentolila S (2004) Interactions of mitochondrial and nuclear genes that affect male gametophyte development. *Plant Cell* 16: S154–S169.

[80] Hartwell LH, Hopfield JJ, Leibler S and Murray AW. From molecular to modular cell biology. *Nature* 402, C47–C52 (1999).

[81] Hayashi T, Rizzuto R, Hajnoczky G, Su TP (February 2009). "MAM: more than just a housekeeper". *Trends Cell Biol.* 19(2): 81–8.

[82] Head B, Griparic L, Amiri M, Gandre-Babbe S et al. 2009. Inducible proteolytic inactivation of OPA1 mediated by the OMA1 protease in mammalian cells. *J Cell Biol* 187: 959–66.

[83] Heggeness MH, Simon M, Singer SJ, 1978. Association of mitochondria with microtubules in cultured cells. *Proc. Natl Acad. Sci. USA* 75 (8), 3863–3866.

[84] Henchcliffe, C and Beal MF. Mitochondrial biology and oxidative stress in Parkinson disease pathogenesis. *Nature Clin. Pract. Neurol.* 4, 600–609 (2008).

[85] Herrmann JM, Neupert W (April 2000). "Protein transport into mitochondria". *Current Opinion in Microbiology.* 3 (2): 210–214.

[86] Hermann GJ, Thatcher JW, Mills JP, Hales KG, et al. 1998. Mitochondrial fusion in yeast requires the transmembrane GTPase Fzo1p. *J Cell Biol* 143: 359–73.

[87] Hideg E, Kobayashi M, Inaba H 1991. Spontaneous ultraweak" light emission from respiring spinach leaf mitochondria. *Biochim. Biophys. Acta* 1098, 27–31.

[88] Hochachka PW (1994) *Muscles as molecular and metabolic machines.* Boca Raton: CRC Press.

[89] Hoppins S, Nunnari J 2009. The molecular mechanism of mitochondrial fusion. *Biochim Biophys Acta* 1793: 20–6.

[90] Hyde BB, Twig G, Shirihai OS 2010. Organellar vs cellular control of mitochondrial dynamics. *Semin Cell Dev Biol* 21: 575–81.

[91] Inaba, H 1988. Super-high sensitivity systems for detection and spectral analysis of ultraweak photon emission from biological cells and tissues. *Experientia* 44 (7), 550–559.

[92] Inoki K, Kim J, Guan KL. AMPK and mTOR in cellular energy homeostasis and drug targets. *Annu Rev Pharmacol toxicol.* 2012;52:381–400.

[93] Ishihara N, Nomura M, Jofuku A, Kato H, et al. 2009. Mitochondrial fission factor Drp1 is essential for embryonic development and synapse formation in mice. *Nat Cell Biol* 11: 958–66.

[94] Ishihara, L and Brayne C. A systematic review of depression and mental illness preceding Parkinson's disease. *Acta Neurol. Scand.* 113, 211–220 (2006). 143.

[95] Isojima Y, Isoshima T, Nagai K, Kikuchi K, Nakagawa H, Ultraweak biochemiluminescence detected from rat hippocampal slices, *NeuroReport* 6:658–660, 1995.

[96] Jelínek F, Pokorný J. Microtubules in biological cells as circular waveguides and resonators, *Electro- magnetobiol* 20:75–80, 2001.

[97] Johnsen S, Widder EA 1999. The physical basis of transparancy in biological tissue: ultrastructure and the minimization of light scattering. *J. Theor. Biol.* 199, 181–198.

[98] Karbowski M, Neutzner A, Youle RJ 2007. The mitochondrial E3 ubiquitin ligase MARCH5 is required for Drp1 dependent mitochondrial division. *J Cell Biol* 178: 71–84.

[99] Kasha M, Pullman B, eds. *Horizons in Biochemistry*. New York: Academic Press. pp 189–225.

[100] Kataoka Y, Cui Y, Yamagata A, Niigaki M, Hirohata T, Oishi N, Watanabe Y, ActivityDependent Neural Tissue Oxidation Emits Intrinsic Ultraweak Photons, *Biochem Biophys Res Commun* 285:1007–1011, 2001.

[101] Kato T. The other, forgotten genome: mitochondrial DNA and mental disorders. *Mol. Psychiatry* 6, 625–633 (2001).

[102] Katz B (1969) *The release of neural transmitter substances.* Springfield, IL: Thomas.

[103] Kawai T, Takahashi K, Sato S, Coban C, Kumar H, Kato H, Ishii KJ, Takeuchi O and Akira S (2005). IPS-1, an adaptor triggering RIG-I- and Mda5-mediated type I interferon induction. *Nat. Immunol.* 6, 981–988.

[104] Kempner, ES and FE Hanson. 1968. Aspects of light production by Pholobacterium fischeri. *J. Bacteriol.* 95: 975-979.

[105] Kirkwood SC et al. Longitudinal personality changes among presymptomatic Huntington disease gene carriers. Neuropsychiatry Neuropsychol. *Behav. Neurol.* 15, 192–197 (2002).

[106] Kitano H. Computational systems biology. *Nature* 420, 206–210 (2002).

[107] Klishin A, Sedova M, Blatter LA. Time-dependent modulationofcapacitativeCa2+ entrysignalsbyplasmamembrane Ca2+ pump in endothelium. *Am. J. Physiol.* 274 (Cell Physiol. 43): C1117—C1128, 1998.

[108] Kneubuhl FK, Sigrist MW 1999. Laser. Teubner, Stuttgart. Lipson SG, Lipson HS, Tannhauser DS, 1995. *Optical Physics,* 3rd Edition. Cambridge University Press, Cambridge.

[109] Kobayashi M, Takeda M, Sato T, Yamazaki Y, Kaneko K, Ito K, Kato H, Inaba H. In vivo imaging of spontaneous ultraweak photon emission from a rat's brain correlated with cerebral energy metabolism and oxidative stress, *Neurosci Res* 34:103–113, 1999.

[110] Kobayashi Masaki (2014) Highly sensitive imaging for ultra-weak photon emission from living organisms; *J Photochemistry and Photobiology B: Biology*, 139, 34-38, ISSN1011-1344; https://doi.org/10.1016/j.jphotobiol.2013.11.011. (http://www.sciencedirect.com/science/article/pii/S1011134413002558).

[111] Kopell NJ, Gritton HJ, Whittington MA, Kramer MA (2014) Beyond the Connectome: The Dynome, *Neuron,* 83:6, 1319-1328,

[112] Kumar S (2005) Molecular clocks: four decades of evolution. *Nat Rev Genet* 6: 654–662.()

[113] Kety SS (1957) The general metabolism of the brain in vivo. In: *Metabolism of the nervous system* (RichterD,ed),London:Pergamon, pp 221–237.

[114] Laloi C, Apel K and Danon A (2004) Reactive oxygen signalling: the latest news. *Current Opinion in Plant Biology* 7: 323–328.

[115] Lamming DW, Ye L, Sabatini DM, Baur JA. Rapalogs and mTOR inhibitors as anti-aging therapeutics. *J Clin Invest.* 2013;123(3):980–989.

[116] Legendre, P, Rosenmund C, Westbrook GL. Inactivation of NMDA channels in cultured hippocampal neurons by intracellular calcium. *J. Neurosci.* 13: 674–684, 1993.

[117] Leist, M, Single B, Castoldi AF, Kuhnle S, Nicotera P. Intracellular adenosine triphosphate (ATP) concentration: a switch in the decision between apoptosis and necrosis. *J. Exp. Med.* 185: 1481–1486, 1997.

[118] Leslie SW, Chandler LJ, Barr EM, Farrar RP (1985) Reduced calcium uptake by rat brain mitochondria and synaptosomes in response to aging. *Brain Res* 329:177–183.

[119] Li JB, Church GM (2013) Deciphering the functions and regulation of brain-enriched A-to-I RNA editing. *Nat Neurosci* 16: 1518–1522.

[120] Linker SB, Marchetto MC, Narvaiza I. (2017), Examining non LTR retro transposons in the context of the evolving primate brain. *BMC Biol* 15:68.

[121] Lipson, SG, Lipson, HS, Tannhauser DS 1995. *Optical Physics,* 3rd Edition. Cambridge University Press, Cambridge.

[122] Li Z, Okamoto K, Hayashi Y and Sheng M. The importance of dendritic mitochondria in the morphogenesis and plasticity of spines and synapses. *Cell* 119, 873–887 (2004).

[123] Lu M, Zhu X-H, Yi Z, Mateescu GD, Chen W. Quantitative assessment of brain glucose metabolic rates using in vivo deuterium magnetic resonance spectroscopy. *J Cerebral Blood Flow & Metabolism.* 2017; doi:10.1177/0271678X1770644.

[124] Lyketsos CG et al. Mental and behavioral disturbances in dementia: findings from the Cache County Study on Memory in Aging. *Am. J. Psychiatry* 157, 708–714 (2000).

[125] Lyketsos CG et al. Neuropsychiatric disturbance in Alzheimer's disease clusters into three groups: the Cache County study. *Int. J. Geriatr. Psychiatry* 16, 1043–1053 (2001).

[126] Manfredi AA, Rovere-Querini P 2010. The mitochondrion – a Trojan horse that kicks off inflammation? *N Engl J Med* 362: 2132–4.

[127] Mannella CA (2006). "Structure and dynamics of the mitochondrial inner membrane cristae". *Biochimica et Biophysica Acta.* 1763 (5–6): 542 548. doi:10.1016/j.bbamcr.2006.04.006.

[128] Makino A, Scott BT, Dillmann WH 2010. Mitochondrial fragmentation and superoxide anion production in coronary endothelial cells from a mouse model of type 1 diabetes. *Diabetologia* 53: 1783–94.

[129] Margineantu DH, Gregory Cox, W, Sundell L, Sherwood SW, et al. 2002. Cell cycle dependent morphology changes and associated mitochondrial DNA redistribution in mitochondria of human cell lines. *Mitochondrion* 1: 425–35.

[130] Mateescu GD, Ye A, Flask CA, Erokwu B, Duerk JL. In vivo assessment of oxygen consumption via deuterium magnetic resonance. *Adv Exp Med Biol.* 2011;701:193 -199, and references cited therein.

[131] Mateescu GD, Ye A, Flask CA, Erokwu B, Twieg M, Gupta K, Griswold M. Novel biomarkers of mitochondrial function: the mitochondrial index and the crossing point of glucose and oxygen consumption curves obtained by in vivo dynamic deuterium magnetic resonance. *Proc Intl Soc Magn Reson Med.* 2015;019.

[132] Maurino VG and Peterhansel C (2010) Photorespiration: current status and approaches for metabolic engineering. *Current Opinion in Plant Biology* 13: 249–256.

[133] *McBride HM, Neuspiel M, Wasiak S. "Mitochondria: more than just a powerhouse". Curr. Biol. 16 (14) (July 25, 2006).: R551–60. doi:10.1016/* j.cub.2006.06.054. PMID 16860735.

[134] Mei W 1994. About the nature of biophotons. *J Biol. Systems* 2 (1), 25–42.

[135] Meylan E, Curran J, Hofmann K, Moradpour D, Binder M, Bartenschlager R and Tschopp J (2005). Cardif is an adaptor protein in the RIG-I antiviral pathway and is targeted by hepatitis C virus. *Nature* 437, 1167–1172.

[136] Mitchell P 1977. Vectorial chemiosmotic processes. *Annu. Rev. Biochem.* 46, 996–1005.

[137] Mitra K, Wunder C, Roysam B, Lin G, et al. 2009. A hyperfused mitochondrial state achieved at G1-S regulates cyclin E buildup and entry into S phase. *Proc Natl Acad Sci USA* 106: 11960–5.

[138] Moncada S, Erusalimsky JD. Does nitric oxide modulate mitochondrial energy generation and apoptosis? *Nat Rev Mol Cell Biol.* 2002;3: 214–220.

[139] Nantes IL, Cilentos G, Bechara EJH, Vercesi AE 1995. Chemiluminescence diphenylacetaldehyde oxidation by mitochondria is promoted by cytochromes and leads to oxidative injury of the organelle. *J. Photochem. Photobiol.* 62 (3), 522–527.

[140] Neuspiel M, Schauss AC, Braschi E, Zunino R et al. 2008. Cargoselected transport from the mitochondria to peroxisomes is mediated by vesicular carriers. *Curr Biol* 18: 102–8.

[141] Nicholls DG, Budd SL (2000) Mitochondria and neuronal survival. *Physiol Rev* 80:315–360.

[142] Nicholls DG. The effective proton conductances of the inner membrane of mitochondria from brown adipose tissue: dependency on proton electrochemical gradient. *Eur. J. Biochem.* 77: 349–356, 1977.

[143] Nicholls DG and Bernson VSM. Inter-relationships between proton electrochemical gradient, adenine nucleotide phosphorylation potential and respiration during substrate-level and oxidative phosphorylation by mitochondria from brown adipose tissue of cold-adapted guinea-pigs. *Eur. J. Biochem.* 75: 601–612, 1977.

[144] Nicotera P and Leist M. Energy supply and the shape of death in neurons and lymphoid cells. *Cell Death Differ.* 4: 435–442, 1997.

[145] Nogales E, Wolf SG, Downing K. Structure of the alpha beta tubulin dimer by electron crystallography, *Nature* 391:199–203, 1998.

[146] Oliver KR, Greene WK (2011) Mobile DNA and the TE-Thrust hypothesis: supporting evidence from the primates. *Mobile DNA* 2:8; https://doi.org/10.1186/1759-8753-2-8.

[147] Pacher P, Hajnoczky G 2001. Propagation of the apoptotic signal by mitochondrial waves. *EMBO J* 20: 4107–21.

[148] Park HJ and Friston K (2013) Structural and functional brain networks: from connections to cognition. *Science* 342, 1238411.

[149] Paulsen, JS, Ready, RE, Hamilton, JM, Mega, MS and Cummings JL Neuropsychiatric aspects of Huntington's disease. *J. Neurol. Neurosurg. Psychiatry* 71, 310–314 (2001).

[150] Perez-Pinzon MA, Mumford PL, Rosenthal M and Sick TJ. Antioxidants, mitochondrial hyperoxidation and electrical recovery after anoxia in hippocampal slices. *Brain Res.* 754: 163– 170, 1997.

[151] Picard M and Burelle Y (2012) Mitochondria: starving to reach quorum? Insight in to the physiological purpose of mitochondrial fusion. *Bioessays* 34, 272–274.

[152] Pichler BJ, Wehrl HF, Judenhofer MS. Positron emission tomography/magnetic resonanceimaging: the next generation of multimodality imaging? *Semin Nucl Med.* 2008;38:199-208.

[153] Pokorný J, Jelínek F, Trkal V, Lamprecht I, Hölzel R (997) Vibrations in Microtubules. *J Biol Phys* 23:171–179, 1997.

[154] Poznik GD, Henn BM, Yee MC, Sliwerska E, Euskirchen GM, Lin AA, Snyder M, Quintana-Murci L, Kidd JM, Underhill PA, Bustamante CD (2013) "Sequencing Y chromosomes resolves discrepancy in time to common ancestor of males versus females". *Science*. 341 (6145): 562–65. doi:10.1126/science.1237619.

[155] Rafiki, A, Gozlan H, Ben-Ari Y, Khrestchatisky M, Medina I. (1997) The calcium-dependent transient inactivation of recombinant NMDA receptor-channel does not involve the high affinity calmodulin binding site of the NR1 subunit. *Neurosci. Lett.* 223: 137–139, 1997.

[156] Rapaport D, Brunner M, Neupert W, Westerman B (1998) Fzo1p is a mitochondrial outer membrane protein essential for the biogenesis of functional mitochonrdia in Saccharomyces cerevisiae. *J Biol Chem* 273: 20150–5.

[157] Reijnders JS, Ehrt U, Weber WE, Aarsland D. and Leentjens AF. A systematic review of prevalence studies of depression in Parkinson's disease. *Mov. Disord.* 23, 183–189 (2008).

[158] Rendong Tang, Jiapei Dai. Biophoton signal transmission and processing in the brain. *Journal of Photochemistry and Photobiology B: Biology, Volume 139,* 5 October 2014, Pages:71-75.

[159] Rolfe DFS, Brown GC (1997). Cellular energy utilization and molecular origin of standard metabolic rate in mammals. *Physiol Rev* 77:731– 758.

[160] Rolfe F and Brand D (1997) The physiological significance of mitochondrial proton leak in animal cells and tissues. *Biosci. Rep.* 17: 9–16, 1997.

[161] Rosenmund C, Feltz A, Westbrook GL (1995) Calciumdependent inactivation of synaptic NMDA receptors in hippocampal neurons. *J. Neurophysiol.* 73: 427–430.

[162] Sadun, AA, Morgia CL and Carelli V (2011). Leber's Hereditary Optic Neuropathy. Curr. Treat. Options Neurol. 13, 109–117 DiMauro S and Schon EA (2003). Mitochondrial respiratory-chain diseases. *N. Engl. J. Med.* 348, 2656–2668.

[163] Sagan L 1967. On the origin of mitosing cells. *J Theor Biol* 14: 255–74.

[164] Schapira AH. Mitochondrial disease. *Lancet* 368, 70–82 (2006).

[165] Sato H, Ellis, GW, Inoue S 1975. Microtubular origin of mitotic spindle form birefringence: demonstration of the applicability of Wiener's equation. *J. Cell. Biol. 67, 501–517.*

[166] Schmucker S and Puccio H (2010). Understanding the molecular mechanisms of Friedreich's ataxia to develop therapeutic approaches. *Hum. Mol. Genet.* 19 (R1), R103–R110.

[167] Schweizer M, Richter C. Nitric oxide potently and reversibly deenergizes mitochondria at low oxygen tension. *Biochem Biophys Res Commun.* 1994;204:169–175.

[168] Scott I 2010. The role of mitochondria in the mammalian antiviral defense system. *Mitochondrion* 10: 316–20.

[169] Seth, RB, Sun L, Ea CK and Chen ZJ (2005) Identification and characterization of MAVS, a mitochondrial antiviral signaling protein that activates NF-kappaB and IRF 3. *Cell* 122, 669–682.

[170] Sibson NR, Dhankar A, Mason GF, Rothman DL, Behar KL, Shulman RG (1998) Stoichiometric coupling of brain glucose metabolism and glutamatergic neuronal activity. *Proc Natl Acad Sci U S A* 95:316–321.

[171] Siesjö B (1978) *Brain energy metabolism.* New York: Wiley.

[172] Sigman M, Dehaene S (2008) Brain mechanisms of serial and parallel processing during dual-task performance. *J Neurosci* 28:7585–7598.

[173] Sik A, Passer BJ, Koonin EV, Pellegrini L 2004. Self-regulated cleavage of the mitochondrial intramembrane-cleaving protease PARL yields Pbeta, a nuclear-targeted peptide. *J Biol Chem* 279: 15323–9.

[174] Silvestri G, Mongini T, Odoardi, F, Modoni A, deRosa G, Doriguzzi C, Palmucci L, Tonali P and Servidei S (2000). A new mtDNA mutation associated with a progressive encephalopathy and cytochrome c oxidase deficiency. *Neurology* 54, 1693–1696.

[175] Skulachev VP. Mitochondrial filaments and clusters as intracellular power-transmitting cables, *Trends Biochem Sci* 26:23–29, 2001.

[176] Smalheiser NR (2014) The RNA-centred view of the synapse: non-coding RNA sand synaptic plasticity. *PhilosTransRSoc BBiolSci* 369:20130504–20130504.

[177] Smits P, Smeitink, J, and van den Heuvel L (2010). Mitochondrial translation and beyond: processes implicated in combined oxidative phosphorylation deficiencies. *J. Biomed. Biotechnol.* 2010, 737385.

[178] Sohal RS, Ku HH, Agarwal S, Forster MJ, Lal H (1994) Oxidative damage, mitochondrial oxidantgeneration and antioxidant defenses during aging and in response to food restriction in the mouse. *Mech Ageing Dev*;74:121–33.

[179] Spencer M 1982. *Fundamentals of Light Microscopy.* Cambridge University Press, Cambridge.

[180] Sporns O (2013) The human connectome: origins and challenges. *Neuroimage* 80, 53–61.

[181] Srere P 1980. The infrastructure of the mitochondrial matrix. *Trends Biochem. Sci.* 5, 120–121.

[182] Steinlechner S et al. Co-occurrence of affective and schizophrenia spectrum disorders with PINK1 mutations. *J. Neurol. Neurosurg. Psychiatry* 78, 532–535 (2007).

[183] Strogatz SH. Exploring complex networks. *Nature* 410, 268–276 (2001).

[184] Suen DF, Norris KL, Youle RJ 2008. Mitochondrial dynamics and apoptosis. *Genes Dev* 22: 1577–90.

[185] Swerdlow RH, Burns JM and Khan SM. The Alzheimer's disease mitochondrial cascade hypothesis. *J. Alzheimers Dis.* 20 (Suppl. 2), 265–279 (2010).

[186] Sydow A et al. Tau-induced defects in synaptic plasticity, learning, and memory are reversible in transgenic mice after switching off the toxic Tau mutant. *J. Neurosci.* 31, 2511–2525 (2011).

[187] Szabadkai G, Simoni AM, Chami M, Wieckowski MR et al. 2004. Drp1-dependent division of the mitochondrial network blocks intraorganellar Ca^{2b} waves and protects against Ca^{2b}-mediated apoptosis. *Mol Cell* 16: 59–68.

[188] Taguchi N, Ishihara N, Jofuku A, Oka T et al. 2007. Mitotic phosphorylation of dynamin-related GTPase Drp1 participates in mitochondrial fission. *J Biol Chem* 282: 11521–9.

[189] Thar R, Kühl M. Propagation of electromagnetic radiation in mitochondria? *Journal of Theoretical Biology,* Volume 230, Issue 2, 2004, Pages 261-270, ISSN 0022-5193, https://doi.org/10.1016/j.jtbi.2004.05.021. (http://www.sciencedirect.com/ science/article/pii/S0022519304002498).

[190] Thar R, Kühl M. Propagation of electromagnetic radiation in mitochondria? *Journal of Theoretical Biology,* Volume 230, Issue 2, 2004, Pages 261-270, ISSN 0022-5193, https://doi.org/10.1016/j.jtbi.2004.05.021. (http://www. sciencedirect.com/science/article/pii/S0022519304002498.

[191] Tondera D, Grandemange S, Jourdain A, Karbowski M et al. 2009. SLP-2 is required for stress-induced mitochondrial hyperfusion. *EMBO J* 28: 1589–600.

[192] Torroni A, Achilli A, Macaulay V, Richards M, Bandelt H (2006) Harvestingthe fruit of the human mtDNA tree. *Trends Genet* 22: 339–345.

[193] Turrens, JF 2003. Mitochondrial formation of reactive oxygen species. *J. Physiol.* 552 (Pt 2), 335–344.

[194] Turner C and Schapira AH. Mitochondrial matters of the brain: the role in Huntington's disease. *J. Bioenerg. Biomembr.* 42, 193–198 (2010).

[195] Twig G, Elorza A, Molina AJ, Mohamed H et al. 2008. Fission and selective fusion govern mitochondrial segregation and elimination by autophagy. *EMBO J* 27: 433–46.

[196] Tymianski M, Charlton MP, Carlen PL, Tator CH. Source specificity of early calcium neurotoxicity in cultured embryonic spinal neurons. *J. Neurosci.* 13: 2085–2104, 1993.

[197] Underhill PA, Kivisild T (2007) Use of Y Chromosome and Mitochondrial DNAPopulation Structure in Tracing Human Migrations. *Annu Rev Genet* 41: 539–564.

[198] Van Den Heuvel MP, Sporns O (2013) Network hubs in the human brain. *Trends Cogn Sci* 17:683–696.

[199] Van Niel CB (1931) "On the morphology and physiology of the purple and green sulfur bacteria". *Arch. Microbiol.* 3: 1–114.

[200] Van Wijk R, Van Wijk EPA, Van Wietmarschen HA, Van der Greef Towards whole-body ultra-weak photon counting and imaging with a focus on human beings: A review. *Journal of Photochemistry and Photobiology B: Biology,* Volume 139, 5 October 2014, Pages 39-46.

[201] Varshney LR, Chen BL, Paniagua E, Hall DH; Chklovskii DB (2011) Sporns, Olaf, ed. *"Structural Properties of the Caenorhabditis elegans Neuronal Network".* *PLoS Computational Biology.* 7 (2).

[202] Vass, Imre, Cser Krisztian (2009). "Janus-faced charge recombinations in photosystem II photoinhibition". *Trends in Plant Science.* 14 (4): 200–205.

[203] Vicario C, Arizmendi C, Malloch G, Clark JB, Medina JM Lactate utilization by isolated cells from early neonatal rat brain. *J. Neurochem.* 57: 1700–1707, 1991.

[204] Vives-Bauza C, Zhou C, Huang Y, Cui M et al. 2010. PINK1-dependent recruitment of Parkin to mitochondria in mitophagy. *Proc Natl Acad Sci USA* 107: 378–83.

[205] Wakabayashi J, Zhang Z, Wakabayashi N, Tamura Y, et al. 2009. The dynaminrelated GTPase Drp1 is required for embryonic and brain development in mice. *J Cell Biol* 186: 805–16.

[206] Wallace DC, Lott MT 2002. Mitochondrial genes in degenerative diseases, cancer and aging. In *Emery and Rimoin's Principles and Practice of Medical Genetics*, ed. DL Rimoin, JM Connor, RE Pyeritz, BR Korf, pp. 299–409. London: Churchill Livingstone

[207] Wallace DC, Lott MT, Brown MD, Kerstann K 2001. Mitochondria and neuro-ophthalmological diseases. In *The Metabolic and Molecular Basis of Inherited Disease*, ed. CR Scriver, AL Beaudet, WS Sly, D Valle, pp. 2425–512. New York: McGraw-Hill.

[208] Wallace DC (2005) A mitochondrial paradigm of metabolic and degenerative diseases, aging, and cancer: A dawn for evolutionary medicine. *Annu Rev Genet.* 39, 359–407.

[209] Wang GJ, Thayer SA. Sequestration of glutamate-induced Ca2+ loads by mitochondria in cultured rat hippocampal neurons. *J. Neurophysiol.* 76: 1611–1621, 1996.

[210] Werth JL and Thayer SA. Mitochondria buffer physiological calcium loads in cultured rat dorsal root ganglion neurons. *J. Neurosci.* 14: 346–356, 1994.

[211] Wiemerslage L, Lee D (2016). "Quantification of mitochondrial morphology in neurites of dopaminergic neurons using multiple parameters". *J Neurosci Methods.* doi:10.1016/j.jneumeth.2016.01.008.

[212] *Wise RR (2006). The structure and function of plastids. (Wise RR, Hoober KJ, eds.) Dordrecht: Springer. pp. 3–21.*

[213] Wong-Riley MTT (1989) Cytochrome oxidase: an endogenous metabolic marker for neuronal activity. *Trends Neurosci* 12:94–101.

[214] Wong-Riley MTT, Anderson B, Liebl W, Huang Z (1998) Neurochemical organization of the macaque striate cortex: correlation of cytochrome oxidase with Na+ K+ ATPase, NADPH-diaphorase, nitric oxide synthetase and N-methyl-D-aspartate receptor subunit I. *Neurosci* 83:1025–1045.

[215] Woolley JD, Khan BK, Murthy NK, Miller BL and Rankin KP. The diagnostic challenge of psychiatric symptoms in neurodegenerative disease: rates of and risk factors for prior psychiatric diagnosis in patients with early neurodegenerative disease. *J. Clin. Psychiatry* 72, 126–133 (2011).

[216] Xu LG, Wang YY, Han KJ, Li LY, Zhai Z and Shu HB (2005). VISA is an adapter protein required for virus-triggered IFN-beta signaling. *Mol. Cell* 19, 727–740.

[217] Xu W, Liu L, Charles IG, Moncada S. Nitric oxide induces coupling of mitochondrialsignallingwiththeendoplasmicreticulumstressresponse. *Nat Cell Biol.* 2004;6:1129–1134.

[218] Yamada Y 2000. Fundamental studies of photon migration in biological tissues and their application to optical tomography. *Opt. Rev.* 7 (5), 366–374.

[219] Yasukawa K, Oshiumi H, Takeda M, Ishihara N et al. 2009.Mitofusin 2 inhibits mitochondrial antiviral signaling. *Sci Signal* 2: ra47.

[220] Youle RJ, Karbowski M 2005. Mitochondrial fission in apoptosis. *Nat Rev Mol Cell Biol* 6: 657–63.

[221] Yu T, Robotham JL, Yoon Y 2006. Increased production of reactive oxygen species in hyperglycemic conditions requires dynamic change of mitochondrial morphology. *Proc Natl Acad Sci* USA 103: 2653–8.

[222] Zuckerkandl E, Pauling L (1962) Molecular disease, evolution, and geneticheterogeneity. In: Loogvali, Eva-Liis; Kivisild, Toomas; Margus, Tõnu; Villems, Richard (2009), O'Rourke, Dennis, ed., "Explaining the Imperfection of the Molecular Clock of Hominid Mitochondria", *PLoS ONE,* 4 (12): e8260, doi:10.1371/journal.pone.0008260, PMC 2794369 , PMID 20041137.

[223] Zunino R, McBride H. 2004. Sumo1 conjugates mitochondrial substrates and participates in mitochondrial fission. *Curr Biol* 14: 340–5.

[224] Zhang Q, Raoof M, Chen Y, Sumi Y et al. 2010. Circulating mitochondrial DAMPs cause inflammatory responses to injury. *Nature* 464:104–7.

[225] Zhang, L et al. (2016) Altered brain energetics induces mitochondrial fission arrest in Alzheimer's Disease. *Sci. Rep.* 6, 18725.

[226] Zubenko GS et al. A collaborative study of the emergence and clinical features of the major depressive syndrome of Alzheimer's disease. *Am. J. Psychiatry* 160, 857–866 (2003).

[227] Zunino R, Braschi E, Xu L, McBride HM 2009. Translocation of SenP5 from the nucleoli to the mitochondria modulates DRP1-dependent fission during mitosis. *J Biol Chem* 284: 17783–95.

In: Focus on Systems Theory Research
Editors: Manuel F. Casanova and Ioan Opris

ISBN: 978-1-53614-561-8
© 2019 Nova Science Publishers, Inc.

Chapter 12

THE NUTRITION SYSTEM AND THE BRAIN

Cosmin Sonea[*] and Ioan Opris, PhD[†]
USAMV Bucharest, Romania

ABSTRACT

Nutrition is the process by which an organism ingests, absorbs, transports, utilizes, and excretes/eliminates food substances. A nutrient is an "essential chemical" in food that supports human/animal/organism's life. Nutrients with their action and interaction may establish a precisely defined balance with respect to health and disease. The nutrition system includes food intake, absorption, assimilation, biosynthesis, catabolism, and excretion/elimination. It deals with the interaction of nutrients and other substances in food in relation to maintenance, growth, health, disease and reproduction. As the nutrition process indicates, the brain with its complex network stretches beyond the enteric neurons, being formed by intrinsic and extrinsic neurons that innervate the gut, enteric glia, and also the sensory epithelial cells, such as the enteroendocrine cells. The structural and functional connectivity of the nutritional system within the brain's connectome, plays a crucial role in the understanding of animal nutrition, foraging, health/disease and survival. This chapter summarizes recent findings on the function of nerve cells in the brain and sensory epithelial cells that mediates signals from the gut to the brain.

---

[*] Corresponding Author: Sonea Cosmin, Department of Veterinary Medicine, University of Agronomical Sciences and Veterinary Medicine, Bucharest, Romania.
[†] Email: ioanopris.phd@gmail.com.

1. INTRODUCTION

Nutrition may be regarded as an interacting system involving all phases of food relationship inherent to an organism. Let's begin with a bit of history.

1.1. History of Human Nutrition

The knowledge that food affects health was first mentioned in the writings of ancient Egyptians and Indians (Beisel, 1991, 1992; Satyaraj et al., 2011). Around 2,500 years ago, Hippocrates, stated "Let food be your medicine and medicine be your food" (Gershon, 1999). Modern nutritional science dates back to the eighteenth century, when the explanation of lymphoid tissue atrophy in malnourished population in England (Beisel, 1991; Satyaraj et al., 2011) suggested an association between nutritional status and immune function.

1.2. Nutrition

Nutrition is the process by which an organism ingests, absorbs, transports, utilizes, and excretes/eliminates food substances. A nutrient is an "essential chemical" in food that supports human/animal/organism's life. There are seven major classes of nutrients: carbohydrates, fats, fibers, minerals, proteins, vitamins, and water. Nutrients with their action and interaction establish a precisely defined balance with respect to health and disease. The "nutritional system includes food intake, absorption, assimilation, biosynthesis, catabolism, and excretion/elimination" (Lean, 2015). It deals with the interaction of nutrients and "other substances in food in relation to maintenance, growth, health, disease" and reproduction of an organism (Lean, 2015). The diet of an organism is what it eats, which is largely determined by the availability and palatability of foods.

1.2.1. Macronutrients vs. Micronutrients.

The macronutrients provide structural material (amino acids from which proteins are built, and lipids from which cell membranes and some signaling molecules are built) and energy. Some of the structural material can be used to generate energy internally which can be measured in joules or calories (sometimes called "kilocalories"). Carbohydrates and proteins provide 17 kJ approximately (4 kcal) of energy per gram, while fats provide 37 kJ (9 kcal) per gram (Berg et al., 2002), though the net energy from either depends on such factors as absorption and digestive effort, which vary substantially from instance to instance. Vitamins, minerals, fiber, and water "do not provide energy, but are required for other reasons" (Berg et al., 2002).

Nutritional deficiencies of essential dietary components, such as vitamins and micronutrients, "alter immune competence and increase the risk of infection" (Verma et al., 2016). The deficiency of adequate macronutrients and selected micronutrients, such as zinc, selenium, iron, copper, and vitamins A, B-6, C, E, leads to immune deficiency-related infections in children (Bendich and Chandra, 1990; Chandra, 1997). Micronutrient deficiencies affect innate immune responses as well as adaptive cellular immune responses (Afacan et al., 2012). The immune response is "dependent on the nutritional components of food intake", which modulates the induction of regulatory *versus* effector response at the gut mucosal level (Satyaraj, 2011).

1.2.2. Animal vs. Plant Nutrition

Animal nutrition focuses on the "dietary needs of animals", primarily those in agriculture and food production, but also in zoos, aquariums, and wildlife management. Carnivore and herbivore diets are contrasting, with "basic nitrogen and carbon proportions" varying for their particular foods. Many herbivores rely on "bacterial fermentation" to create digestible nutrients from indigestible plant cellulose, while "carnivores must eat animal meats to obtain certain vitamins or nutrients", their bodies cannot otherwise synthesize. (*https://www.nationalgeographic.org/encyclopedia/herbivore/*)

Plant nutrition is the study of the chemical elements that are necessary for plant growth (Allen et al., 2010). There are several principles that apply to plant nutrition. Some elements are directly involved in plant metabolism. However, this principle does not account for the so-called beneficial elements, whose presence, while not required, have clear positive effects on plant growth. A nutrient that is able to limit plant growth according to "Liebig's law of the minimum") (i.e., growth being controlled by the scarcest resource) is considered an essential plant nutrient if the plant cannot complete its full life cycle without it. There are 16 essential plant soil nutrients, besides the three major elemental nutrients carbon and oxygen that are obtained by photosynthetic plants from carbon dioxide in air, and hydrogen, obtained from water.

1.3. Processed Foods

These foods are obtained by the transformation of cooked ingredients into food by physical or chemical means. Food processing typically involves activities such as mincing and macerating, liquefaction, emulsification, and cooking (such as boiling, broiling, frying, or grilling); pickling, pasteurization; and canning or other packaging.

Primary-processing such as dicing, slicing, freezing or drying when leading to secondary products are also included.

2. THE GUT-BRAIN CONNECTION AND THE CONNECTOME

The digestive system is "innervated through its connections with the central nervous system (CNS) and by the enteric nervous system (ENS) within the wall of the gastrointestinal tract" (see Figure 1). The ENS "works in concert with" CNS reflex and command centers and with neural pathways that pass through sympathetic ganglia to control digestive function (Furness et al., 2014).

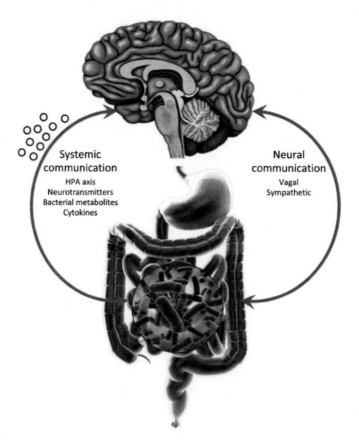

Figure 1. The Gut-Brain Connection. The connection between the central nervous system (CNS; upper) and by the enteric nervous system (ENS: lower). Systemic communications occur between CNS and ENS. HPA axis is a complex set of relationships and signals between the hypothalamus, the pituitary gland and the adrenals. Neural communication involves Vagal Sympathetic nerve. With permission from https://www.garmaonhealth.com/gut-bacteria-for-brain-health/gut-brain-connection/.

There is bidirectional information flowing between the ENS and CNS and between the ENS and sympathetic prevertebral ganglia (Furness et al., 2014).

- it is evident that the neural network stretches beyond enteric neurons. It is formed by both intrinsic and extrinsic neurons innervating the gut, enteric glia, and innervated sensory epithelial cells, such as enteroendocrine cells.
- a new neural connection has been reported between sensory cells of the gut epithelium and the nervous system that mediates signals from the gut to the brain.
- how the gut senses its environment, relays those signals to the brain, and how the brain influences the gut.
- gut-brain connection provides a pathway for how the body handles food.

2.2.1. The Enteric Nervous System

The enteric nervous system (ENS) is one of the main parts of the autonomic nervous system (ANS) and "consists of a "mesh-like system of neurons" that governs the function of the gastrointestinal tract" (Furness, 2008). ENS is also called the "second brain", likely because it is capable of acting independently to the sympathetic and parasympathetic nervous systems, although it may be "influenced" by these two. The ENS in humans consists of about 500 million neurons (Furness, 2008), five times as many as the one hundred million neurons in the human spinal cord (Rakhilin et al., 2016). ENS is embedded in the lining of the gastrointestinal system, beginning in the esophagus and extending down to the anus (Rakhilin et al., 2016).

The ENS neurons are distributed in many thousands of small ganglia (Figure 2), the majority being collected into two types of ganglia: myenteric (Auerbach's) and submucosal (Meissner's) plexuses (Furness et al., 2014). The myenteric plexus (MP) forms a continuous network that extends from the upper esophagus to the internal anal sphincter. Submucosal ganglia and connecting fiber bundles form plexuses just in the small and large intestines (not in the stomach and esophagus). The connections between the ENS and CNS are carried by the vagus and pelvic nerves and sympathetic pathways. Neurons also project from the ENS to prevertebral ganglia, the gallbladder, pancreas and trachea. ENS and CNS roles differ considerably along the digestive tract. The striated muscle esophageal movements are determined by neural pattern generators in the CNS.

The CNS has a key role in monitoring the state of the stomach, by controlling its contractile activity and acid secretion through vago-vagal reflexes. In contrast, the ENS in the small intestine and colon contains full reflex circuits, including sensory neurons, interneurons and several classes of motor neuron, through which muscle activity, transmucosal fluid fluxes, local blood flow and other functions are controlled. The CNS has control of defecation, via the defecation centers in the lumbosacral spinal cord. The importance of the ENS is emphasized by the life-threatening effects of some ENS neuropathies. By way of contrast, removal of vagal or sympathetic connections within the gastrointestinal tract has minor effects on GI function. The ENS "integrates many sensory signals" to control and maintain normal gut functions (Neunlist and Schemann, 2014). Nutrients are one of the "prominent" factors which determine the "chemical milieu" in the lumen and, after absorption, also within the gut wall (Neunlist and Schemann, 2014). Enteric neurons contain the molecular "machinery" to respond specifically to nutrients.

These transporters and receptors are "not expressed exclusively" in the ENS but "are also present" in other cells such as enteroendocrine cells (EECs) and extrinsic sensory nerves, signaling satiety or hunger. Glucose, amino acids and fatty acids all activate enteric neurons, as suggested by enhanced c-Fos expression or spike discharge (Neunlist and Schemann, 2014). These excitatory effects are the "result of a direct neuronal activation" but also "involve the activation of EECs which, upon activation by luminal nutrients, release mediators such as ghrelin, cholecystokinin or serotonin". The presence or absence of nutrients in the intestinal lumen "induces" long-term changes in "neurotransmitter expression, excitability, neuronal survival and ultimately impact upon gut motility, secretion or intestinal permeability". Together with EECs and vagal nerves, the ENS must be recognized as an "important player" initiating concerted responses to nutrients (Neunlist and Schemann, 2014).

2.2.2. The Gut-Brain Axis

The gastrointestinal tract (GIT) and the nervous system, both central (CNS) and enteric (ENS), are involved in bidirectional "extrinsic communication" by parasympathetic and sympathetic nerves, each comprising efferent fibers such as cholinergic and noradrenergic, respectively, and afferent sensory fibers required for gut-brain signaling (Konturek et al., 2004). Afferent nerves are "equipped with multiple sensors at their terminals in the gut" that are related to visceral mechano-chemo- and noci-receptors. The excitation of these afferent nerves may "trigger" a variety of visceral reflexes regulating GIT functions, including appetitive behavior (Konturek et al., 2004). Relevant to GIT, food intake "depends upon many influences" from the CNS, as well as from body energy stores (adipocytes) that express and release leptin in "proportion to fat stored and acting in long-term regulation of food intake" (Konturek et al., 2004). Leptin acts via receptors (Ob-R) present in afferent visceral nerves and the hypothalamic arcuate nucleus (ARC), whose neurons are "capable of expressing and releasing" neuropeptide Y (NPY) and agouti related protein (AgRP) that "triggers the ingestive behavior" through the paraventricular nucleus (PVN). In addition to such long-term regulation, a "short-term version of regulation" is acting on a meal-to-meal basis. This, more immediate regulation, is "secured by several gut hormones", like cholecystokinin (CCK), peptides YY (PYY) and oxyntomodulin (OXM), that are "released from the endocrine intestinal cells". The latter factors act via G-protein coupled receptors (GPCR) either on afferent nerves or directly on ARC neurons, which in turn inhibit expression and release of food-intake stimulating NPY and AgRP. The end result is that "satiety is induced through inhibition" of the PVN (Konturek et al., 2004).

The "bidirectional" communication between the brain and the GIT, namely the "brain–gut axis" is based on a complex system, including the vagus nerve, but also sympathetic (via the prevertebral ganglia), endocrine, immune, and humoral links as well as the influence of gut microbiota (Carabotti et al., 2015). This complex interaction serves to regulate gastrointestinal homeostasis and to connect emotional and cognitive areas of the brain with gut functions (Carabotti et al., 2015). The ENS produces more than 30 neurotransmitters and has more neurons than the spinal chrod. Hormones and peptides that the ENS releases into the blood circulation cross the blood–brain barrier (e.g., ghrelin) and can act synergistically with the vagus nerve, for example to regulate food intake and appetite (Hagemann et al., 2003).

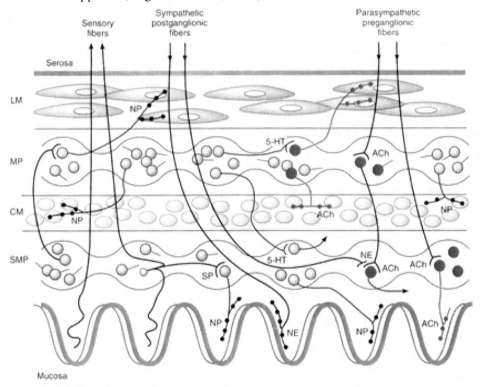

Figure 2. The enteric nervous system (LM, longitudinal muscle layer; MP, myenteric plexus; CM, circular muscle layer; SMP, submucosal plexus; ACh, acetylcholine; NE, norepinephrine; NO, nitric oxide; NP, neuropeptides; SP, substance P; 5-HT, serotonin. With Permission from Katzung BG, Basic and Clinical Pharmacology, 10th edition, The McGraw-Hill company).

The brain–gut axis is becoming increasingly important as a "therapeutic target" for gastrointestinal and psychiatric disorders, such as inflammatory bowel disease (IBD) (Bonaz et al., 2017), depression (Verma et al., 2011), and posttraumatic stress disorder (PTSD) (Verma et al., 2011). The gut is an important "control center of the immune system". In effect, the vagus nerve has immunomodulatory properties (Goverse et al., 2016). As a result, this nerve plays important roles in the relationship between the gut, the brain, and inflammation. There are new "treatment options" for modulating the brain–gut axis, for example, vagus nerve stimulation (VNS) and meditation techniques. Moreover, the vagus nerve also represents an "important link between nutrition and psychiatric, neurological and inflammatory diseases" (Verma et al., 2011).

The gut-brain axis is involved in a multitude of physiological processes including satiety, food intake, regulation of glucose and fat metabolism, insulin secretion and bone metabolism (Romijn et al., 2008). Regardless of whether we emphasize bottom-up or top-bottom pathways, it is a bi-directional communication system, comprised of neural pathways, such as the enteric nervous system (ENS), vagus, sympathetic and spinal nerves, and humoral pathways, which include cytokines, hormones, and neuropeptides as signaling molecules. Recent evidence, arising from animal models, supports: i) a role of microbes as signaling components in the gut-brain axis, ii) a role of bacteria (commensals, probiotics, and pathogens) as key modulators of gut-brain communication, and iii) the role of microbes, including commensals, probiotics and gastrointestinal pathogens, in bottom-up pathways of communication in the gut-brain axis (Bercik et al., 2012).

The gastrointestinal system can be considered the "gateway for food entry" in the body. Rather than being a "passive player", it is now clear that gut strongly influences feeding behavior and contributes to the maintainance of energy balance (Cuomo et al., 2011). The GIT plays a role in the control of food intake, by "focusing on the interplay existing between the enteric nervous system and gastrointestinal hormones" and their ability to modulate digestive motility and sensitivity (Cuomo et al., 2011). The gut hormones, together with nervous signals, likely contribute to the "regulation of energy balance and modulation of food intake" through the control of digestive motility and sensations (Cuomo et al., 2011).

The microorganisms residing within our gut form part of a complex multidirectional communication network with the brain known as the microbiome-gut-brain axis, playing a role in modulating neurodevelopment and behavior (Sherwin et al., 2016). Under homeostatic conditions, and in response to internal and external stressors, the bacterial commensals of our gut can signal to the brain through a variety of mechanisms to influence processes such neurotransmission, neurogenesis, microglia activation, and ultimately modulate behavior (Sherwin et al., 2016).

2.2.3. The Vagus Nerve as a Link between Gut and Brain

The Vagus Nerve (VN) carries an "extensive range of signals from the digestive system and organs to the brain and vice versa" (Rosas-Ballina et al., 2011). The VN is the "tenth cranial nerve, extending from its origin in the brainstem through the neck and the thorax down to the abdomen" (Rosas-Ballina et al., 2011). Because of its long path through the human body, it has also been described as the "wanderer nerve" (Rosas-Ballina et al., 2011). The "VN exits from the medulla oblongata in the groove between the olive and the inferior cerebellar peduncle, leaving the skull through the middle compartment of the jugular foramen". In the neck, the "VN provides required innervation

The Nutrition System and the Brain   267

to most of the muscles of the pharynx and larynx", which are responsible for swallowing and vocalization. In the thorax, it "provides the main parasympathetic supply to the heart and stimulates a reduction in the heart rate".

In the intestines, the "VN regulates the contraction of smooth muscles and glandular secretion". "Preganglionic neurons of vagal efferent fibers emerge from the dorsal motor nucleus of the VN located in the medulla, and innervate the muscular and mucosal layers of the gut both in the lamina propria and in the muscularis externa" (Rosas-Ballina et al., 2011). The "celiac branch supplies the intestine from proximal duodenum to the distal part of the descending colon" (Rosas-Ballina et al., 2011). The "abdominal vagal afferents, include mucosal mechano-receptors, chemoreceptors, and tension receptors in the esophagus, stomach, and proximal small intestine, and sensory endings in the liver and pancreas". The "sensory afferent cell bodies are located in the nodose ganglia and send information to the nucleus tractus solitarii (NTS)" (see Figure 2). The NTS projects the vagal sensory information to several regions of the CNS such as the locus coeruleus (LC), the rostral ventrolateral medulla, the amygdala, and the thalamus (See Verma et al., 2011). The vagus nerve is "responsible for the regulation of internal organ functions, such as digestion, heart rate, and respiratory rate, as well as vasomotor activity, and certain reflex actions, such as coughing, sneezing, swallowing, and vomiting" (See Rosas-Ballina et al., 2011). Its activation leads to the release of acetylcholine (ACh) at the synaptic junction with secreting cells, intrinsic nervous fibers, and smooth muscles (see Rosas-Ballina et al., 2011). ACh binds to nicotinic and muscarinic receptors and stimulates muscle contractions in the parasympathetic nervous system. Animal studies have demonstrated the remarkable "regeneration capacity of the vagus nerve". For example, "subdiaphragmatic vagotomy induced transient withdrawal and restoration of central vagal afferents as well as synaptic plasticity in the NTS" (See Rosas-Ballina et al., 2011).

2.2.4. The Brain-Gut Connectome

We propose to look at the nutritional system as a massively interacting system of "interconnected multistage and multiscale networks that encompass hidden mechanisms by which nutrition, microbiome, metabolism, genetic predisposition, and the immune system interact together" and with the brain to delineate health and disease.

(a) The *connectome of the human brain*. The "connectome" is the brain's wiring diagram, in terms of connections between neurons and between brain regions.

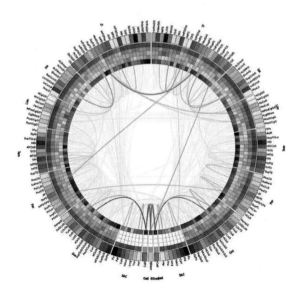

A neat technique for visualizing connections, is based on the "circular representation of human cortical networks" for subject and population-level connectomic visualization (Irimia et al. (2012)). Such "connectograms" use MRI scans, and image processing. But what does it mean? The outermost ring shows the various brain regions arranged by lobe (fr — frontal; ins — insula; lim — limbic; tem — temporal; par — parietal; occ — occipital; nc — non-cortical; bs — brain stem; CeB — cerebellum) and further ordered anterior-to-posterior. The "color map" of each region is "lobe-specific and maps the color of each regional parcellation". In other words, the "outer ring is just a list of brain regions", each with an assigned color. The "inner rings tell us about those regions". Proceeding inward towards the center of the circle, these measures are: total grey matter (GM) volume, total area of the surface associated with the GM–WM interface (at the base of the cortical ribbon), mean cortical thickness, mean curvature and connectivity per unit volume. For non-cortical regions, only average regional volume is shown. So, each of the five inner rings displays data about one aspect of brain anatomy, for each of the regions. The colors are a heat map of the numbers. Finally, the "lines between regions represent the degrees of connectivity between regions via white matter tracts", as measured with diffusion tensor imaging: The links represent the computed degrees of connectivity between segmented brain regions. Links shaded in blue represent DTI tractography pathways in the lower third of the distribution of FA, green lines the middle third, and red lines the top third (see text for details).

Gut Connectome

The enteric nervous system has been studied thus far as an isolated unit. As researchers probe deeper into the function of this system, it is evident that the neural network stretches beyond enteric neurons (Bohórquez and Lidle, 2015). It is formed by both intrinsic and extrinsic neurons innervating the gut, enteric glia, and innervated sensory epithelial cells, such as enteroendocrine cells. This summarizes recent knowledge on function and disease of nerves, glia, and sensory epithelial cells of the gut in eight distinctive articles. The timing and growing knowledge for each individual field calls for an appropriate term encompassing the entire system. This neuronal ensemble is called the "gut connectome" and summarizes the work from a food sensory perspective.

Neurochemical Connectome

The rat neurochemical connectome is fundamental for "exploring neuronal information processing" (Noori et al., 2017). By using advanced data mining, supervised machine learning, and network analysis, Noori's study integrated over fifty years of neuroanatomical investigations into a multiscale, multilayer neuro-chemical connectome of the rat brain (Noori et al., 2017). This "neurochemical connectivity database (ChemNetDB) is supported by comprehensive systematically-determined receptor distribution maps". The rat connectome has an onion-type structural organization and shares a number of structural features with mesoscale connectomes of mouse and macaque. Furthermore, the extreme values of graph theoretical measures (e.g., degree and betweenness) are associated with deep brain structures such as amygdala, bed nucleus of the stria terminalis, dorsal raphe, and lateral hypothalamus, which regulate primitive, yet fundamental functions, such as circadian rhythms, reward, aggression, anxiety, and fear. The ChemNetDB is a freely available resource for systems analysis of motor, sensory, emotional, and cognitive information processing.

Connectome genetics seeks to uncover how genetic factors shape brain functional connectivity (Mechling et al., 2016); Mechling and colleagues tested whether the sole targeted deletion of the mu opioid receptor gene (Oprm1) alters the brain connectome in living mice (Mechling et al., 2016). Analysis of combined resting-state fMRI diffusion tractography showed pronounced modifications of functional connectivity with only minor changes in structural pathways. Fine-grained resting-state fMRI mapping, graph theory, and intergroup comparison revealed Oprm1-specific hubs and captured a "unique gene-to-network signature". Strongest perturbations occurred in connectional patterns of pain/aversion-related nodes, including the mu receptor-enriched habenula node. This data demonstrated that the main receptor for morphine predominantly shapes the so-called reward/aversion circuitry, with major influence on negative affect centers. Schlegel et al., {2016) used Electron Microscopy based reconstruction to generate the entire connectome of hugin-producing neurons in the Drosophila larval CNS. These authors demonstrated that hugin neurons use synaptic transmission in addition to peptidergic neuromodulation and identified acetylcholine as a key transmitter. Hugin neuropeptide and acetylcholine are both necessary for the regulatory effect on feeding. Subtypes of hugin neurons connect chemosensory to endocrine system by combinations of synaptic and peptide-receptor connections (Schlegel et al., 2016). It was further proposed that hugin neurons are part of a physiological control system that has been conserved at the functional and molecular level.

3. THE INTERPLAY BETWEEN NUTRITION, MICROBIOME, METABOLISM AND IMMUNE SYSTEM

The field of nutrition, so far, has not been investigated from the viewpoint of a "massively interacting system of interconnected networks" (Verma et al., 2016). Here, based on the systematic of Verma et al., (See Figure 4) we review the "essence of interactions" between the four key players– nutrition, microbiome, metabolism, and the immune system (Verma et al., 2016). Recent findings (Klingelhoefer et al., 2015) support the role of altered gut microbiome involved in influencing the activity of enteric neurons in Parkinson's disease patients (Klingelhoefer et al., 2015; Verma et al., 2016).

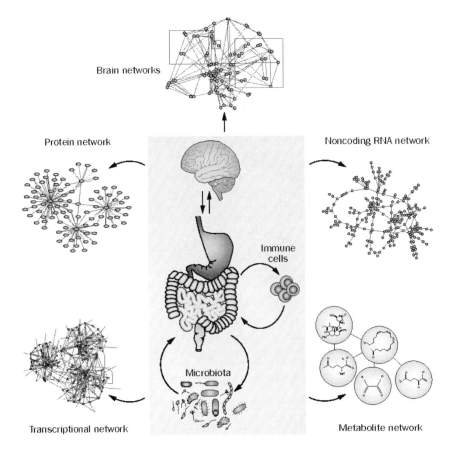

Figure 3. Systems-based interactions between central and peripheral components of the brain–gut axis can be studied at the level of the genome, epigenome, transcriptome, proteome, metabolome and brain connectome. With permission from Verma et al., 2016.

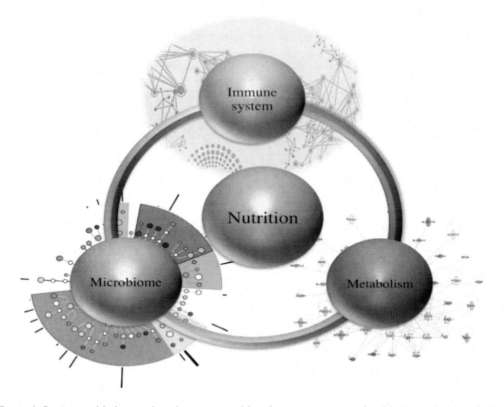

Figure 4. Systems-wide interactions between nutrition, immune system, microbiome, and metabolism. With permission from Verma et al., 2016.

3.1. Nutrition *vs.* Immune System

As showed by Verma et al., (2016), nutrient deficiencies affect important innate immune responses, as well as adaptive cellular immune responses (Afacan et al., 2011). The immune response depends on the nutritional components of food intake, which "modulates the induction of regulatory versus effector response" at the gut mucosal level (Satyaraj, 2011). Current immune deficiency cases are also "the result of increased stress, increased caloric intake, obesity, autoimmunity, allergic disorders", in an aging population, which does not necessarily relate to under-nutrition (Satyaraj, 2011). Thus, an unbalanced nutrition, unhealthy lifestyle choices, limited physical activity, and the polluted environment, in general, compromise the host immune response, thereby increasing possibility to a wide range of diseases. The nutritional status of an individual is a key determinant of the "susceptibility" of the immune system to infection and disease (Kau et al., 2011; Clemente et al., 2012). For example, during an infection, the host requirements for energy substrates and nutrients increase fast in the presence of invading microorganisms or in an "immune-mediated disease that involves proliferation of immune cell subsets" (Verma et al., 2016). However, it is well known that "infectious agents reduce the motivation for voluntary food intake due to the stimulation of leukocytes to produce inflammatory cytokines" (Verma et al., 2016). The immune cells use the cytokines to provide information to other physiological systems, including the brain that modulates the food intake (Johnson, 1998; Dantzer et al., 2008). The increased metabolic demands are utilized to increase body temperature (e.g., fever) (Dantzer, 2001) required for the proliferation of the immune cells during "elimination of an infectious pathogen". The growth, survival, and differentiation of the immune cells "depend on glucose metabolism" as a source of energy, which has a huge impact on our health (Palmer et al., 2015).

3.2 Nutrition *vs.* Microbiome

The ability of gut microbiota to "communicate with the brain and thus modulate behavior" is emerging as an exciting concept in health and disease (Verma et al., 2016). The enteric microbiota interacts with the host to form essential relationships that govern homeostasis (Cryan and O'Mahony, 2011). Despite the unique "enteric-bacterial fingerprint" of each individual, there appears to be a certain balance that provides health benefits. It is, therefore, reasonable to imagine that "a decrease in the desirable gastrointestinal bacteria will lead to deterioration in gastrointestinal, neuroendocrine or immune relationships and ultimately disease" (Verma et al., 2016). Studies in mice, exploring the impact of the enteric microbiota on the host (especially on the central nervous system), demonstrate that "germ-free mice display alterations in stress-responsivity, central neurochemistry and behavior indicative of a reduction in anxiety in comparison to conventional mice" (see Verma et al., 2016). This suggests that "specific modulation of the enteric microbiota may be a useful strategy for stress-related disorders and for modulating the co-morbid aspects of gastrointestinal disorders such as irritable bowel syndrome and inflammatory bowel disease" (Verma et al., 2016).

Role of the Microbiome in Shaping a Healthy Immune System

Microbiome plays a crucial role in shaping the functions of the immune system thereby providing a protective mechanism to fight against infection. The "commensal bacteria" help in maintaining the balance with the foreign (often pathogenic) bacteria, by "modulating" the components of host innate immune system. A "dysregulation of homeostasis" between host and gut microbes leads to dysbiosis, which can give rise to pathogenic states, such as inflammatory bowel disease (IBD) (Vermeire et al., 2003; Viladomiu et al., 2013). A "change in the composition of gut microbes has been associated with development of asthma in animal models". A recent study by Arrieta et al. (Arrieta et al., 2015) "demonstrated that infants who exhibit transient gut microbial dysbiosis during the early days of life are at high risk of asthma". Another study by Fonseca et al. showed that during the post resolution of infection stage from Yersinia pseudotuberculosis, the signals derived from the "gut microbiota" aided in the maintenance of inflammatory mesentery remodeling and "restoration of mucosal immunity" (Fonseca et al., 2015).

The intestinal immune system, thus, plays an important role in maintaining the "balance of commensal and foreign microorganisms inside the gut along with keeping the diversity of the commensal microorganisms" (Verma et al., 2016). However, due to high bacterial densities inside the gut, the task is "challenging" as compared to other organs and tissues. The immune system has adopted certain ways, such as "immunological tolerance, by diverting various resources to segregate the microbiome on the luminal side of the epithelial barrier" (Hooper, 2009). Probiotics have been shown to "beneficially modulate the intestinal ecosystem" (Trop, 2014). However, both probiotics and prebiotics can influence the "composition of the intestinal microflora" and alter the "metabolic composition of the microbiome" (Bassaganya-Riera et al., 2012). In fact, in cases of dysbiosis, the possibility of "manipulating the gut bacterial composition by using probiotic bacteria" has already been explored as a promising therapeutic intervention against inflammatory bowel disease (Bassaganya-Riera et al., 2012). There is increasing evidence that host-microbe interactions play a "key role in maintaining homeostasis" (Borre et al., 2014). Alterations in gut microbial composition is associated with marked changes in behaviors relevant to mood, pain and cognition, establishing the critical importance of the bi-directional pathway of communication between the microbiota and the brain in health and disease. Dysfunction of the microbiome-brain-gut axis has been "implicated in stress-related disorders such as depression, anxiety and irritable bowel syndrome and neurodevelopmental disorders such as autism". (Borre et al., 2014).

3.3 Nutrition *vs.* Metabolism

Multiple "bacterial genomes modulate the metabolic reactions" inside the body exemplified by the production of short-chain fatty acids (SCFAs), an essential component of host health (Verma et al., 2016). Humans lack enzymes required for digestion of dietary fibers (den Besten, 2013). The microbial community inside the gut ferments these undigested carbohydrates for energy storage. As already mentioned, the "fermentation results in a wide variety of lipid molecules", including oleic acid and SCFAs (den Besten, 2013) such as butyrate, propionate, acetate, that provide the colon with "energy required during metabolic demands as well as regulatory signals that help in the maintenance of homeostasis" (Verma et al., 2016). Along with being a local nutrient source for colonocytes, "SCFAs regulate energy homeostasis by stimulating lectin production in adipocytes" as well as, glucagon-like peptide secretion by the intestinal endocrine cells (Verma et al., 2016). The SCFAs also "regulate neutrophil function and migration, inhibit inflammatory cytokine-induced expression of vascular cell adhesion molecule-1, and increase the expression of tight junction proteins in the colon epithelia" (Verma et al., 2016). Overall, they affect a "wide range of host processes", including energy utilization, host–microbe signaling, epithelial cell integrity, and gut mobility (Musso et al., 2011). Oleic acid is a commonly found dietary component and is also a "microbial metabolism" product. Increased concentrations of oleic acid are found within Parabacteroides (Sakamoto et al., 2006), and oral treatment with commensal Parabacteroides distasonis has been shown to significantly reduce the severity of intestinal inflammation in murine models of acute and chronic colitis (Kverka et al., 2011). Thus, it is important to understand whether the diet-derived products of "microbial metabolism" are released under similar conditions in the presence of varying food substrates that may include proteins, carbohydrates, and fat (Verma et al., 2016). The host metabolome is a "rich" resource for studying metabolic function of the gut microbiome.

3.4. The Link between Nutrition, Metabolism, Immune System and Microbiome

Understanding the relationship between immune system, microbiome, and metabolism regulated by nutrition (as shown in Figure 4) will assist in targeting the nutrition components, while recognizing their systems-wide effects (Verma et al., 2016). This would lead to "identification of emerging properties of this complex system and utilization of the newly derived information and knowledge for improved health outcomes". Microbes are important components of the human ecosystem, and they "account for approximately 100 trillion", including both the ones residing outside as well as inside the human body (Dave et al., 2012, Whitman et al., 1998). The gut microbiome is a key player in "regulating the defense responses and metabolism, thereby contributing toward shaping the immune responses (regulatory or effector) and aiding in the maturation of the immune system" (Verma et al, 2016). The various "physiological factors" responsible for differences in genetic elements of the microbiome within a host include diet, geographical location, and environmental interaction (Turnbaugh et al. 2007). The interactions between the gut microbiome, immune system, metabolism, and nutrition are "crucial determinants of health outcomes".

Diet and nutritional status are the key players in defining the composition and function of the gut microbiome as well as the host immune response. A comprehensive understanding of nutritional quality of the dietary interventions (Marion-Letellier, 2009) that "modulate" the components of the gut microbiota and mucosal immune responses can prove useful for maintenance of health. A systems-level framework that integrates various *in vitro* and *in vivo* models, including human data, can facilitate the systems-wide mechanistic insights (Borenstein, 2012).

4. NUTRITION AND REWARD

Nutrition and reward are two key functions of the brain (Sonea et al., 2017). Nutrition and reward use "food" intake that represents the energy source for all vital functions of an organism. However, pleasure or hedonic reward/nutrition (Figure 5) has two opposite facets, a) reinforced consumption of palatable food - obesity (fear for hunger), and b) motivated and reinforced starving – anorexia nervosa = hedonic for hunger. The mechanisms of reward and decision-making use a network of brain regions including the orbitofrontal and the anterior cingulate cortex (Neubert et al., 2015).

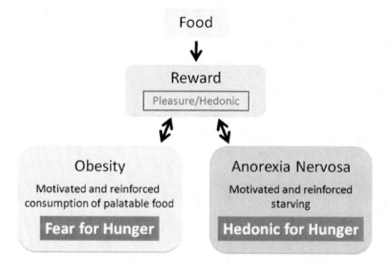

Figure 5. Diagram of food reward.

4.1. Reinforced Consumption of Palatable Food or Obesity

Obesity may be also regarded as fear for hunger. Few studies have focused on whole-brain networks in obesity and binge eating disorder (BED). A recent study used multi-echo resting-state functional magnetic resonance imaging (rsfMRI) combined with a data-driven graph theory approach to assess brain network characteristics in obesity (Baek et al., 2017). Obese subjects exhibited significantly reduced global and local network efficiency as well as decreased modularity compared with healthy controls, showing disruption in small-world and modular network structures. In regional metrics, the putamen, pallidum and thalamus exhibited significantly decreased nodal degree and efficiency in obese subjects. Obese subjects also showed decreased connectivity of cortico-striatal/cortico-thalamic networks associated with putaminal and cortical motor regions. These findings were significant with ME-ICA with limited group differences observed with conventional denoising or single-echo analysis. It was also found that "disruption" in global network properties and motor cortico-striatal networks in obesity consistent with habit formation theories. The findings of Baek et al., (2017) highlight the role of network properties in pathological food misuse as possible biomarkers and therapeutic targets. Novel therapies targeting the orexin system for sleep disorders, are also used for obesity and drug addiction (Sakurai and Mieda 2011).

4.2. Motivated and Reinforced Starving or Anorexia Nervosa

Anorexia may be also regarded as a hedonic/pleasure for hunger. Anorexia nervosa (AN) and body dysmorphic disorder (BDD) frequently co-occur and have several overlapping phenomenological features (Zhang et al., 2016). Zhang and colleagues compared "modular organization of brain structural connectivity" in individuals with BDD weight-restored AN and healthy controls (HC). AN showed "abnormal modularity" involving frontal, basal ganglia and posterior cingulate nodes. There was a trend in BDD for similar abnormalities, but "no significant differences compared with AN". Abnormal network organization patterns in AN, "partially shared" with BDD, may have implications for understanding integration between reward and habit/ritual formation, as well as conflict monitoring/error detection.

5. NUTRITION AND DISEASE

For humans, a healthy nutrition/diet includes preparation of food and storage methods that preserve nutrients from oxidation, heat or leaching, and that reduce risk of foodborne illness. An unhealthy diet can cause deficiency-related diseases such as

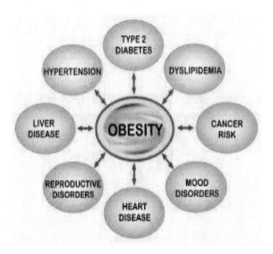

Figure 6. Nutrition and disease.

blindness, anemia, scurvy, preterm birth, stillbirth and cretinism, or nutrient excess health-threatening conditions such as obesity and metabolic syndrome; and such common chronic systemic diseases as cardiovascular disease, diabetes, and osteoporosis. Under-nutrition can lead to wasting in acute cases, and the stunting of marasmus in chronic cases of malnutrition (Figure 6). The field of nutrition primarily focuses on the role of diet and its nutritional contents in disease prevention.

Gut Microbiome Impacts Human Brain Health

Here are some of the ways that the gut microbiome impacts the function of our brain:

1. Structural bacterial components such as lipopolysaccharides provide low-grade tonic stimulation of the innate immune system (Galland, 2014). Excessive stimulation due to bacterial dysbiosis, small intestinal bacterial overgrowth, or increased intestinal permeability may produce systemic and/or central nervous system inflammation.
2. Bacterial proteins may cross-react with human antigens to stimulate dysfunctional responses of the adaptive immune system.
3. Bacterial enzymes may produce neurotoxic metabolites such as D-lactic acid and ammonia. Even beneficial metabolites such as short-chain fatty acids may exert neurotoxicity.
4. Gut microbes can produce hormones and neurotransmitters that are identical to those produced by humans. Bacterial receptors for these hormones influence microbial growth and virulence.
5. Gut bacteria directly stimulate afferent neurons of the enteric nervous system to send signals to the brain via the vagus nerve. Through these varied mechanisms, gut microbes shape the architecture of sleep and stress reactivity of the hypothalamic-pituitary-adrenal axis (Galland, 2014). They influence memory, mood, and cognition and are clinically and therapeutically relevant to a range of disorders, including alcoholism, chronic fatigue syndrome, fibromyalgia, and restless legs syndrome. Their role in multiple sclerosis and the neurologic manifestations of celiac disease is being studied. Nutritional tools for altering the gut microbiome therapeutically include changes in diet, probiotics, and prebiotics (Galland, 2014).

The ability of stress to modulate the microbiota and also for microbiota to change the set point for stress sensitivity are being unraveled (Sherwin et al., 2016). Dysregulation of the gut microbiota composition has been identified in several psychiatric disorders, including depression (Sherwin et al., 2016). This has led to the concept of bacteria that have a beneficial effect upon behavior and mood (psychobiotics) being proposed for potential therapeutic interventions. Understanding the mechanisms by which the bacterial commensals of our gut are involved in brain function may lead to the development of novel microbiome-based therapies for these mood and behavioral disorders.

5.1. Malnutrition

Malnutrition is defined as insufficient, excessive, or imbalanced consumption of nutrients by an organism. The gastrointestinal (GI) system is responsible for the digestion and absorption of ingested food and liquids (Greenwood-Van Meerveld et al., 2017). The major factors affecting GI physiology and function, include the intestinal microbiota, chronic stress, inflammation, and aging with a focus on the neural regulation of the GI tract and an emphasis on basic brain-gut interactions that serve to modulate the GI tract. GI diseases refer to diseases of the esophagus, stomach, small intestine, colon, and rectum. The major symptoms of common GI disorders include recurrent abdominal pain and bloating, heartburn, indigestion/dyspepsia, nausea and vomiting, diarrhea, and constipation. GI disorders rank among the most prevalent disorders, with the most common including esophageal and swallowing disorders, gastric and peptic ulcer disease, gastroparesis or delayed gastric emptying, irritable bowel syndrome (IBS), and inflammatory bowel disease (IBD). Many GI disorders are difficult to diagnose and their symptoms are not effectively managed. Thus, basic research is required to drive the development of novel therapeutics. One approach is to enhance our understanding of gut physiology and pathophysiology especially as it relates to gut brain communications since they have clinical relevance to a number of GI complaints and represent a therapeutic target for the treatment of conditions including inflammatory diseases of the GI tract such as IBD and functional gut disorders such as IBS.

5.2. Cancer

Cancer is a common disease in developing countries. According to the International Agency for Research on Cancer, "In the developing world, cancers of the liver, stomach and esophagus were more common, often linked to consumption of carcinogenic preserved foods, such as smoked or salted food, and parasitic infections that attack organs." Developed countries "tended to have cancers linked to affluence or a 'Western lifestyle' — cancers of the colon, rectum, breast and prostate — that can be caused by obesity, lack of exercise, diet and age (Lakhan and Vieira, 2008).

5.3. Mental Disorders

Among the mental disorders involving nutrition we can mention here are: Alzheimer disease, major depression, bipolar disorder, schizophrenia, and obsessive-compulsive disorder. Attention-deficit/hyperactivity disorder (ADHD) and conditions involving excessive eating (e.g., obesity, binge/loss of control eating) are increasingly prevalent within pediatric populations. Correlational and some longitudinal studies have suggested inter-relationships between these disorders (Seymour et al., 2015). In addition, a number of common neural correlates are emerging across conditions, e.g., functional abnormalities within circuits subserving reward processing and executive functions.

Various neuropsychiatric disorders, especially addictions, feature impairments in risky decision making (Kohno et al., 2014). Maladaptive decision making by methamphetamine users may reflect circuit-level dysfunction, underlying deficits in task-based activation (Kohno et al., 2014). Heightened resting-state connectivity within the mesocorticolimbic system, coupled with reduced prefrontal cortical connectivity, may create a bias toward reward-driven behavior over cognitive control in methamphetamine users. Interventions to improve this balance may enhance treatments for stimulant dependence and other disorders that involve maladaptive decision making.

Anhedonia, defined as the reduced ability to experience pleasure, is a key feature to multiple psychiatric disorders and "causes substantial disability" (Sharma et al., 2017). Anhedonia "severity" appears related to reward deficits in specific neural networks. The authors identified "foci of dysconnectivity" associated with "reward responsivity" in the nucleus accumbens, the default mode network (DMN), and the cingulo-opercular network. Reward deficits were associated with "decreased connectivity between the nucleus accumbens and the DMN" and "increased connectivity between the nucleus accumbens and the cingulo-opercular network". In addition, "impaired reward responsivity" was associated with DMN "hyperconnectivity and diminished connectivity between the DMN and the cingulo-opercular network.

The brain is an organ greatly influenced by the substances present in the diet (Bourre, 2004). Dietary regulation of blood glucose level (via ingestion of food with a low glycemic index ensuring a low insulin level) improves the quality and duration of intellectual performance. The nature of the amino acid composition of dietary proteins contributes to good cerebral function; tryptophan plays a special role. Many indispensable amino acids present in dietary proteins help to elaborate neurotransmitters and neuromodulators. Omega-3 fatty acids provided the first coherent experimental demonstration of the effect of dietary nutrients on the structure and function of the brain. Consequently, the nature of polyunsaturated fatty acids (in particular omega-3) present in formula milks for infants (premature and term) conditions the visual and cerebral abilities, including intellectual abilities. Moreover, dietary omega-3 fatty acids are certainly involved in the prevention of some aspects of cardiovascular disease (including at the level of cerebral vascularization), and in some neuropsychiatric disorders, particularly depression, as well as in dementia, notably Alzheimer's disease.

5.4. Metabolic Syndrome

Metabolic syndrome is a clustering of at least three of the five following medical conditions: abdominal obesity, high blood pressure, high blood sugar, high serum triglycerides and low high-density lipoprotein levels. Metabolic syndrome is associated with the risk of developing cardiovascular disease and type 2 diabetes (Kaur, 2014). In the US about a quarter of the adult population have metabolic syndrome, and the prevalence increases with age, with racial and ethnic minorities being particularly affected (Beltrán-Sánchez et al., 2013; Falkner and Cossrow, 2014). Insulin resistance, metabolic syndrome, and prediabetes are closely related to one another and have overlapping aspects. The syndrome is thought to be caused by an underlying disorder of energy utilization and storage.

6. CONCLUSION

Although the communication between gut microbiota and the CNS are not fully elucidated, neural, hormonal, immune and metabolic pathways have been suggested. Thus, the notion of microbiome-brain-gut axis is emerging, suggesting that microbiota-modulating strategies may be a tractable therapeutic approach for developing novel treatments for CNS disorders. The discussed results suggest that "patterns" of connectivity among large-scale networks within the brain-gut connectome are critical to the neurobiology of nutrition mechanism and its dysfunctions.

6.1. Future of Nutrition

It remains to be studied how, for instance, nutrient-induced changes in the ENS may influence additional gut functions such as intestinal barrier repair, intestinal epithelial stem cell proliferation differentiation, and also, the signalling of extrinsic nerves to brain regions which control food intake (Neunlist and Schemann, 2014). An understanding of the interaction between networks can help design better strategies for primary prevention for diseases, such as PD, which show the involvement of gut–brain axis in the disease pathogenesis (Klingelhoefer et al., 2015). Such investigation requires modeling tools, informatics techniques, and major computational resources in order to gain a better understanding of the mechanisms by which the four key players interact, to delineate health and disease (Klingelhoefer et al., 2015).

6.1.1. Mathematical and Computational Modeling

The vast aspects of this interconnected network operate on the basis of complex regulatory networks that can be analyzed in a well-defined manner using mathematical and computational modeling (Verma et al. 2016). The recent modeling frameworks applied include the use of (1) ordinary differential equations (ODEs) that are used for cancer immunology, natural killer cell responses, B cell responses (naive and memory), T regulatory cell dynamics and T cell responses; (2) partial differential equations are used for modeling age-structured and spatiotemporal models; (3) stochastic differential equations account for noise and sporadic events, (4) agent-based models account for probabilistic uncertainty in biological interaction, and (5) advanced machine-learning algorithms that correlate cellular and molecular events to changes in health and disease outcomes.

6.2. Challenges of Nutrition in the Context of Increased Population in 2050

It is estimated that demand of feeding a population will increase up to nine billion people needing food by 2050, which necessitates the need for devising methods that not only meet the demand but also ensure continuous wholesome food supply (Kau et al., 2011).

REFERENCES

Afacan, NJ; Fjell, CD; Hancock, RE. A systems biology approach to nutritional immunology-focus on innate immunity. *Mol Aspects Med*, (2012), 33(1), 14–25. doi:10.1016/j.mam.2011.10.013.

Allen, V. Barker; David, J. Pilbeam. *Handbook of Plant Nutrition*. CRC Press, 2010, p. Preface.

Arrieta, MC; Stiemsma, LT; Dimitriu, PA; Thorson, L; Russell, S; Yurist-Doutsch, S; et al. Early infancy microbial and metabolic alterations affect risk of childhood asthma. *Sci Transl Med*, (2015), 7(307), ra152–307. doi:10.1126/scitranslmed.aab2271.

Baek, K; Morris, LS; Kundu, P; Voon, V. Disrupted resting-state brain network properties in obesity: decreased global and putaminal cortico-striatal network efficiency. *Psychol Med.*, 2017 Mar, 47(4), 585-596.

Bassaganya-Riera, J; Viladomiu, M; Pedragosa, M; De Simone, C; Carbo, A; Shaykhutdinov, R; et al. Probiotic bacteria produce conjugated linoleic acid locally in the gut that targets macrophage PPAR gamma to suppress colitis. *PLoS One*, (2012), 7(2), e31238. doi:10.1371/journal.pone.0031238.

Bassaganya-Riera, J; Hontecillas, R. Dietary CLA and n-3 PUFA in inflammatory bowel disease. *Curr Opin Clin Nutr Metab Care*, (2010), 13(5), 569. doi:10.1097/MCO.0b013e32833b648e.

Bassaganya-Riera, J; Viladomiu, M; Pedragosa, M; De Simone, C; Hontecillas, R. Immunoregulatory mechanisms underlying prevention of colitis- associated colorectal cancer by probiotic bacteria. *PLoS One*, (2012), 7(4), e34676. doi:10.1371/journal.pone.0034676.

Bassaganya-Riera, J; DiGuardo, M; Viladomiu, M; de Horna, A; Sanchez, S; Einerhand, AW; et al. Soluble fibers and resistant starch ameliorate disease activity in interleukin-10-deficient mice with inflammatory bowel disease. *J Nutr*, (2011), 141(7), 1318–25. doi:10.3945/jn.111.139022.

Beltrán-Sánchez, H; Harhay, MO; Harhay, MM; McElligott, S. Prevalence and trends of metabolic syndrome in the adult U.S. population, 1999–2010. *Journal of the American College of Cardiology.*, (2013), 62 (8), 697–703.

Beisel, WR. The history of nutritional immunology. *J Nutr Immunol*, (1991), 1(1), 5–40.

Beisel, WR. History of nutritional immunology: introduction and overview1. *J Nutr*, (1992), 122(3S), 591.

Bendich, A; Chandra, RK. Micronutrients and immune functions. *Ann N Y Acad Sci*, (1990), 587, 3–320. doi:10.1111/j.1749-6632.1990.tb00144.x.

Bercik, P; Collins, SM; Verdu, EF. Microbes and the gut-brain axis. *Neurogastroenterol Motil.*, (2012), 24(5), 405-13.

Berg, J; Tymoczko, JL; Stryer, L. *Biochemistry (5th ed.)*. San Francisco: W.H. Freeman., p. 603, (2002).

den Besten, G; van Eunen, K; Groen, AK; Venema, K; Reijngoud, DJ; Bakker, BM. The role of short-chain fatty acids in the interplay between diet, gut microbiota, and host energy metabolism. *J Lipid Res*, (2013), 54(9), 2325–40. doi:10.1194/jlr.R036012.

Bohórquez, DV; Liddle, RA. The gut connectome: making sense of what you eat. *J Clin Invest.*, (2015), 125(3), 888-90.

Bonaz, B; Sinniger, V; Pellissier, S. *Vagus nerve stimulation: a new promising therapeutic.*

Borenstein, E. Computational systems biology and in silico modeling of the human microbiome. *Brief Bioinform*, (2012), 13(6), 769–80. doi:10.1093/bib/ bbs022.

Borre, YE; Moloney, RD; Clarke, G; Dinan, TG; Cryan, JF. The impact of microbiota on brain and behavior: mechanisms & therapeutic potential. *Adv Exp Med Biol.*, (2014), 817, 373-403.

Bourre, JM. The role of nutritional factors on the structure and function of the brain: an update on dietary requirements. *Rev Neurol* (Paris)., (2004), 160(8-9), 767-92.

Chandra, RK. Nutrition and the immune system: an introduction. *Am J Clin Nutr*, (1997), 66(2), 460S–3S.

Clemente, JC; Ursell, LK; Parfrey, LW; Knight, R. The impact of the gut microbiota on human health: an integrative view. *Cell*, (2012), 148(6), 1258–70. doi:10.1016/j.cell.2012.01.035.

Common Methods of Processing And Preserving Food. Streetdirectory.com., April 7, 2015.

Cryan, JF; O'Mahony, SM. The microbiome-gut-brain axis: from bowel to behavior. *Neurogastroenterol Motil.*, (2011), 23(3), 187-92.

Cuomo, R; D'Alessandro, A; Andreozzi, P; Vozzella, L; Sarnelli, G. Gastrointestinal regulation of food intake: do gut motility, enteric nerves and entero-hormones play together? *Minerva Endocrinol.*, (2011), 36(4), 281-93.

Dantzer, R; O'Connor, JC; Freund, GG; Johnson, RW; Kelley, KW. From inflammation to sickness and depression: when the immune system subjugates the brain. *Nat Rev Neurosci*, (2008), 9(1), 46–56. doi:10.1038/nrn2297.

Dantzer, R. Cytokine-induced sickness behavior: mechanisms and implications. *Ann N Y Acad Sci*, (2001), 933(1), 222–34. doi:10.1111/j.1749-6632.2001. tb05827.x.

Dave, M; Higgins, PD; Middha, S; Rioux, KP. The human gut microbiome: current knowledge, challenges, and future directions. *Transl Res*, (2012), 160(4), 246–57. doi:10.1016/j.trsl.2012.05.003.

Falkner, B; Cossrow, ND. Prevalence of metabolic syndrome and obesity-associated hypertension in the racial ethnic minorities of the United States. *Current Hypertension Reports.*, (2014), 16 (7), 449.

Food Processing Lesson Plan Johns Hopkins Bloomberg School of Public Health. April 7, 2015.

Fonseca, DM; Hand, TW; Han, SJ; Gerner, MY; Glatman Zaretsky, A; Byrd, AL; et al. Microbiota-dependent sequelae of acute infection compromise tissue-specific immunity. *Cell*, (2015), 163(2), 354–66. doi:10.1016/j.cell.2015.08.030.

Furness, JB. The Enteric Nervous System. John Wiley & Sons., (2008), pp. 35–38.

Furness, JB; Callaghan, BP; Rivera, LR; Cho, HJ. The enteric nervous system and gastro-intestinal innervation: integrated local and central control. *Adv Exp Med Biol.*, 2014, 817, 39-71.

Galland, L. The gut microbiome and the brain. *J Med Food.*, (2014), 17(12), 1261-72.

Romijn, JA; Corssmit, EP; Havekes, LM; Pijl, H. *Gut-brain axis Curr Opin Clin Nutr Metab Care.*, (2008), 11(4), 518-21.

Gershon, MD. *The Second Brain: A Groundbreaking New Understanding of Nervous Disorders of the Stomach and Intestine*, Harper Perennial., 1999.

Greenwood-Van Meerveld, B; Johnson, AC; Grundy, D. Gastrointestinal Physiology and Function. *Handb Exp Pharmacol.*, (2017), 239, 1-16.

Greicius, G; Arulampalam, V; Pettersson, S. A CLA's act: feeding away inflammation. *Gastroenterology*, (2004), 127(3), 994–6. doi:10.1053/j.gastro.2004.07.038.

Hooper, LV. Do symbiotic bacteria subvert host immunity? *Nat Rev Microbiol*, (2009), 7(5), 367–74. doi:10.1038/nrmicro2114.

Irimia, A; Chambers, MC; Torgerson, CM; Van Horn, JD. Circular representation of human cortical networks for subject and population-level connectomic visualization. *NeuroImage*, (2012), 60(2), 1340-51.

Johnson, R. Immune and endocrine regulation of food intake in sick animals. *Domest Anim Endocrinol*, (1998), 15(5), 309–19. doi:10.1016/ S0739-7240(98)00031-9.

Kau, AL; Ahern, PP; Griffin, NW; Goodman, AL; Gordon, JI. Human nutrition, the gut microbiome and the immune system. *Nature*, (2011), 474(7351), 327–36. doi:10.1038/nature10213.

Kaur, J. *A comprehensive review on metabolic syndrome.* Cardiology Research and Practice., 2014, 943162.

Klingelhoefer, L; Reichmann, H. Pathogenesis of Parkinson disease – the gut brain axis and environmental factors. *Nat Rev Neurol*, (2015), 11(11), 625–36. doi:10.1038/ nrneurol.2015.197.

Kohno, M; Morales, AM; Ghahremani, DG; Hellemann, G; London, ED. Risky decision making, prefrontal cortex, and mesocorticolimbic functional connectivity in methamphetamine dependence. *JAMA Psychiatry.*, (2014), 71(7), 812-20.

Konturek, SJ; Konturek, JW; Pawlik, T; Brzozowski, T. Brain-gut axis and its role in the control of food intake. *J Physiol Pharmacol.*, (2004), 55(1 Pt 2), 137-54.

Kverka, M; Zakostelska, Z; Klimesova, K; Sokol, D; Hudcovic, T; Hrncir, T; et al. Oral administration of Parabacteroides distasonis antigens attenuates experimental murine colitis through modulation of immunity and microbiota composition. *Clin Exp Immunol*, (2011), 163(2), 250–9. doi:10.1111/j.1365-2249.2010.04286.x.

Lean, MiEJ (2015). "Principles of Human Nutrition". Medicine. 43 (2): 61–65. doi:10.1016/j.mpmed.2014.11.009.

Marion-Letellier, R; Déchelotte, P; Iacucci, M; Ghosh, S. Dietary modulation of peroxisome proliferator-activated receptor gamma. *Gut*, (2009), 58(4), 586–93. doi:10.1136/gut.2008.162859.

Mechling, AE; Arefin, T; Lee, HL; Bienert, T; Reisert, M; Ben Hamida, S; Darcq, E; Ehrlich, A; Gaveriaux-Ruff, C; Parent, MJ; Rosa-Neto, P; Hennig, J; von Elverfeldt, D; Kieffer, BL; Harsan, LA. Deletion of the mu opioid receptor gene in mice reshapes the reward-aversion connectome. *Proc Natl Acad Sci U S A.*, (2016), 113(41), 11603-11608.

Musso, G; Gambino, R; Cassader, M. Interactions between gut microbiota and host metabolism predisposing to obesity and diabetes. *Annu Rev Med*, (2011), 62, 361–80. doi:10.1146/annurev-med-012510-175505.

National Geographic. https://www.nationalgeographic.org/encyclopedia/herbivore/.

Neubert, FX; Mars, RB; Sallet, J; Rushworth, MF. Connectivity reveals relationship of brain areas for reward-guided learning and decision making in human and monkey frontal cortex. *Proc Natl Acad Sci U S A.*, (2015), 112(20), E2695-704. doi: 10.1073/ pnas.1410767112.

Neunlist, M; Schemann, M. Nutrient-induced changes in the phenotype and function of the enteric nervous system. *J Physiol.*, (2014), 592(14), 2959-65.

Noori, HR; Schöttler, J; Ercsey-Ravasz, M; Cosa-Linan, A; Varga, M; Toroczkai, Z; Spanagel, R. A multiscale cerebral neurochemical connectome of the rat brain. *PLoS Biol.*, (2017), 15(7), e2002612.

Palmer, CS; Ostrowski, M; Balderson, B; Christian, N; Crowe, SM. Glucose metabolism regulates T cell activation, differentiation, and functions. *Front Immunol*, (2015), 6, 1. doi:10.3389/fimmu.2015.00001.

Rakhilin, N; Bradley, Barth; Jiahn, Choi; Nini, L. Muñoz; Subhash, Kulkarni; Jason, S. Jones; David, M. Small; Yu-Ting, Cheng; Yingqiu, Cao; Colleen, LaVinka; Edwin, Kan; Xinzhong, Dong; Michael, Spencer; Pankaj, Pasricha; Nozomi, Nishimura; Xiling, Shen. Simultaneous optical and electrical *in vivo* analysis of the enteric nervous system. *Nature Communications*, 2016, 7, 11800.

Rosas-Ballina, M; Olofsson, PS; Ochani, M; Valdés-Ferrer, SI; Levine, YA; Reardon, C; Tusche, MW; Pavlov, VA; Andersson, U; Chavan, S; Mak, TW; Tracey, KJ. Acetylcholine-synthesizing T cells relay neural signals in a vagus nerve circuit. *Science*, (2011), 334(6052), 98-101.

Sakamoto, M; Benno, Y. Reclassification of Bacteroides distasonis, Bacteroides goldsteinii and Bacteroides merdae as Parabacteroides distasonis gen. nov., comb. nov., Parabacteroides goldsteinii comb. nov. and Parabacteroides merdae comb. nov. *Int J Syst Evol Microbiol*, (2006), 56(7), 1599–605. doi:10.1099/ijs.0.64192-0.

Sakurai, T; Mieda, M. Connectomics of orexin-producing neurons: interface of systems of emotion, energy homeostasis and arousal. *Trends Pharmacol Sci.*, (2011), 32(8), 451-62.

Satyaraj, E. Emerging paradigms in immunonutrition. *Top Companion Anim Med*, (2011), 26(1), 25–32. doi:10.1053/j.tcam.2011.01.004.

Schlegel, P; Texada, MJ; Miroschnikow, A; Schoofs, A; Hückesfeld, S; Peters, M; Schneider-Mizell, CM; Lacin, H; Li, F; Fetter, RD; Truman, JW; Cardona, A; Pankratz, MJ. Synaptic transmission parallels neuromodulation in a central food-intake circuit. *Elife.*, (2016), 5. pii: e16799. doi: 10.7554/eLife.16799.

Seymour, KE; Reinblatt, SP; Benson, L; Carnell, S. Overlapping neurobehavioral circuits in ADHD, obesity, and binge eating: evidence from neuroimaging research. *CNS Spectr.*, (2015), 20(4), 401-11.

Sharma, A; Wolf, DH; Ciric, R; Kable, JW; Moore, TM; Vandekar, SN; Katchmar, N; Daldal, A; Ruparel, K; Davatzikos, C; Elliott, MA; Calkins, ME; Shinohara, RT; Bassett, DS; Satterthwaite, TD. Common Dimensional Reward Deficits Across Mood and Psychotic Disorders: A Connectome-Wide Association Study. *Am J Psychiatry.*, (2017), 174(7), 657-666.

Sherwin, E; Rea, K; Dinan, TG; Cryan, JF. A gut (microbiome) feeling about the brain. *Curr Opin Gastroenterol.*, 2016 Mar, 32(2), 96-102.

Sonea, C; Opris, AL; Casanova, MF; Constantinescu, MV; Opris, I. Mind the Reward: Nutrition vs. Addiction Chapter 26 In *Physics of the mind and brain disorders: Advances in Electrostimulation Therapies*, edited by Dr. Ioan Opris and Manuel F Casanova, in Springer Series in Neural Systems, Springer Nature, (2017), 469-489.

Trop, TK. Intestinal microbiota, probiotics and prebiotics in inflammatory bowel disease. *World J Gastroenterol*, (2014), 20(33), 11505. doi:10.3748/wjg. v20.i33.11505.

Turnbaugh, PJ; Ley, RE; Hamady, M; Fraser-Liggett, CM; Knight, R; Gordon, JI. The human microbiome project. *Nature*, (2007), 449(7164), 804–10. doi:10.1038/ nature06244.

Verma, M; Hontecillas, R; Abedi, V; Leber, A; Tubau-Juni, N; Philipson, C; Carbo, A; Bassaganya-Riera, J. Modeling-Enabled Systems Nutritional Immunology. *Front. Nutr.*, (2016), 3, 5. doi: 10.3389/fnut.2016.00005.

Vermeire, S; Noman, M; Van Assche, G; Baert, F; Van Steen, K; Esters, N; et al. Autoimmunity associated with anti-tumor necrosis factor α treatment in Crohn's disease: a prospective cohort study. *Gastroenterology*, (2003), 125(1), 32–9. doi:10.1016/S0016-5085(03)00701-7.

Viladomiu, M; Hontecillas, R; Yuan, L; Lu, P; Bassaganya-Riera, J. Nutritional protective mechanisms against gut inflammation. *J Nutr Biochem*, (2013), 24(6), 929–39. doi:10.1016/j.jnutbio.2013.01.006.

Whitman, WB; Coleman, DC; Wiebe, WJ. Prokaryotes: the unseen majority. *Proc Natl Acad Sci U S A*, (1998), 95(12), 6578–83. doi:10.1073/pnas.95.12.6578.

Ye, L; Liddle, RA. Gastrointestinal hormones and the gut connectome. *Curr Opin Endocrinol Diabetes Obes.*, (2017), 24(1), 9-14.

Zhang, A; Leow, A; Zhan, L; GadElkarim, J; Moody, T; Khalsa, S; Strober, M; Feusner, JD. Brain connectome modularity in weight-restored anorexia nervosa and body dysmorphic disorder. *Psychol Med.*, (2016), 46(13), 2785-97.

In: Focus on Systems Theory Research
Editors: Manuel F. Casanova and Ioan Opris

ISBN: 978-1-53614-561-8
© 2019 Nova Science Publishers, Inc.

Chapter 13

A MODULAR APPROACH TO THE ORGANIZATION OF BRAIN FUNCTIONS

Ioan Opris, PhD[1,2,*], Estate M. Sokhadze, PhD[3],
Emily L. Casanova, PhD[3],
Cosmin Sonea[2] and Manuel F. Casanova, MD[3]

[1]Department of Neurological Surgery, Miami Project to Cure Paralysis,
University of Miami, Miller School of Medicine, Miami, FL, US
[2]Department of Veterinary Medicine,
University of Agronomical Sciences and Veterinary Medicine,
Bucharest, Romania
[3]Department of Developmental Behavioral Pediatrics,
University of South Carolina School of Medicine Greenville,
Greenville Health System, SC, US

ABSTRACT

The operation of brain functions occurs in ensembles of neurons from different laminae of cortical columns, modular networks composed of microcircuits, modules and the hubs of the brain's connectome. This involves the integration of information by distributed networks of neurons that generate engrams, and complex functional sequences, such as the *perception-to-action cycle*. The functions of the brain are considered to be the byproduct of the integration of perceptual prefrontal cortical signals processed in supra-granular cortical layers, the action-related information from the infra-

---

* Corresponding Author Email: ixo82@med.miami.edu.

granular layers, and the reward signals originating in the midbrain. Cortical modules and their connections are the building blocks of this complex hierarchical circuitry that performs the behavioral act. They follow a logic (from both structural and functional perspectives) labelled as the power of two permutation logic. Future investigations of the brain's microcircuits by computational, structural, and physiological approaches, lead to new insights and paradigm-shifting ideas regarding the emergence of the human mind.

1. INTRODUCTION

This chapter is intended to examine the modular nature of neural processing that underlies the emergence of human brain functions. We discuss the operation of microcircuits, such as neurons in different laminae of cortical columns, modular networks composed of microcircuits, and the hubs of the brain's connectome. This involves the integration of information by distributed networks of neurons that generate engrams, cognitive functions, and complex functional sequences, such as the *perception-to-action cycle*. The functions of the brain are considered as the product of the integration of perceptual prefrontal cortical signals processed in supra-granular cortical layers, action-related information represented in infra-granular layers, and reward signals originating in the midbrain. The cortical modules and their connections are the building blocks of this complex hierarchical circuitry that performs the behavioral act. They follow a logic (both from structural and functional perspectives) that has been labelled the power of two permutation logic (Xie et al., 2016).

Overall, determining the foundation of human cognition is a challenging task, but neuroscientists are making progress in our understanding of neuronal mechanisms regarding knowledge, perception, and learning. Investigations of the relationship between different brain structures and cognitive functions are bringing us closer to understanding the mind (Goldman-Rakic, 1995, 1996; Mountcastle, 1997; DeFelipe, 2011; Arnsten, 2013; Opris and Casanova, 2014). We also emphasize the importance of bidirectional information flow in cortico-cortical and thalamo-cortical loops, which integrate *bottom-up* and *top-down* communications between the brain areas.

The higher brain functions integrated in the "mind" can be regarded as the ability of human beings to reason and think. The necessary skill sets for these operations include perception, memory, judgment, thinking, volition, and language. The human mind can be described as a complex process that utilizes, among others, reasoning, thoughts, imagination, and recognition in order to generate complex behaviors, actions, and subjective states, such as feelings and emotions. The mind encompasses myriads of mental processes whose details we cannot consciously monitor. Conscious mental processes emerge from this vast unconscious processing. In terms of localization, many authors consider the *prefrontal cortex* (PFC) to be the seat of the mind because of its representation of higher brain functions, including memory and cognition. Indeed, the paramount role of PFC in cognition has been demonstrated in lesion studies both in humans and monkeys (Bauer and Fuster, 1976; Funahashi et al., 1989, 1993).

2. ANATOMICAL SUBSTRATE OF BRAIN FUNCTION: FROM MICROCIRCUITRY TO CONNECTOME

The anatomical organization of the brain is the key towards understanding the emergence of the mind, from the microscopic level (DeFelipe, 2011) and up to the macroscopic, large-scale level of neuroanatomy.

2.1. Cortical Microcircuitry

Functional specialization of the brain starts with microcircuits that form modules. A modular network can be partitioned into subsets of nodes (modules) that are densely interconnected internally but only sparsely to other subsets (Chunga et al., 2016). In the cortex, modules are composed of vertical arrangements of cortical neurons, called

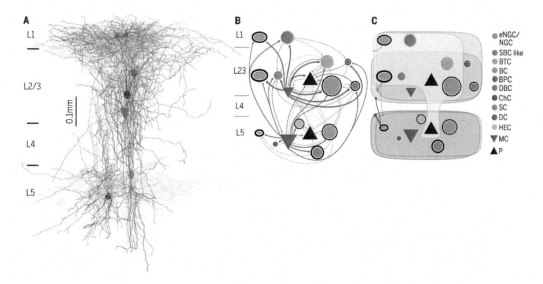

Figure 1. Connections between morphologically distinct types in neocortex (A) Simultaneous octuple whole-cell recording to study connectivity followed by morphological reconstruction. (B) Synaptic connectivity between morphologically distinct types of neurons, including pyramidal (P) neurons. (C) Connectivity from NGCs to other cell types. This connectivity is believed to be nonsynaptic and mediated by volume transmission. Martinotti cell, MC; neurogliaform cell, NGC; basket cell, BC; single-bouquet cell-like cell, SBC-like; bitufted cell, BTC; bipolar cell, BPC, double-bouquet cell, DBC; chandelier cell, ChC; shrub cell, SC; horizontally elongated cell, HEC; deep-projecting cell, DC (With permission from Jiang et al., 2015).

minicolumns (Szentágothai and Arbib, 1975; Mountcastle, 1997; Jiang et al., 2016) (Figure 1). Within the minicolumns, cortical neurons are wired into six horizontal layers (or laminae): three supra-granular layers (L1-L3), a granular layer (L4) and two infra-granular layers (L5/L6). The granular layer receives sensory input via the thalamus (Constantinople and Bruno, 2013).

The supra-granular layers consist of small pyramidal neurons that form vertical connections with the larger pyramidal neurons of the infra-granular layers that generate most of the output from cerebral cortex to other parts of the central nervous system (Buxhoeveden and Casanova, 2002). According to this three-stratum functional module, infra-granular layers execute the associative computations elaborated in supra-granular layers (Buxhoeveden and Casanova, 2002; Casanova et al., 2011). Interestingly, the PFC, that has a crucial role in cognition, has a thicker layer 2/3 than sensory or motor cortices.

2.2. Brain's Connectome

As it is well known, the human brain is a complex biophysical system consisting of approximately 86 billion neurons (Herculano-Houzel, 2009), each one interconnected to others by thousands of synapses (Andersen, 1990), that result in over one hundred trillion synaptic connections. The composite of all neural connections of the brain is called the *connectome*. The connectome's pathways between forebrain and neocortex are referred to as a *connectivity matrix* (Murray and Shanahan, 2012). The connectome's structure and function can be analyzed using mathematical methods developed for complex networks, for example graph-theoretical methods. With these approaches, topological features of the connectome can be described, such as sparse networks and meso-level microcircuits that define cortical modularity (Opris and Casanova, 2014). Within these topologies, dynamical neural states can be described as spatial arrangement of electrical activity.

The main components of the hierarchical architecture of the brain include *cortical modules* (layers and minicolumns), subcortical nuclei (basal ganglia and thalamus) and brainstem structures (midbrain, pons, and medulla). These structures process sensory inputs, including vision, auditory information, touch, smell, and taste. The end results of neural processing are manifested as overt motor behaviors of different complexity, such as eye and/or limb movements, speech and covert cognitive states, such as perception, awareness, memory and decision making processes.

2.3. Functional Connectomics: Default Mode vs. Executive Control Networks

In large-scale neuronal networks, neural activity is distributed across all brain regions (Bar et al., 2016). Specific spatio-temporal neuronal patterns occur at rest and during cognitive tasks. The networks exhibiting patterns of activity at rest (in the absence of external task demands) are known as the *default mode network* (DMN), while the networks exhibiting patterns of activity during cognitive control tasks are known as the *executive control network* (ECN; Figure 2).

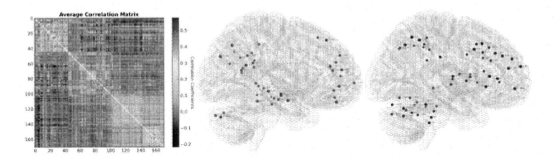

Figure 2. Default mode *vs* Executive control networks. *Left:* A group average 171 × 171 correlation matrix calculated from 154 subjects and organized by modules (Modules I to IV from left upper to right lower corner). BOLD signal time courses were extracted from 171 unsmoothed cortical and subcortical regions. Matrix was subsequently partitioned using the spectral partitioning method. *Center:* DMN in red color and *Right:* ECN in blue color. Graphs theoretical (GT) analysis of the default module network The GT analysis of the whole-brain network based on the average BOLD time courses of voxels within 171 ROIs as extracted from unsmoothed functional data. The optimal solution of the graph partitioning led to four functionally distinct modules: the executive-control (I), the salience (II), the default mode network (Module III), and visual (IV) networks (Taken with permission from Bar et al., 2016).

DMN includes a set of midline and inferior parietal regions in the absence of most external task demands, but are associated with cognitive processes that require internally-directed or self-generated thoughts, such as mental simulation and perspective/future thinking (Young et al., 2016). ECN activation is shown within the lateral prefrontal cortex, a core hub of the executive control system. ECN is engaged during cognitive tasks that require externally-directed attention, such as working memory, relational integration, response inhibition, and task-set switching. ECN brain networks are linked to the top-down control of attention and cognition. Cognitive functions, like *creative thinking* recruits brain regions associated with both cognitive control and spontaneous imaginative processes (Young et al., 2016). These complex functions implicate regions within large-scale networks, including the ECN and the DMN. Despite their apparent cooperation, the DMN and ECN tend to act in opposition; the activation of one network typically corresponding to suppression of the other. This antagonistic relationship is thought to reflect opposing modes of attention, with ECN activity indicating focused external attention and DMN activity indicating spontaneous interoception.

2.4. Modularity

The modular (community) structure of the network is identified by optimizing a network-based modularity metric that takes into account the direction of network edges (Leicht and Newman, 2008). The metric belongs to a family of modularity measures (e.g., Newman and Girvan, 2004) that quantifies the density of edges present within communities (given a network partition) relative to what would be expected if edges were distributed uniformly. A spectral optimization technique is applied to identify the partition for which the modularity metric was maximized. (Harriger et al., 2012) Optimization of a network-based modularity metric (Leicht and Newman, 2008) resulted in a partition of the network into 5 structural modules, with a value of the modularity measure $Q = 0.362$. Intra-modular edges accounted for 58% of all connections, resulting in an average within-module connection density of 0.191 *versus* a between-module density of 0.037. Figure 3A displays the macaque cortex connection matrix, with the regions rearranged to show the individual modules. In addition, within each module, nodes are ranked according to their degree (sum of in-degree and out-degree).

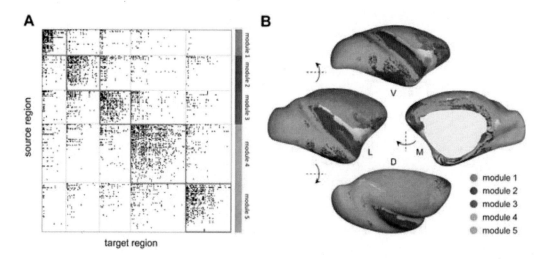

Figure 3. Connection matrix and network modules. (A) Binary connection matrix comprising 242 regions and 4090 directed projections. Regions are arranged by *module assignment,* and within each module they are ranked by their degree (sum of in-degree and out-degree). The node ordering and module assignments are reported in the Supplementary Information. (B) Surface rendering of the inflated right hemisphere of macaque cortex, with surface regions color-coded by to their module assignments. Some points on the surface corresponded to multiple cortical regions since multiple schemes for regional parcellations were used for surface mapping. This could lead to multiple module assignment for a given surface point. In case of multiple assignments, regions were colored according to a majority rule, choosing the mode of the distribution of module assignments. In the case of a tie, a module was chosen at random from the tied set, resulting in a mottled appearance. Surface plots at left and right show lateral (L) and medial (M) views; plots at top and bottom show ventral (V) and dorsal (D) views. (With permission from Harriger et al., 2012).

This node arrangement shows that regions of macaque cortex exhibit a broad distribution of node degrees, previously characterized as exponential (Modha and Singh, 2010), and that high-degree nodes are encountered in each of the 5 modules. A rendering of the spatial layout of these modules on an inflated surface plot of the macaque cortex is shown in Figure 3B. Structural modules mainly consist of spatially contiguous regions comprising frontal/orbitofrontal ("module 1"), inferior temporal ("module 2"), frontal/superior temporal ("module 3"), prefrontal/motor/somatosensory ("module 4"), and occipital/visual/prefrontal regions ("module 5").

3. MODULAR SUBSTRATE OF BRAIN FUNCTIONS: FROM MICROCIRCUITRY TO MACRO-NETWORKS

Modularity is a key characteristic of structural and functional brain circuits/networks across multiple domains and scales of the connectome (Sporns and Betzel, 2016). Anatomical modules generally reflect functional associations among neurons within cortical areas (microcircuit modularity) and between brain regions (network modularity). Structural modules are often spatially compact, whereas functional modules can be more widely distributed and fluctuate in relation to cognitive states. Modular organization may confer increased robustness and more flexible learning, help to conserve wiring cost, and promote functional specialization and complex brain dynamics. Clune et al., (2013) argue that modularity has evolved as a by-product of strong selection pressure on reducing the cost of connections in networks. Indeed, the notion that wiring cost is a major constraint on the layout of (structural) brain networks has a long history in neuroscience. In addition to the spatial layout of nodes and hubs, specific functional constraints, such as network's processing efficiency, were found to be important in supporting the idea that brain network topology is shaped by a trade-off between spatial and functional factors (Bullmore and Sporns 2012).

3.1. Prefrontal Cortex Is an Integrative Hub of the Connectome

3.1.1. Prefrontal Cortical Connections

Distinct domains of the PFC in primates have a set of connections suggesting that they have different roles in cognition, memory, and emotion. The prefrontal cortical hub-related edges: temporal, parietal, limbic, striatal, thalamic, brainstem, inter-hemispheric, etc. Dense connections between the prefrontal cortical hub and other cortical/subcortical nodes may thus provide short communication relays, efficient neural communication, and robustness of inter-hub communication (van der Heuvel and Sporns, 2013).

3.1.2. Prefrontal-Parietal Connections

Parietal-prefrontal connections are assumed to have a role for the short-term maintenance of visuo-spatial information as part of the *reverberatory circuit* in which feedback projections from PFC serve to maintain excitation of parietal-to-prefrontal feed-forward pathways (Chafee and Goldman-Rakic, 1998).

3.1.3. Prefrontal-Temporal/Hippocampal Connections

Several communication channels link the dlPFC and the hippocampus via the parahippocampal gyrus, subiculum, presubiculum, and adjacent transitional cortices (Goldman-Rakic et al., 1984). These prefrontal projections carry highly specific information for memory consolidation into the hippocampus, whereas the reciprocal projections may allow retrieval by PFC of memories stored in the hippocampus. Recent evidence points to an indirect pathway from the HPC to the mPFC, via midline thalamic *nucleus reuniens*, that play a role in spatial/emotional memory processing (Jin & Maren, 2015).

3.1.4. Cortico-Striatal and Thalamo-Cortical Connections

Direct evidence for a parallel organization of cortico-striatal-thalamo-cortical loops has been recently provided for the human brain (Jeon et al., 2014; Santos et al., 2014). Functional specificity is reflected within the cortico-subcortical loops substantiated by parallel networks (motor, oculomotor, cognitive, and limbic). Such functional specificity depends on varying levels of cognitive hierarchy, as well as on their pattern of connectivity. Higher levels of activations emerge in the ventro-anterior part of the PFC, the head of the caudate nucleus, and the *ventral anterior* nucleus (VA) in the thalamus, while lower levels of activation were located in the posterior region of the PFC, the body of the caudate nucleus, and the *medial dorsal* nucleus (MD) of the thalamus.

3.1.5. Callosal Connections

The *corpus callosum* is a bundle of neural fibers along the longitudinal fissure beneath the fronto-parietal cortex used for communication across hemispheres. Inter-hemispheric interaction (via layer 3) is posited to aid attentional processing (both when attention is conceptualized as a resource and as a selective mechanism for gating sensory information) because it allows for a division of labor across the hemispheres, and for parallel processing, so that operations performed in one hemisphere can be isolated from those executed in the other.

3.1.6. Prefrontal-Brainstem Connection

The brainstem reticular formation is mainly connected to the PFC, particularly to the lateral PFC and ventro-medial PFC (Jang and Kwon, 2015). Also, the *locus coeruleus* and its noradrenergic projections to the frontal lobe provide important contributions to the modulation of cognition and emotion (Sara, 2009). The mPFC provides a potent excitatory influence on neurons of the locus coeruleus (Jodoj et al., 1998). The fact that inactivation of the mPFC suppressed locus coeruleus firing, indicates that the mPFC also provides a resting tonic excitatory influence on locus coeruleus activity. The richly interconnected prefrontal cortical circuits, we discussed above, are part of the brain's functional connectome that integrates cortical signals from *sensory* (visual, auditory, touch, taste, and smell perception), *cognitive* (attention, memory, decision making, intention, free will, language), emotional (fear, joy, anger, etc) and *motor* (skeleto-motor, oculomotor, pupil dilation) neural systems to support the emergence of mind. Brain hubs are formed by central interconnection nodes across distributed microcircuits, loops, and networks (van den Heuvel et al., 2013). PFC is a crucial integrative hub over multiple domains of the connectome, while the mind is the byproduct of such complex integrative processes involving sensory, motor, memory, and reward signals. It is noteworthy how cortical modularity provides flexibility to the emergence of mind by complex logic permutations of neural inputs.

3.2. Noninvasive Neuromodulation of the Connectome

Transcranial magnetic stimulation (TMS) is a powerful tool for the *in vivo* manipulation of brain network activity. Using data from the Human Connectome Project, Opitz et al., (2016) have shown an example of implementation focused on the dorsolateral prefrontal cortex (PFC). Three distinct dorsolateral PFC stimulation zones were identified, differing with respect to the network to be affected (default, frontoparietal) and sensitivity to coil orientation. A key challenge for TMS targeting is the specificity of the networks. Detection analyses suggested that depending on the specific location within dorsolateral PFC, one of two key networks is affected by stimulation. However, significant "collateral stimulation" is likely to occur, depending on location and orientation. To address this concern, the stimulus locations across participants were reduced to 9 zones (oriented in a 3×3 grid on dorsolateral PFC) and created a network connectivity profile for each zone using the 7-intrinsic connectivity network (ICN) parcellation of the brain established by Yeo et al., (2011).

As indicated by the detection analyses (Figure 4), the networks expected to be stimulated were dominated by either the FPN (ICN 2) or the DN (ICN 3); specifically, ICN 2 was dominant for the networks expected to be stimulated at lateral of dorsolateral PFC locations (Z1, Z2, Z4, Z5) while ICN3 was most prominent for medial and posterior locations.

Beyond the FPN and DN, the dorsal attention network (ICN1) as well as the ventral attention network (ICN7) was represented in the expected functional connectivity maps depending on location, though to a lesser extent. Next, were repeated analyses at each possible orientation. As expected, overlap between the predicted functional connectivity maps for TMS and the 4 ICNs (ICN1, ICN2, ICN3, ICN7) varied across both orientations and positions. For example, the FPN (ICN 2) was preferentially associated with posterior–anterior coil positions, whereas the default network (ICN3) showed preferential associations with a 45 degrees to midline orientation.

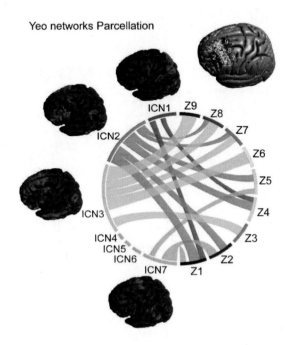

Figure 4. Overlap of TMS networks with established intrinsic connectivity networks. The relative overlap between the TMS functional connectivity maps with the seven ICNs changes depending on the spatial location. For anterior locations (Z1, Z2, Z4, Z5), the frontal–parietal network (ICN 2) shows the strongest overlap. For medial and posterior regions (Z3, Z6, Z7, Z8, Z9), the default network (ICN 3) shows the strongest overlap with TMS networks. Dorsal (ICN 1) and ventral (ICN 7) attention networks show moderate overlap in frontal locations while other networks (ICN 4: limbic network, ICN 5: visual network, ICN 6: somato-motor network) are not being targeted at any of the investigated coil locations. From Opitz et al. (2016) Neuroimage 127:86-96.

4. Emergence of Brain Functions in the Prefrontal Cortical Hub

4.1. Cognitive Functions

4.1.1. Perception to Action Cycle

The "perception-to-action cycle" has been described by Joaquin Fuster as a "circular flow of information" between a subject (animal or human) and its environment a sensory-guided sequence of "actions" that is goal oriented (Quintana and Fuster, 1999; Tishby and Polani, 2011). In Figure 5 illustrates the perception to action network during sound perception and speech production (Schomers and Pulvermüller, 2016). It is in this manner that each behavioral action performed by an animal/human modifies its environment through a top-down executive network from PFC to motor effectors. Actions modify the animal's own perception of the environment in a bottom-up processing sequence through the perceptual network hierarchy, until the goal is achieved (Fuster, 2012; Cutsuridis et al., 2011). Cerebral cortical modules mediate the interactions between the environment and the perceptual-executive systems of the brain (Figure 5). In fact, the inter-laminar prefrontal cortical microcircuits are assumed to bind perceptual and executive control signals to guide goal-driven behavior (Lebedev and Wise, 2002; Opris et al., 2013).

Opris and his colleagues compared neuron firing recorded simultaneously in PFC layers 2/3 and 5/6 and caudate-putamen of Rhesus monkeys, trained in a spatial vs. object, rule-based match-to-sample task (Opris et al., 2013).

They found that, during perception and executive selection phases of the task, cell firing in the localized prefrontal layers and caudate-putamen region exhibited similar location preferences on spatial-trials, but not on object-trials. Then, by stimulating the prefrontal infra-granular-layers with patterns previously derived from supra-granular-layers, it produced stimulation-induced spatial preference in percentage correct performance on spatial trials, similar to neural tuning (Opris et al., 2013). These inter-laminar prefrontal microcircuits may play crucial roles to the perception-to-action cycle by bridging perception circuits in supra-granular cortical layers with selection and executive function in infra-granular layers (Opris et al., 2013).

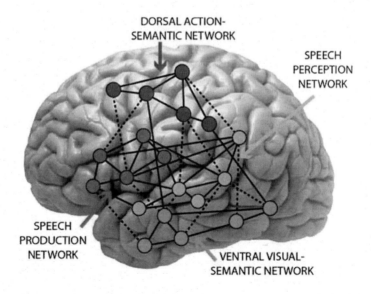

Figure 5. Perception to action cycle. Action-perception circuit for integrative speech production, perception and semantic understanding. From Schomers MR and Pulvermüller F (2016).

4.1.2. Memory Connectome

Functional insight into the cognitive role of PFC in working memory came from single unit recordings (Fuster and Alexander, 1971; Funahashi et al., 1989), in prefrontal cortical cells displaying persistent, sustained levels of neuronal firing during the retention delay period, in tasks that required the monkey to retain information over a short period of time (see Figure 6). This sustained activity (representing a *signature* for working memory) is thought to provide a "bridge across time" between the stimulus cue (e.g., the location of a light stimulus) and its contingent response (e.g., a later delayed saccade to the remembered location of light stimulus). These results have been supported by functional neuroimaging studies in humans that have shown lateral PFC activity during performance on delay response tasks (for review, see Curtis and D'Esposito, 2003). For example, in a functional magneto-resonance imaging (fMRI) study, using an oculomotor delay task similar to that used in monkey studies, it was observed, but also that the magnitude of the activity correlated positively with the accuracy of the memory-guided saccade that followed later (Curtis et al., 2004). Individual variation in working memory has been associated with multiple behavioral and health features including cognitive and physical traits and lifestyle choices. In this context, we used sparse canonical correlation analyses (sCCAs) to determine the covariation between brain imaging metrics of WM-network activation and connectivity and nonimaging measures relating to sensorimotor processing, affective and nonaffective cognition, mental health and personality, physical health and lifestyle choices derived from 823 healthy participants derived from the Human Connectome Project. Modular sparse canonical correlation analyses were implemented to test the covariation of each neuroimaging module to each of the behavioral modules (Figure 6). The behavioral–health and neuroimaging data sets showed significant interdependency. Variables with positive correlation to the neuroimaging variate represented higher physical endurance and fluid intelligence as well as better function in multiple higher-order cognitive domains. Negatively correlated variables represented indicators of suboptimal cardiovascular and metabolic control and lifestyle choices such as alcohol and nicotine use.

Mnemonic (working memory) activity underlying persistent neural activity has been hypothesized to be sustained by synaptic reverberation in a recurrent circuit (Wang, 2001). Neural circuitry may involve reverberatory thalamo-cortical (Wang, 2001) and inter-laminar loops (Takeuchi et al., 2011; Opris et al., 2011-2013). Ben-Yakov and Dudai (2011) established that the hippocampus plays a role in the maintenance of working memory. The authors of this study identified, by fMRI, a bilateral hippocampus activity starting immediately after the presentation of stimuli. Maintenance of working memory by the hippocampus may be part of the long-term memory maintenance process that involves reverberation of neural activity through the cortico-hippocampal-thalamic loop.

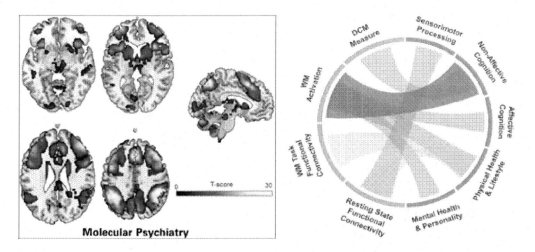

Figure 6. Left. Supra-threshold clusters of activation in the 2-back task. Data derived from the entire sample (n = 823); Po0.05 with family-wise error (FWE) voxel-wise correction and minimum k = 30 voxels. Right. Modular sparse canonical correlation analysis. The connections between the modules are sized based on the r-values. Yellow connections indicate significant associations at P < 0.05; orange connections indicate significant associations at P < 0.01; red connections indicate significant associations at P < 0.001. DCM, dynamic casual modeling; WM, working memory (From Moser et al., 2017).

4.1.3. Decision Making and Executive Control

As populations of neurons carry a large variety of signals correlated with external sensory events, internal mental states or impending behavioral responses, these signals are encoded, decoded, and remapped at several stages of the perception-to-action cycle, in order to provide the most appropriate course of action (Shadlen, 1998; Quintana, 1999; Fuster, 2000, 2001; Opris et al., 2013). Decision making is a cognitive process with several features: (1) accumulation of sensory evidence (Shadlen, 2001; Ratclif, 2002), (2) integration of sensory signals, reward expectation and cognitive information (Curtis et al., 2004), (3) weighing of the options by comparisons between a subject's expected reward and prior experience (Schall, 1999; Opris and Bruce, 2005), and (4) the selection of behavioral response (Zhang et al., 2012). The flow of decision signals is depicted as a rise to threshold process described by the psychological diffusion model of decision (Ratcliff et al., 2011). Ratcliff and colleagues hypothesized that buildup/prelude neurons in *superior colliculus* (SC) and in *frontal eye fields* (FEF) are part of a mechanism that implements the accumulation of sensory evidence in a decision process. They compared neural firing rates to the paths of evidence accumulation for the diffusion process and found that collicular buildup /prelude activity closely follows the trajectory of the decision process described by a diffusion model (Ratcliff et al., 2011). Minicolumns in the PFC (Opris and Casanova, 2014) are interconnected to each other through horizontal 'long range' projections in layer 2/3 (Kritzer and Goldman-Rakic, 1995; Rao et al., 1999) and interlaminar mini-loops (Weiler et al., 2008; Takeuchi et al., 2011). The loop is then

300 *Ioan Opris, Estate M. Sokhadze, Emily L. Casanova et al.*

closed ('reverberatory loops') through projections to the subcortical basal ganglia nuclei and thalamus (Alexander et al., 1986; Swadlow et al., 2002).

Such 'reverberatory loops' may be regarded as the 'basic functional unit' of cognitive/executive mechanism because they: (1) combine incoming signals of the different input layers (Casanova et al., 2007); (2) store mnemonic information through feedback connections in 'persistent' spiking activity (Wang, 2012); and (3) compare input signals to a threshold criterion triggering an output response (selection), which constitutes the ability to make a decision (Ratcliff et al., 2003). Thus, a cortical minicolumn with integrative, selective, and threshold abilities can play the role of a *decision module* (Opris and Casanova 2014).

4.2. Emergence of Brain Function and the Power of Two Permutation Logic

A recent article by the group of Joe Tsien (Xie et al., 2016) proposed an elegant solution to the problem of how neuronal assemblies perform computations. These authors proposed that brain computations are performed by computational building blocks, called *functional computational motifs* (FCMs). Processing of information by FCMs eventually generates all higher brain functions. The principles of FCM operation are based on the theory of connectivity previously proposed by the same group (Tsien, 2015a,b; Li et al., 2016). The theory of connectivity defines mathematical rules that govern the organization of microcircuits and neuronal assemblies. This connectivity architecture incorporates specific-to-general computational connections that, according to Tsien and his colleagues, underlie the emergence of knowledge and adaptive behaviors. These researchers argue that FCMs obey the power-of-two-based permutation logic described by the equation $N = 2^i - 1$, where N is the number of projection-neuron cliques and i is the number of inputs. The set of cliques represents all possible permutations of specific-to-general input configurations. It follows from the permutation rule that each FCM contains principal projection neurons that receive very specific inputs and the neurons receive multiple convergent inputs. This neuronal composition covers all possible patterns defined by the power-of-two-based permutation logic (Figure 7A, B left panel). The proposed connectivity and computation rules explain how information is represented by neural assemblies that utilize specific input coding, assemblies that perform combinatorial operations, and assemblies with generalized representation properties. motivation, behaviors, and consciousness.

The proposed computational architecture agrees well with what we known about microcircuitry of cortical layers. Tsien and his colleagues describe the corresponding computational modules as cortical FCMs. In cortical FCMs, the power-of-two-based computational logic is implemented as a gradient of specific-to-general processing units across cortical laminae (Tsien, 2015a; Li et al., 2016). The connectivity is random in superficial laminae, i.e., L2/3, and nonrandom in deep laminae, i.e., L5/6, where the superficial laminae project. The random connectivity and specific encoding in superficial cortical layers facilitates such neural computations as extraction of novel patterns and sparse encoding of patterns. The non-randomness and generalized encoding in the deep layers facilitate various types of feedback control including control of emotions.

Tsien and his colleagues obtained convincing experimental evidence favoring their theoretical framework. They conducted experiments in mice, where they used tetrode arrays to record signals from cortical neurons located in L2/3 and L5/6 (Figures 7 right panel). The mice were exposed to four types of fearful events: (1) an air puff applied to the mouse's back, (2) an "earthquake" induced by shaking the chamber where the animal was placed, (3) "free-fall in the elevator" produced by placing the animal in a box, and then lifting and dropping the box, and (4) electric foot-shock. After the authors examined different types of neuronal responses to these stimuli, they found that of the total of 197 neurons recorded in L2/3, about 65% exhibited specific responses to only one stimulus type. A much smaller proportion, 1%, responded to all four stimuli and therefore belongs to the general clique. Responses to three stimuli were observed in 14% of the recorded neurons. Two-events neurons constituted 20% of the recorded sample (Figures 7 C,E). The recordings from the neurons located in L5/6 showed a different pattern of responses (Figure 7D). Here, a much smaller proportion of neurons (20%) were selective to one stimulus only, whereas 23% of the neurons responded to all four stimuli. About 55% of the L5/6 neuronal sample responded to either three or four events (compared to just 15% in L2/3). Thus, superficial laminae clearly contained mostly specific cliques, whereas the deep laminae contained mostly general cliques. The authors interpreted these findings as an evidence of a vertical implementation of FCM governed by the power-of-two-based permutation logic.

These and additional experiments of Tsien's group convincingly demonstrated that the power-of-two logic is found in many cortical and subcortical areas and in several animal species. Moreover, they showed that the logic applies to various modalities and physiological functions, including neural processing of emotional, appetitive, and social signals. The logic was even preserved if NMDA receptors, known to be important for memory and plasticity, which were deleted after postnatal development, indicating that the brain's computational architecture is preconfigured and does critically depend on learning. Finally, they found that modulatory DA neurons follow simpler logical rules. Overall, these findings support power-of-two-based permutation logic as a fundamental computational rule employed by the brain. The seemingly simple mathematical rule explains neural computations across a broad range of species, from the simplest nervous systems to very complex.

The computational logic proposed by Tsien and his colleagues is probably applicable to the human brain, as well, even though it contains 86 billion neurons (Herculano-Houzel, 2009) each of which having many thousands of synapses (Andersen, 1990).

302 Ioan Opris, Estate M. Sokhadze, Emily L. Casanova et al.

Given such an enormous complexity, it is very important that we search for unifying computational principles that govern such a network. In this context, the theoretical considerations and experimental findings of Tsien's group definitely represent a step in the right direction.

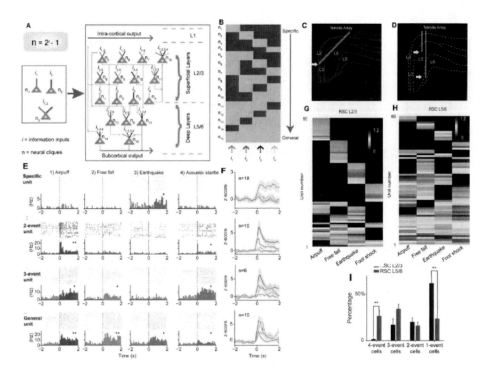

Figure 7. Emergence of the mind follows a power of two permutation logic for governing the specific-to-general wiring and computational logic of cell assemblies. (A) The logic is applicable from the simplest circuits to the high level human brain function. Implementation of the power-of-two-based computational logic is shown in the cortex via various cliques across laminae. In the 6-layered cortex, the layer 4 hosts most of the specific cliques while in the 3-layered cortex (illustrated here), there is no layer 4. As such, the cortex is divided into the L1, the superficial layers (L2/3) which preferentially host low-level combinatorial cells, and deep layers (L5/6) which host more high-level combinatorial cells. The implementation of this power-of-two-based logic can be repeatedly utilized as cortical expansion occurred over evolution. (B) Schematic "bar-code" illustrates the specific-to-general cell-assembly activation patterns, which can be measured by electrodes or imaging techniques, from the 15 distinct neural cliques (N1–15), processing four distinct inputs (i1, i2, i3, i4). The orange color represents the stimulus-triggered activation above the baseline state (in blue). The arrow on the right side illustrates the number of distinct neural cliques exhibiting specific, sub-combinatorial, as well as generalized, responsiveness. Specific neural cliques encode specific features, whereas various permutation rule-based neural cliques encode various convergent patterns, representing relational memories and generalized concepts. This ensemble activation pattern allows pattern-separation, pattern-categorization, and pattern-generalization of various experiences at the cognitive level. (C, D) Histological confirmation of recording tetrode location in the layers L2/3 (in C) and L5/6 (in D) of the retrosplenial cortex (RSC). (E) Specific cells firing in response to air puff, free fall, earthquake and acoustic starle. (F) The population response of the cells to the same events as in E. (G, H) Hierarchical clustering plot revealed that the general four-event clique and three-event cliques constituted a larger proportion. (I) There are significant differences in the distributions of specific c vs. general cells between L2/3 and L5/6. (With permission from Xie et al., 2016).

5. BRAIN DISORDERS AND THE CONNECTOME

Autism spectrum disorder (ASD) is increasingly considered a connectivity disorder (Zhang and Raichle, 2010). Early studies focused on region-specific differences in activation during tasks, with more recent inquiry using resting state fMRI concentrated in seed-based techniques (Hull et al., 2016) and low order models.

5.1. Autism Spectrum Disorder

De Lacy et al., (2017) looked at the clinical populations with ASD using a high-order model to achieve fine spatial and temporal scale, applying ten advanced outcome measures to maximize power. They characterized connectivity within networks, between networks and at the aggregated network system level and compared connectivity motifs across steady-state and dynamic FNC. A more granular picture of the structure of functional connectivity in ASD is shown in Figure 4. Here, the 6 state, 30TR-size window solution is displayed (Figure 8 left), with the full set of state transition matrices

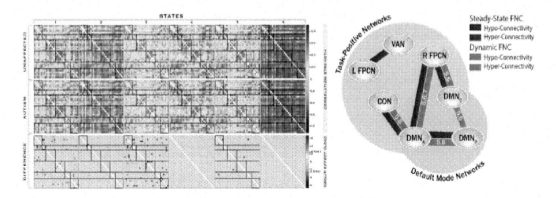

Figure 8. Left: Dynamic functional connectivity across brain states in controls and subjects with ASD. Distinct, stable brain states exist within the aggregated resting state timecourses each with a specific FNC pattern. Each 33× 33 network matrix is composed of Pearson pairwise correlations (color scale) between the 33 networks identified in the group independent component analysis for all subjects, decomposed into individual states using k-means clustering. We computed 9 permutations of this analysis with the 6 state, 30TR-size window solution shown here. Dynamic connectivity in control subjects ('Unaffected') is compared to that in individuals with ASD ('Autism') and significant group effects ('Difference') displayed for each individual state (log scale). Significant pairwise differences in FNC for each state are displayed, corrected for multiple comparisons at alpha =0.05 to control FDR. Right: The control network connectome in ASD. A web of abnormal functional connectivity affecting brain control networks is centered on the right fronto-parietal control network and default mode network in autism. We superimpose pairwise disruption visible in the steady-state and dynamic connectomes (with the specific dynamic state in which dFNC findings appear noted as a number within the line connection) to illustrate the importance of analyzing dynamic connectivity in building an integrated understanding of the differences in connectivity in this complex neuropsychiatric disorder. From de Laci et al., 2017.

for control subjects in the sensitivity analysis available for comparing the effects of parameter variation. Analysis of group effects ('Difference') shows significant (corrected for multiple comparisons at alpha = 0.05 to control FDR) pairwise differences in multiple states. As in steady-state FNC, a mix of abnormally decreased and increased correlation is evident in control network pairings with decreased connectivity more common among domain specific networks. While it is difficult to attribute specific behaviors or tasks that may be associated with individual brain states identified in dynamic resting-state analysis, we note that disruption to the overall configuration of pairwise correlations is most common in certain states. In these states there is more diffuse anticorrelation, particularly in the relationships among network systems vs. within systems, and between the control network vs. sensorimotor and visual groups. In particular, the right fronto-parietal control network is anticorrelated with most other TPN members. When comparing findings in a high-order model and large, varied subject group, several specific network connections are prominent, such as deficits in the right fronto-parietal DMNA, right fronto-parietal-DMNC, and cingulo-opercular-DMNA circuits, and in the DMNA-DMNP axis proved quite robust (Figure 8 right), and may link mechanistically to the disrupted state change tempo that was identified in autism.

5.2. Alzheimer Disease

Alzheimer's disease (AD) is known to be associated not only with regional gray matter damages, but also with abnormalities in functional integration between brain regions. Dai et al., (2015) looked into the intrinsic functional connectivity patterns of whole-brain networks in AD patients *vs.* healthy controls (HCs). They found that AD selectively targeted highly connected hub regions (in terms of nodal functional connectivity strength) of brain networks, involving the medial and lateral prefrontal and parietal cortices, insula, and thalamus. This impairment was connectivity distance-dependent (Euclidean), with the most prominent disruptions appearing in the long-range connections (e.g., 100–130 mm). Moreover, AD also disrupted functional connections within the default-mode, salience and executive-control modules, and connections between the salience and executive-control modules (See Figure 9 A). These disruptions of the connectivity hub and the modular integrity are significantly correlated with the patients' cognitive performance. Finally, the nodal connectivity strength in the posteromedial cortex exhibited a highly discriminative power in distinguishing individuals with AD from HCs.

A Modular Approach to the Organization of Brain Functions   305

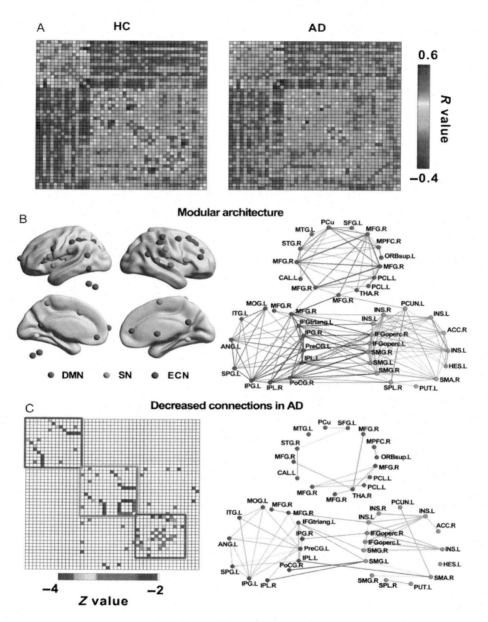

Figure 9. Modular analysis of the brain functional network. (A) Correlation matrices among 47 ROIs are shown for the HC (left panel) and AD(right panel) groups. (B) Surface (left panel) and topological (right panel) representations of the modular architecture of the brain networks in the HC group. Three modules were identified, the DMN (red colors), SN (green colors) and ECN (blue colors). The red nodes outside the brain are the regions of cerebellum. The within-module nodes and edges aremarked in the same color. The intermodule connections are marked with black lines. Notably, 4 nodes (2 in magenta and 2 in yellow) on the surfaces did not belong to the DMN, SN, or ECN in the modular detection and therefore were not shown in the right panel. (C) Matrix (left panel) and topological (right panel) representations of AD-related functional connectivity decreases. Blue and cyan lines represent AD-related decreases in inter- and intramodule connections, respectively. Notably, between-group statistical comparisons were restricted to positive correlations of either the HC or AD group. DMN, default-mode network; SN, salience network; ECN, executive-control network; HC, healthy control; AD, Alzheimer's disease.From Dai et al. (2014).

Taken together, Dai and colleagues' results emphasize AD-related degeneration of specific brain hubs, thus providing novel insights into the pathophysiological mechanisms of connectivity dysfunction in AD and suggesting the potential of using network hub connectivity as a diagnostic biomarker. The correlation matrix with 47 rows and 47 columns for each group (Figure 9A) is further decomposed into 3 major modules the DMN, the salience network (SN), and the executive control network (ECN; Figure 9B). Notably, the modular structure of the HC group was highly similar to that of the AD group. Furthermore, was found that functional connectivities exhibited AD-related decreases, categorized as 88.3% intra-module and 11.7% intermodule connections (Figure 9C). These intra-module disconnections primarily belonged to the ECN (22/60, 36.6%), followed by the SN (19/60, 31.7%) and the DMN (12/60, 20%). Intermodule disconnections were located between the SN and ECN. Only one connection—between the left middle occipital gyrus and the left calcarine fissure and surrounding cortex— exhibited a significant increase in the AD group relative to the HC group. Correlation matrix with 47 rows and 47 columns for each group (Figure 9A) and further decomposed them into 3 major modules (the DMN, the salience network (SN), and the executive control network (ECN; Figure 9B).

CONCLUSION

To conclude, the human mind relies on the laminar-columnar arrangement of the neurons in the cerebral cortex that enable the emergence of various features of the mind, such as attention, memory, decision making, and motor planning. We foresee that future investigations of the brain's microcircuits (DeFelipe, 2010b; Opris and Casanova, 2014), including computational, structural, and physiological approaches, will lead to new insights and paradigm-shifting ideas regarding the emergence of the human mind. Although the complexity of human brain circuits is immense, getting to the essence of mind is a feasible task.

REFERENCES

Alderson-Day B., Weis S., McCarthy-Jones S., Moseley P., Smailes D., Fernyhough C. (2016) The brain's conversation with itself: neural substrates of dialogic inner speech, *Soc. Cogn. Affect. Neurosci.*, 11: 110-20.10.1093/scan/nsv094.

Allman, J. Hakeem A. Nimchinsky E., Hof P. (2006) The Anterior Cingulate Cortex, *Annals of the New York Academy of Sciences*, 935: 107-17.

Arnsten A. F. (2013) The neurobiology of thought: the groundbreaking discoveries of Patricia Goldman-Rakic1937-2003, *Cereb Cortex*, 23 (10): 2269-81. doi: 10.1093/cercor/bht195.

Bär K-J, de la Cruz F, Schumann A, Koehlera S, Sauera H, Critchley H, Wagnera G. (2016) Functional connectivity and network analysis of midbrain and brainstem nuclei. NeuroImage 134(2016) 53–63.

Bauer, R. H. and Fuster, J. M. (1976) Delayed-matching and delayed-response deficit from cooling dorsolateral prefrontal cortex in monkeys, *Q. J. Exp. Psychol.* B, 90, 293-302.

Beul S. F., Grant S., Hilgetag C. C. (2015) A predictive model of the cat cortical connectome based on cytoarchitecture and distance, *Brain. Struct. Funct.*, 220: 3167-3184. doi: 10.1007/s00429-014-0849-y.

Burgess, P. W., Dumontheil, I., & Gilbert, S. J. (2007) The gateway hypothesis of rostral prefrontal cortex (area 10) function, *Trends in Cognitive Science*, 11(7): 290-8.

Cajal S. R. (1899) Estudios sobre la corteza cerebral humana I: corteza visual. *Rev. Trim. Microgr.* 4, 1-63. Translated in: DeFelipe, J., and Jones, E. G. (1988). Cajal on the Cerebral Cortex. New York: Oxford University Press.

Chafee M. V. and Goldman-Rakic, P. S. (1998) Matching patterns of activity in primate prefrontal area 8a and parietal area 7ip neurons during a spatial working memory task, *J. Neurophysiol,* 79: 2919-2940.

Chunga A. W., Schirmerb M. D., Krishnanc M. L., Ballc G., Aljabarc P., Edwardsc, A. D. Montana G. (2016) Characterising brain network topologies: A dynamic analysis approach using heat kernels, *NeuroImag*e 141: 490-501.

Curtis, C. E. and D'Esposito, M. (2003) Persistent activity in the prefrontal cortex during working memory, *Trends. Cogn. Sci.* 7: 415-423.

Curtis, C. E., Rao, V. Y. and D'Esposito, M. (2004) Maintenance of spatial and motor codes during oculomotor delayed response tasks, *J. Neurosci.*, 24: 3944-3952.

Dai, Z., Yan, C., Li, K., Wang, Z., Wang, J., Cao, M., et al. (2014). Identifying and mapping connectivity patterns of brain network hubs in Alzheimer's disease. *Cereb. Cortex* 25, 3723–3742. doi:10.1093/cercor/bhu246

DeFelipe J. (2011) The evolution of the brain, the human nature of cortical circuits, and intellectual creativity, *Front. Neuroanatomy,* 5 (29): 1-17. doi: 10.3389/fnana.2011.00029.

de Lacy N, Doherty D, King BH, Rachakonda S, and Calhoun VD (2017) Disruption to control network function correlates with altered dynamic connectivity in the wider autism spectrum. *NeuroImage*: Clinical, 15:513–524.

D'Esposito M. (2007) From cognitive to neural models of working memory, *Phil. Trans. R. Soc. B,* 362, 761-772.

Falk D., Hildebolt C., Smith K., Morwood M. J., Sutikna T., Brown P., Jatmiko, Saptomo E. W., Brunsden B., Prior F. (2005) *The brain of LB1, Homo floresiensis, Science,* 308 (5719): 242-5. doi:10.1126/science.1109727 PMID 15749690.

Funahashi S., Bruce C. J. and Goldman-Rakic, P. S. (1989) Mnemonic coding of visual space in the monkey's dorsolateral prefrontal cortex, *J. Neurophysiol.,* 61: 331-349.

Funahashi S., Bruce C. J. and Goldman-Rakic P. S. (1993) Dorsolateral prefrontal lesions and oculomotor delayed response performance: evidence for mnemonic "scotomas", *J. Neurosci.,* 13: 1479-1497.

Fuster J. M. & Alexander G. E. (1971) Neuron activity related to short-term memory, *Science,* 173: 652-654.

Fuster J. M. (2000) Executive frontal functions, *Exp. Brain Res.,* 133: 66 – 70.

Fuster, J. M. (2001) The prefrontal cortex-an update: time is of the essence, *Neuron,* 30: 319-333.

Fuster J. M. Bodnar, M. Kroger, J. K. (2000) Cross-modal and cross-temporal association in neurons of frontal cortex, *Nature,* 405: 347-351.

Gilbert, J., Spengler, S., Simons, J. S, Steele, J. D., Lawrie, S. M., Frith, C. D., Burgess, P. W. (2006) Functional specialization within rostral prefrontal cortex (area 10): a meta-analysis, *Journal of Cognitive Neuroscience,* 18 (6): 932-948.

Goldman-Rakic P. S. (1996) The prefrontal landscape: implications of functional architecture for understanding human mentation and the central executive, Philos. *Trans. R. Soc. Lond. B Biol. Sci.,* 351 (1346): 1445-53.

Grillner S., Markram H., De Schutter E., Silberberg G., LeBeau F. (2005) Microcircuits in action – from CPGs to neocortex, *Trends in Neurosciences,* 28 (10): 525-33.

Harriger L, van den Heuvel MP, Sporns O (2012) Rich Club Organization of Macaque Cerebral Cortex and Its Role in Network Communication. *PLoS ONE* 7(9): e46497. doi:10.1371/journal.pone.0046497.

He M., Tucciarone J., Lee S. H., Nigro M. J., Kim K., Levine J. M., Kelly S. M., Krugikov I., Wu P., Chen Y., Gong L., Hou Y., Osten P., Rudy B., and Huang Z. J. (2016) Strategies and tools for combinatorial targeting of GABAergic neurons in mouse cerebral cortex, *Neuron,* 91: 1228-1243, 2016. doi: http://dx.doi.org/10.1016/j.neuron.2016.08.021.

Jacobs B., Schall M., Prather M., Kapler E., Driscoll L., Baca S., Jacobs J., Ford K., Wainwright M., Treml M. (2001) Regional dendritic and spine variation in human cerebral cortex: a quantitative Golgi study, *Cereb. Cortex,* 11 (6): 558-71. doi:10.1093/cercor/11.6.558 PMID 11375917.

Jiang X, Shen S, Cadwell CR, Berens P, Sinz F, Ecker AS, Patel S, Tolias AS (2015) Principles of connectivity among morphologically defined cell types in adult neocortex. Science. 350(6264):aac9462. doi: 10.1126/science.aac9462.

Jodoj E., Chiang C., Aston-Jones G. (1998) Potent excitatory influence of prefrontal cortex activity on noradrenergic locus coeruleus neurons, *Neuroscience,* 83 (1): 63-79.

Knowlton, B. J., Morrison, R. G., Hummel, J. E., Holyoak, K. J. (2012) A neurocomputational system for relational reasoning, *Trends in Cognitive Sciences,* 16 (7): 373-381. doi:10.1016/j.tics.2012.06.002.

Koechlin E. and Hyafil A. (2007) Anterior prefrontal function and the limits of human-decision making, *Science,* 318: 594-598.

Lebedev M. A., Messinger A., Kralik J. D., Wise S. P. (2004) Representation of Attended Versus Remembered Locations in Prefrontal Cortex, *PLoS Biol.* 2 (11): e365. doi:10.1371/journal.pbio.0020365.

Lebedev M. A., Wise S. P. (2002) Insights into seeing and grasping: distinguishing the neural correlates of perception and action, *Behav. Cogn. Neurosci. Rev.,* 1(2): 108-29.

Limb C. J., Braun A. R. (2008) Neural Substrates of Spontaneous Musical Performance: An fMRI Study of Jazz Improvisation, *PLoS ONE* 3(2): e1679. doi:10.1371/journal.pone.0001679.

Mansouri F. A., Buckley M. J., Mahboubi M., Tanaka K. (2015) Behavioral consequences of selective damage to frontal pole and posterior cingulate cortices, *Proc. Natl. Acad. Sci. USA,* 112 (29): E3940-9. doi: 10.1073/pnas.1422629112.

Mayse J. D., Nelson G. M. Avila I., Gallagher M. & Lin S.-C. (2015).Basal forebrain neuronal inhibition enables rapid behavioral stopping, *Nature Neuroscience,* 18: 1501-1508.

McFarland N. R., Haber S. N. (2002) Thalamic relay nuclei of the basal ganglia form both reciprocal and nonreciprocal cortical connections, linking multiple frontal cortical areas, *J. Neurosci,* 22: 8117-32.

Moser DA, Doucet GE, Ing A, Dima D, Schumann G, Bilder RM, Frangou S. (2017) An integrated brain-behavior model for working memory *Mol Psychiatry.* doi: 10.1038/mp.2017.247.

Mountcastle V. B. (1997) The columnar organization of the neocortex, *Brain,* 120 (4): 701-22.

Murray S. (2012) The brain's connective core and its role in animal cognition, Philos. *Trans. R. Soc. Lond. B Biol. Sci.,* 367 (1603): 2704-2714. doi: 10.1098/rstb. 2012.0128.

Ongür D., Ferry A. T., Price J. L. (2003) Architectonic subdivision of the human orbital and medial prefrontal cortex, *J. Comp. Neurol.,* 460 (3): 425-49. doi:10.1002/cne.10609 PMID 12692859.

Opris I. and Casanova M. F. (2014) Prefrontal cortical minicolumn: from executive control to disrupted cognitive processing, *Brain,* 137 (7): 1863-75. doi: 10.1093/brain/awt359.

Opris I., Barborica A., Ferrera V. P. (2005) Microstimulation of dorsolateral prefrontal cortex biases saccade target selection, *J. Cogn. Neurosci.*, 17 (6): 893-904.

Opris I., Santos L. M., Song D., Berger T. W., Gerhardt G. A., Hampson R. E., and Deadwyler S. A. (2013) Prefrontal cortical microcircuits bind perception to executive control, *Scientific Reports*, 3: 2285.

Opris I. Popa I. L., Casanova M. F. (2015) Prefrontal Cortical Microcircuits of Executive Control. Chapter 10. In *"Recent Advances on the Modular Organization of the Cerebral Cortex,"* Editor(s): Manuel F Casanova and Ioan Opris, Springer, Netherlands. pp. 157-179.

Opris I., Ferrera V. P. (2014) Modifying cognition and behavior with electrical microstimulation: implications for cognitive prostheses, *Neurosci. Biobehav. Rev.*, 47: 321-35. doi: 10.1016/j.neubiorev.2014.09.003.

Opris I., Hampson R. E., Stanford T. R., Gerhardt G. A., Deadwyler S. A. (2011) Neural activity in frontal cortical cell layers: evidence for columnar sensorimotor processing, *J. Cogn. Neurosci.*, 23: 1507-1521.

Opris I., Hampson R. E., Gerhardt G. A., Berger T. W., Deadwyler S. A. (2012) Columnar processing in primate pFC: Evidence for executive control microcircuits, *J. Cogn. Neuro.*, 24 (12): 2334-47.

Opris I., Fuqua J. L., Huettl P., Gerhardt G. A., Berger T. W., Hampson R. E., Deadwyler S. A. (2012) Closing the loop in primate prefrontal cortex: Inter-laminar processing, *Frontiers in Neural Circuits*, 6: 88. doi: 10.3389/fncir.2012.00088.

Opris I., Santos L. M., Song D., Berger T. W., Gerhardt G. A., Hampson R.,E. and Deadwyler S. A. (2013) Prefrontal cortical microcircuits bind perception to executive control, *Scientific Reports,* 3: 2285. doi:10.1038/srep02285.

Opris I., Santos L. M., Gerhardt G. A., Song D., Berger T. W., Hampson R. E. and Deadwyler S. A. (2015) Distributed Encoding of Spatial and Object Categories in Primate Hippocampal Microcircuits, *Front. Neurosci.*, 9: 317. doi: 10.3389/fnins.2015.00317.

Opris I., Casanova M. F. (2014) Prefrontal cortical minicolumn: from executive control to disrupted cognitive processing, *Brain,* 137 (7): 1863-75. doi: 10.1093/brain/awt359.

Opris I., Fuqua J. L., Gerhardt G. A., Hampson R. E., Deadwyler S. A. (2015) Prefrontal cortical recordings with biomorphic MEAs reveal complex columnar-laminar microcircuits for BCI/BMI implementation, *J. Neurosci. Methods*, 15 (244): 104-13.

Opris I., Gerhardt G. A., Hampson R. E., Deadwyler S. A. (2015) Disruption of columnar and laminar cognitive processing in primate prefrontal cortex following cocaine exposure, *Front. Syst. Neurosci.*, 9: 79. doi: 10.3389/fnsys.2015.00079.

Opris, I. (2013) Inter-laminar microcircuits across the neocortex: repair and augmentation, Front. Syst. Neurosci., 7: 80. doi: 10.3389/fnsys.2013.00080.

Optiz, A., Fox, M. D., Craddock, R. C., Colcombe, S., and Milham, M. P. (2016). An integrated framework for targeting functional networks via transcranial magnetic stimulation. *Neuroimage* 127, 86–96. doi: 10.1016/j.neuroimage.2015.11.040

Packer A. M. and Yuste R. (2011) Dense, Unspecific Connectivity of Neocortical Parvalbumin-Positive Interneurons: A Canonical Microcircuit for Inhibition? *Journal of Neuroscience,* 31 (37): 13260-13271; doi: https://doi.org/10.1523/JNEUROSCI.3131-11.2011.

Penfield W., Jasper H. (1954) *Epilepsy and the Functional Anatomy of the Brain.* London: Churchill Livingstone.

Petrides M., Pandya D. N. (2007) Efferent association pathways from the rostral prefrontal cortex in the macaque monkey, *J Neurosci.,* 27 (43): 11573-86. doi:10.1523/JNEUROSCI.2419-07.2007 PMID 17959800.

Quintana J., Fuster, J. M. (1999) From perception to action: temporal integrative functions of prefrontal and parietal neurons, *Cereb. Cortex,* 9 (3): 213- 221.

Ramnani N., Owen A. M. (2004) Anterior prefrontal cortex: insights into function from anatomy and neuroimaging, *Nat. Rev. Neurosci.,* 5 (3): 184-94. doi:10.1038/nrn1343 PMID 14976518.

Rao, S. C., Rainer, G., Miller, E. K. Integration of what and where in the primate prefrontal cortex, *Science,* 276 (1997): 821- 824.

Ratcliff, R. (1978) A theory of memory retrieval, *Psychol. Rev.,* 85: 59-108.

Ratcliff, R. (2001) Putting noise into neurophysiological models of simple decision making, *Nat. Neurosci.,* 4: 336-337.

Ratcliff, R. (2002) A diffusion model account of response time and accuracy in a brightness discrimination task: fitting real data and failing to fit fake but plausible data, Psychon. *Bull. Rev.,* 9: 278- 291.

Ratcliff, R., Tuerlinckx, F. (2002) Estimating parameters of the diffusion model: approaches to dealing with contaminant reaction times and parameter variability, *Psychon. Bull. Rev.,* 9: 438- 481.

Ratcliff R., Hasegawa Y. T., Hasegawa, R. P., Childers, R., Smith, P. L. and Segraves M. A. (2011) Inhibition in Superior Colliculus Neurons in a Brightness Discrimination Task? *Neural Comput.,* 23 (7): 1790-1820.

Reddi, B. A., Carpenter, R. H. (2000) The influence on urgency on decision time, *Nat. Neurosci.,* 3: 827-830.

Santos L., Opris I., Hampson R., Godwin D. W., Gerhardt G., Deadwyler S. (2014) Functional dynamics of primate cortico-striatal networks during volitional movements, *Front. Syst. Neurosci,* 8: 27.10.3389/fnsys.2014.00027.

Sara S. J. (2009) The locus coeruleus and noradrenergic modulation of cognition. Nature *Reviews Neuroscience* 10: 211-223. doi: 10.1038/nrn2573.

Schall, J. D. (1999) Weighing the evidence: how the brain makes a decision, *Nat. Neurosci.,* 2: 108-109.

Schall, J. D. (2001) Neural basis of deciding, choosing and acting, Nat. Rev., *Neurosci.*, 2: 33-42.

Schall, J. D. (2002) The neural selection and control of saccades by the frontal eye field, Philos. *Trans. R. Soc. London, B Biol. Sci.*, 357: 1073-1082.

Schomers MR and Pulvermüller F (2016) Is the Sensorimotor Cortex Relevant for Speech Perception and Understanding? An Integrative Review. Front. Hum. Neurosci., 21 September 2016 | https://doi.org/10.3389/fnhum.2016.00435.

Semendeferi K., Armstrong E., Schleicher A., Zilles K., Van Hoesen G. W. (2001) Prefrontal cortex in humans and apes: a comparative study of area 10, *Am. J. Phys. Anthropol.*, 114 (3): 224-41. doi:10.1002/ajpa.20947 PMID 11241188.

Shadlen M. N., Newsome W. T. (1998) The variable discharge of cortical neurons: implications for connectivity, computation, and information coding, *J. Neurosci.*, 18: 3870- 3896.

Shadlen M. N., Newsome W. T. (2001) Neural basis of a perceptual decision in the parietal cortex (area LIP) of the rhesus monkey, *J. Neurophysiol.*, 86: 1916-1936

Sporns O. and Betzel R. F. (2016) Modular Brain Networks, *Annu. Rev. Psychol.*, 67: 613-640. doi: 10.1146/annurev-psych-122414-033634.

Tierney P. L., Thierry A. M., Glowinski J., Deniau J. M., Gioanni Y. (2008) Dopamine modulates temporal dynamics of feedforward inhibition in rat prefrontal cortex in vivo, *Cereb. Cortex.*, 18 (10): 2251-62. doi: 10.1093/cercor/bhm252.

Tishby N. and Polani D. (2011) Information Theory of Decisions and Actions. p. 601-636. In: *Perception-Action Cycle. Models, Architectures, and Hardware*. Eds. Cutsuridis V, Hussain A and Taylor JG. Springer Series in Cognitive and Neural Systems.

Tsujimoto S., Genovesion A., Wise S. P. (2010) Evaluating self-generated decisions in frontal pole cortex of monkeys, *Nature Neurosci.*, 13: 120-126 doi:10.1038/nn.2453.

van den Heuvel M. P. and Sporns O. (2011) Rich-club organization of the human connectome, *J. Neurosci.*, 31 (44): 15775-86. doi: 10.1523/JNEUROSCI.3539-11.2011.

Wallis J. D. (2010) Polar exploration, *Nat Neurosci.*, 13 (1): 7-8. doi:10.1038/nn0110-7 PMID 20033080.

Wang, X. -J. (2002) Probabilistic decision making by slow reverberation in cortical circuits, *Neuron*, 36: 955-968.

Wise, S. P., Murray, E. A., Gerfen, C. R. (1996) The frontal cortex-basal ganglia system in primates, *Crit. Rev. Neurobiol.*, 10: 317- 356.

Xie, K., Fox, G. E., Liu, J., Lyu, C., Lee, J. C., Kuang, H., et al. (2016). Brain Computation is organized via power-of-two-based permutation logic. *Front. Syst. Neurosci.* 10:95. doi: 10.3389/fnsys.2016.00095

Young C. B., Raz G., Everaerd D., Beckmann C. F., Tendolkar I., Hendler T., Fernández G. and Hermans E. J. (2016) Dynamic Shifts in Large-Scale Brain Network Balance As a Function of Arousal, *Journal of Neuroscience*, 37 (2): 281-290.

Zhang J., Hughes L. E., Rowe J. B. (2012) Selection and inhibition mechanisms for human voluntary action decisions, *Neuroimage*, 63 (1): 392-402. doi: 10.1016/j.neuroimage.2012.06.058.

Modha DS, Singh R (2010) Network architecture of the long-distance pathways in the macaque brain. *Proc Natl Acad Sci USA* 107: 13485–13490.

Leicht EA, Newman MEJ (2008) Community structure in directed networks. *Phys Rev Lett* 100: 118703.

Newman MEJ, Girvan M (2004) Finding and evaluating community structure in networks. *Phys Rev E* 69: 026113.

ABOUT THE EDITORS

Manuel F. Casanova, MD
University of South Carolina School of Medicine Greenville, SC, US
Professor of Biomedical Sciences
SMART State Endowed Chair in Translational Neurotherapeutics
Greenville Health System, SC, US
Research Director of the Developmental Behavioral Pediatric Fellowship
SMART State Endowed Chair in Translational Neurotherapeutics
Clinical Faculty at Clemson University, SC, US
School of Health Research
Email: manuel.casanova@louisville.edu

Ioan Opris, PhD
The Miami Project to Cure Paralysis
University of Miami Miller School of Medicine
Lois Pope LIFE Center, LPLC
Miami, FL, US
Email: ixo82@med.miami.edu

INDEX

A

A priori knowledge, 27, 29

accreditation and quality measurement systems, 115

aging, 50, 51, 55, 59, 60, 61, 62, 63, 64, 65, 69, 70, 71, 72, 73, 74, 75, 76, 77, 78, 79, 80, 140, 141, 215, 217, 218, 222, 223, 229, 230, 232, 248, 250, 251, 254, 256, 271, 278

algorithm, 101, 102, 110, 113, 114, 134, 137, 141

Alzheimer Disease (AD), 72, 140, 141, 304, 305, 306

annotation, 133, 135

antioxidants, 50, 66, 67, 68, 69, 70, 71, 72, 75, 76, 253

apical dendrites, 216

architecture of systems problem solving, 4, 46

autism, 164, 208, 220, 273, 303, 304, 307

axonal bundles, 216

B

basal ganglia, 209, 276, 290, 300, 309, 312

bias, 1, 2, 12, 16, 20, 26, 27, 30, 32, 35, 38, 43, 44, 45, 279

biochemical reactions, 132, 135, 225, 231

bioconstructs, 50

biomarker, 141, 306

biomass, 136, 143, 147

biophotons, 221, 237, 238, 239, 240, 252

bioreliability, 50, 52, 57, 71

biotechnology, 133, 144, 146, 218

bottom-up processing, 208, 297

brain hemispheres, 97

C

cancer, 59, 127, 132, 136, 139, 140, 142, 144, 145, 147, 149, 150, 192, 199, 200, 201, 202, 204, 231, 243, 256, 278, 281, 282

cell, 55, 56, 59, 60, 62, 65, 66, 67, 68, 69, 71, 72, 73, 75, 77, 133, 135, 137, 139, 140, 141, 142, 143, 144, 145, 149, 150, 194, 203, 204, 205, 206, 210, 211, 212, 217, 218, 219, 220, 221, 222, 223, 224, 225, 226, 227, 228, 229, 230, 231, 232, 235, 236, 238,239, 242, 243, 244, 245, 246, 247, 248, 249, 250, 251, 252, 254, 255, 256, 257, 260, 267, 271, 273, 280, 281, 283, 285, 289, 297, 302, 308, 310

cerebral cortex, vi, 205, 208, 209, 210, 211, 212, 213, 216, 217, 218, 219, 245, 290, 306, 307, 308, 310

Chinese philosophy, 25

complex network, 81, 97, 132, 255, 259, 290

complex systems, v, 4, 8, 53, 81, 89, 92, 97, 98, 99, 118, 126, 171, 172, 173, 176, 177, 178, 179, 180, 181, 182, 183, 187, 188, 189, 194

complex systems theory, v, 171, 172, 176, 177, 178, 179

computational modeling and simulation, 172, 173, 179, 181, 182

constraint-based, 131, 132, 133, 135, 139, 148, 150

constraint-bound systems, 30

context, 1, 2, 8, 9, 10, 13, 14, 15, 16, 17, 18, 19, 27, 30, 31, 32, 33, 34, 38, 40, 42, 43, 44, 45, 46, 62, 84, 116, 126, 131, 137, 138, 141, 143, 148, 149,

318 *Index*

150, 180, 181, 183, 194, 196, 198, 201, 208, 211, 229, 241, 251, 281, 298, 302

context dependence, 1

context-based, 131, 137, 138

core actors, 14, 15, 16, 17, 18, 20, 21, 40, 41, 42, 43, 45

Crick, Francis, 206

D

data integration, v, 131, 133, 137, 143

database, 141, 144, 146, 269

determinism, 50

diabetes, 132, 140, 149, 192, 251, 277, 280, 284, 286

disease, 76, 123, 125, 131, 133, 138, 140, 141, 147, 150, 172, 183, 184, 186, 187, 188, 192, 193, 194, 195, 196, 197, 198, 199, 200, 201, 202, 204, 225, 230, 231, 232, 233, 234, 235, 242, 244, 245, 247, 248, 249, 250, 251, 253, 254, 255, 256, 257, 258, 259, 260, 265, 267, 269, 270, 271, 272, 273, 276, 277, 278, 279, 280, 281, 282, 284, 286, 304, 305, 307

disorder, 161, 220, 233, 234, 265, 275, 276, 279, 280, 286, 303

dorsolateral prefrontal cortex, 211, 295, 307, 308, 310

drug target, 70, 131, 133, 138, 139, 140, 141, 142, 143, 144, 147, 150, 249

dynom/dynome, vi, 221, 235, 240, 241, 250

dyslexia, 208, 217, 220

dyslexic, 208, 218

E

electrical-information analogies, 81

emergencies, 81

emergent phenomena, 207

Emx2, 211

entanglement, 81, 87, 91, 92, 97

entanglement swapping, 92

enzyme, 55, 56, 57, 58, 66, 69, 73, 79, 132, 133, 136, 139, 143, 227, 230, 231, 232, 246

evolution, 53, 75, 84, 93, 133, 140, 149, 152, 164, 165, 166, 167, 168, 169, 170, 178, 179, 205, 207, 209, 210, 218, 222, 241, 244, 245, 246, 250, 257, 302, 307

F

failures, 36, 49, 50, 51, 53, 54, 55, 56, 58, 64, 66, 67, 71, 72, 123, 179

Feynman path diagram, 92

flux, 53, 93, 94, 95, 96, 100, 132, 134, 135, 136, 138, 140, 141, 144, 146, 148, 223

flux balance analysis (FBA), 135, 136, 139, 144, 146

Fourier transform, 86, 89

free energy principle, 151, 152, 158, 161, 168, 169

free radicals, 50, 64, 65, 66, 67, 68, 69, 70, 73, 74, 76, 77, 79, 246

G

gene expression, 70, 131, 137, 138, 139, 140, 141, 142, 148, 223, 235

genetics, 50, 194, 256, 269

genome-scale metabolic model (GEM), v, 131, 132, 133, 134, 135, 136, 137, 138, 139, 141, 142, 143, 144, 145, 147, 148, 149, 150

genotype-phenotype relationship, 132, 138, 146

goal-setter, 1, 20, 23, 27, 30, 31, 38, 42, 43

goal-setting, 1, 3, 4, 10, 14, 15, 16, 17, 18, 20, 22, 23, 24, 25, 26, 27, 29, 30, 32, 34, 35, 38, 44, 45, 47

goal-value, 9, 10, 11, 12, 13, 14, 15, 17, 18, 19, 20, 21, 22, 23, 24, 25, 26, 27, 28, 29, 30, 31, 32, 34, 35, 36, 37, 38, 39, 40, 41, 42, 43, 44, 45

good enough, 1, 14, 37, 38, 39, 40, 44, 45

gyrator, 95, 96, 100

H

Hegelian inquiring systems, 8

hierarchical recursive organization, 151, 152, 169

high-throughput, 137, 138

holistic, 115, 116, 122, 123, 133, 140, 172, 176, 178, 206, 212

holistic health care systems, 115

holistic healthcare systems relationship model, 122

I

information action, 81, 94

information analogies, 81, 94, 95, 97

information capacitance, 85

Index

information content, 82, 83, 84, 85, 86, 90, 91, 92, 93, 94, 96, 97, 98
information energy, 97
information flow, 82, 83, 84, 85, 86, 88, 90, 91, 92, 93, 94, 96, 97, 98, 262, 288
information gate, 82, 83, 87, 89
information impedance, 85, 86
information inductance, 85
information memcapacitor, 94
information memelement, 81, 93
information meminductor, 94
information memristor, 94
information power, 81, 82, 90, 91, 97, 99
information resistance, 85
information resonance, 92
inquiring systems, 6, 7, 8, 46, 47
integrated systems, 115
interference, 65, 81, 89, 97, 198
interpersonal synchrony, 152, 168, 170
intuition, 1, 22, 25, 26, 34, 39, 44, 210
isotropy, 217

K

Kantian inquiring systems, 7
kinetic, 60, 132, 133, 144, 193
knowledge, 1, 2, 7, 8, 9, 11, 12, 14, 22, 24, 25, 26, 27, 29, 30, 31, 33, 34, 35, 36, 39, 42, 44, 45, 47, 59, 68, 82, 83, 84, 92, 95, 96, 97, 98, 102, 117, 138, 139, 142, 175, 178, 193, 194, 200, 202, 206, 207, 237, 241, 260, 269, 274, 283, 288, 300
knowledge-based action, 96, 97
Kronecker product, 87

L

Landau-Kleffner syndrome, 213, 218
law-bound systems, 30
Leibnizian inquiring systems, 7
life testing, 50, 72
limbic system, 209, 210
Lockean inquiring systems, 7
longevity, 50, 60, 61, 62, 63, 65, 66, 71, 73, 76, 79, 232
long-haul truck drivers, 171, 172

M

magnetic – information analogies, 81, 95
malfunctions, 49, 51, 57, 58, 60, 67, 71, 141
Markov blankets, 159, 162, 163, 164, 165, 169, 170
metabolism, 50, 57, 65, 71, 75, 76, 132, 133, 136, 137, 139, 140, 141, 143, 146, 147, 148, 149, 196, 222, 224, 225, 227, 232, 234, 238, 240, 243, 248, 250, 251, 254, 261, 266, 267, 270, 271, 272, 273, 274, 282, 284, 285
metabolite, 132, 136, 235
metamodeling, 5, 47
mindsets, 124
minicolumns, 205, 207, 208, 212, 213, 214, 216, 217, 218, 290, 299
mitochondria, vi, 53, 55, 57, 58, 67, 68, 70, 76, 221, 222, 223, 224, 225, 226, 227, 228, 229, 230, 231, 232, 233, 234, 235, 236, 237, 238, 239, 240, 242, 244, 245, 246, 247, 248, 250, 251, 252, 253, 254, 255, 256, 257, 258
multiple subpial transection, 213, 218

N

neomammalam complex, 209
network, 75, 96, 99, 124, 132, 133, 134, 135, 142, 144, 145, 147, 148, 149, 150, 160, 185, 223, 224, 225, 235, 237, 239, 240, 241, 247, 255, 256, 263, 266, 268, 269, 275, 276, 279, 281, 289, 291, 292, 293, 295, 296, 298, 302, 303, 304, 305, 306, 307, 308, 313
neuropil, 217
non-alcoholic fatty liver disease (NAFLD), 140, 141, 149, 150

O

obesity, 132, 140, 141, 183, 184, 186, 187, 188, 271, 275, 277, 278, 279, 280, 281, 283, 284, 285
objective function, 131, 135, 136, 139, 143, 146, 147
occupational safety, 172, 182
of general system theory, 206
omics data, 138, 142
organism, 60, 61, 62, 66, 68, 70, 71, 132, 133, 135, 162, 165, 191, 193, 194, 195, 196, 199, 200, 201, 207, 223, 227, 238, 239, 240, 241, 259, 260, 275, 278

320 *Index*

oxygen, 50, 55, 57, 58, 59, 64, 65, 66, 68, 69, 71, 73, 74, 77, 78, 136, 223, 225, 227, 228, 229, 231, 236, 242, 245, 250, 251, 254, 255, 257, 261

P

pathway, 133, 140, 141, 205, 245, 252, 263, 273, 294
Pauli exclusion principle, 91
Pax6, 211
phenotype, 134, 145, 208, 285
physical-information analogies, 81, 93, 97, 98, 99
preliminary knowledge, 6, 27, 29, 30, 31, 32, 33, 34, 35, 36, 37, 38, 39, 42, 43, 44
preventive maintenance, 50, 56, 58, 60, 69, 71
program, 50, 51, 60, 66, 71, 74, 120, 172, 187, 191, 193, 195, 241
prophylaxis, 50, 56, 67, 68
pyramidal cells, 216, 217

Q

quantum complex network, 97
quantum entanglement, 91, 99
quantum informatics, 81
quantum system theory, 81, 98

R

reconstruction, 99, 131, 132, 133, 134, 142, 143, 144, 145, 146, 147, 148, 149, 150, 269, 289
reductionism, 172, 173, 174, 175, 176, 177, 179, 183, 191, 193, 194, 196, 202, 203, 206, 207, 220
reductionist approach, 177, 179, 193, 206
reliability, v, 49, 50, 51, 52, 53, 55, 56, 57, 58, 59, 60, 61, 62, 63, 65, 66, 67, 70, 71, 72, 73, 74, 78, 79, 80, 100
reptilian complex, 209
robustness, v, 49, 50, 51, 60, 66, 70, 72, 74, 75, 78, 136, 293

S

science, iv, viii, 2, 3, 5, 6, 22, 24, 25, 26, 33, 35, 46, 47, 51, 74, 79, 80, 99, 100, 101, 115, 117, 118, 119, 120, 125, 126, 127, 128, 129, 150, 169, 185, 186, 187, 188, 191, 193, 203, 204, 206, 209, 218, 228, 240, 247, 250, 252, 253, 255, 256, 260, 285, 307, 308, 309, 311
self-organization, viii, 81, 96, 98, 100, 120, 152, 153, 156, 157, 159, 164, 168, 169, 170, 191, 201, 202, 204, 205, 217
Shannon entropy, 88
Singerian inquiring systems, 8
solution space, 132, 135, 136
steady-state, 135, 136, 303, 304
stochastic, 50, 51, 52, 58, 61, 62, 66, 71, 74, 75, 80, 132, 229, 281
superoxide radicals, 57, 58, 63, 71, 73
system alliance, 84
system context, 1
system design, 1, 2, 3, 4, 5, 6, 8, 9, 10, 11, 12, 13, 14, 15, 16, 17, 18, 19, 20, 21, 22, 23, 24, 26, 27, 29, 30, 31, 32, 33, 34, 35, 36, 37, 38, 39, 40, 41, 42, 43, 44, 45, 46, 188
system design methodologies, 1
system designer, 1, 4, 5, 6, 12, 14, 15, 16, 17, 18, 19, 20, 21, 23, 24, 26, 27, 30, 31, 32, 33, 34, 35, 36, 37, 38, 39, 40, 42, 44, 45
system theory, vii, 81, 96, 100, 119, 128, 207
systems biology, 49, 50, 51, 67, 70, 74, 131, 133, 143, 144, 147, 250, 281, 282
systems engineering, 3, 14, 32, 47, 100, 128
systems medicine, v, 131, 133, 138, 139, 144, 147
systems paradigms, 9
systems theory, iv, vi, vii, 2, 25, 47, 71, 74, 78, 79, 101, 117, 119, 122, 124, 126, 128, 151, 152, 153, 154, 157, 159, 169, 170, 177, 178, 179, 182, 205, 206, 209, 218
systems thinking, v, 46, 47, 115, 116, 117, 118, 119, 121, 122, 123, 124, 125, 127, 128, 177, 178, 184, 185
systems-oriented event analysis (SOEA) method, 123, 124

T

tissue-specific, 131, 137, 138, 140, 148, 149, 283
topological, 132, 290, 305
Triune brain, 209, 210, 218
Triune brain model, 209
truth, 1, 6, 7, 8, 9, 11, 15, 25, 36, 38, 40, 41, 42

V

variational neuroethology, 152, 165, 166, 168
ventricular zone, 210
von Neumann entropy, 87, 88, 90

W

Warburg effect, 139, 140, 149
wave information capacitance, 89
wave information content, 88
wave information flow, 87
wave information impedance, 88
wave information inductance, 88
wave information power, 90
wave information resistance, 88
wave probabilistic functions, 81, 86, 87, 88, 90, 99, 100

Z

z-transform, 85

THE LIFE AND TIMES OF THE WORLD'S MOST FAMOUS MATHEMATICIANS

AUTHORS: Ann F. Varela (Eastern New Mexico University, New Mexico, USA); Michael F. Shaughnessy (Eastern New Mexico University, Portales, New Mexico, USA)

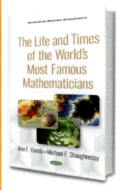

SERIES: Mathematics Research Developments

BOOK DESCRIPTION: In this book, the lives and discoveries of various mathematicians will be explored and examined, so as to provide some insight into various mathematical functions and operations.

HARDCOVER ISBN: 978-1-53613-975-4
RETAIL PRICE: $195

SINGLE VARIABLE INTEGRAL AND DIFFERENTIAL CALCULUS IN A NUTSHELL WITH ELEMENTS OF CRITICAL THINKING

AUTHORS: Ranis Ibragimov and Pirooz Mohazzabi (University of Wisconsin-Parkside, WI, USA)

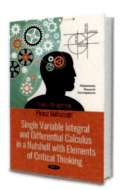

SERIES: Mathematics Research Developments

BOOK DESCRIPTION: This book presents a variety of calculus problems concerning different levels of difficulty with technically correct solutions and methodological steps that look also correct, but that have obviously wrong results (like $0 = 1$). Those errors are aimed to be resolved by applying critical thinking (i.e., reasonable, reflective, responsible, and skillful thinking).

HARDCOVER ISBN: 978-1-53614-047-7
RETAIL PRICE: $195

Quaternion Matrix Computations

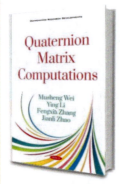

Authors: Musheng Wei, Ying Li, Fengxia Zhang and Jianli Zhao (Liaocheng University, Shandong, P. R. China)

Series: Mathematics Research Developments

Book Description: In this monograph, the authors describe state-of-the-art real structure-preserving algorithms for quaternion matrix computations, especially the LU, the Cholesky, the QR and the singular value decomposition of quaternion matrices, direct and iterative methods for solving quaternion linear systems, generalized least squares problems, and quaternion right eigenvalue problems.

Hardcover ISBN: 978-1-53614-121-4
Retail Price: $160

Simulated Annealing: Introduction, Applications and Theory

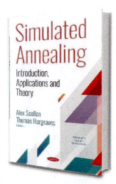

Editors: Alex Scollen and Thomas Hargraves

Series: Mathematics Research Developments

Book Description: The opening chapter of this book aims to present and analyze the application of the simulated annealing algorithm in solving parameter optimization problems of various manufacturing processes.

Hardcover ISBN: 978-1-53613-674-6
Retail Price: $195